Notice

Medicine is an ever-changing science. As new research and clinical experience broaden our knowledge, changes in treatment and drug therapy are required. The authors and the publisher of this work have checked with sources believed to be reliable in their efforts to provide information that is complete and generally in accord with the standards accepted at the time of publication. However, in view of the possibility of human error or changes in medical sciences, neither the authors nor the publisher nor any other party who has been involved in the preparation or publication of this work warrants that the information contained herein is in every respect accurate or complete, and they disclaim all responsibility for any errors or omissions or for the results obtained from use of the information contained in this work. Readers are encouraged to confirm the information contained herein with other sources. For example and in particular, readers are advised to check the product information sheet included in the package of each drug they plan to administer to be certain that the information contained in this work is accurate and that changes have not been made in the recommended dose or in the contraindications for administration. This recommendation is of particular importance in connection with new or infrequently used drugs.

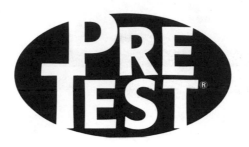

Clinical Vignettes for the USMLE Step 2

PreTest® Self-Assessment and Review

Third Edition

McGraw-Hill
Medical Publishing Division

New York   Chicago   San Francisco   Lisbon   London   Madrid   Mexico City
Milan   New Delhi   San Juan   Seoul   Singapore   Sydney   Toronto

A O4238S

W B 18

Clincal Vignettes for the USMLE Step 2

1 2 3 4 5 6 7 8 9 0   DOC/DOC   0 9 8 7 6 5 4 3

ISBN 0-07-138886-9

This book was set in Berkeley by North Market Street Graphics.
The editor was Catherine A. Johnson.
The production supervisor was Phil Galea.
Project management was provided by North Market Street Graphics.
RR Donnelley was printer and binder.

This book is printed on acid-free paper.

Cataloging-in-Publication data is on file for this title at the Library of Congress.

Contents

Preface

The current format of the United States Medical Licensing Examination (USMLE) Step 1 emphasizes clinical vignettes as the primary test questions. The examination is 400 questions, broken into eight blocks of 50 questions each. Examinees have one hour to complete each block.

Clinical Vignettes for the USMLE Step 1: Third Edition parallels this format. The book contains 400 clinical-vignette-style questions covering the basic sciences and was assembled based on the published content outline for the USMLE Step 1. The questions are divided into eight blocks of 50 questions. As on the Step 1 exam, each block tests the examinee in all basic science areas. Halfway through each block, a stopwatch set at 30 minutes is included to remind the examinee of the one-hour limit. Answers are in the second half of the book. Each answer is accompanied by a concise but comprehensive explanation and is referenced to a key textbook or journal article for further reading.

The questions in this book were culled from the seven PreTest® Basic Science books. The publisher acknowledges and thanks the following authors for their contributions to this book:

Pediatrics: Robert J. Yetman, MD
Psychiatry: Debra Klamen, MD
Medicine: Steven L. Berk, MD and William R. Davis, MD
Sergey: Norman Snow, MD
Neurology: David Anschel, MD
Physical Diagnosis: Jo Ann Reteguiz, MD
Obstetrics and Gynecology: Michelle Wylen, MD

McGraw-Hill
September 2003

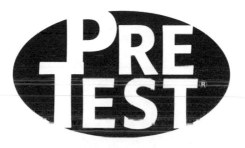

Clinical Vignettes for the USMLE Step 2

PreTest® Self-Assessment and Review

BLOCK 1

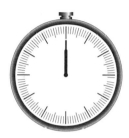

Questions

1-1. A 37-year-old postal worker from Atlantic City, New Jersey, presents to the emergency room with the chief complaint of dry cough for several days. He has fever, malaise, dyspnea on exertion, and pleuritic chest pain. He has experienced mild nausea and diffuse abdominal pain. He has been in good health otherwise and has no recent travel history. No contacts have been ill. Physical examination is remarkable for a temperature of 101.4°F and decreased breath sounds at the lung bases bilaterally. Chest radiograph reveals pleural effusions and a widened mediastinum. Which of the following is the most likely diagnosis?

a. Pneumonic plague
b. Tularemia
c. Hemorrhagic fever
d. Inhalation anthrax
e. Hantavirus pulmonary syndrome

1-2. After being struck on the head by a four-by-four, a previously serious and dependable construction worker starts making inappropriate sexual remarks to his co-workers, is easily distracted, and loses his temper over minor provocations. What part of his brain has been damaged?

a. Occipital lobe
b. Temporal lobe
c. Limbic system
d. Basal ganglion
e. Frontal lobe

1-3. A 68-year-old hypertensive man undergoes successful repair of a ruptured abdominal aortic aneurysm. He receives 9 L Ringer's lactate solution and four units of whole blood during the operation. Two hours after transfer to the surgical intensive care unit, the following hemodynamic parameters are obtained:

Systemic blood pressure (BP): 90/60 mmHg
Pulse: 110/min
Central venous pressure (CVP): 7 mmHg
Pulmonary artery pressure: 28/10 mmHg
Pulmonary capillary wedge pressure: 8 mmHg
Cardiac output: 1.9 L/min
Systemic vascular resistance: 35 Woods units (normal is 24 to 30 Woods units)
PaO_2: 140 kPa (FiO_2: 0.45)
Urine output: 15 mL/h (specific gravity: 1.029)
Hematocrit: 35%

Proper management now calls for

a. Administration of a diuretic to increase urine output
b. Administration of a vasopressor agent to increase systemic blood pressure
c. Administration of a fluid challenge to increase urine output
d. Administration of a vasodilating agent to decrease elevated systemic vascular resistance
e. A period of observation to obtain more data

1-4. A 35-year-old woman has noticed that over the past 3 to 5 months she has had some difficulties with balance, particularly when she closes her eyes. On examination, she has decreased hearing in her left ear and also left body dysdiadochokinesia. Her physician orders a head CT. Given this CT scan, which was obtained without contrast enhancement, the physician must assume that the posterior fossa mass at the arrow is

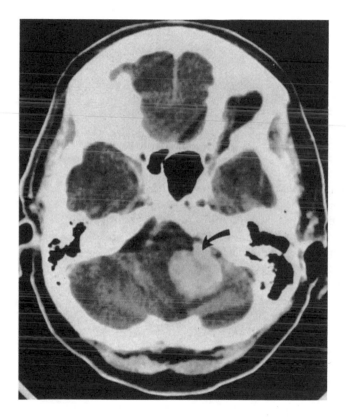

a. Normal
b. Calcified
c. Highly vascular
d. Granulomatous
e. Highly cystic

1-5. You see a healthy 40-year-old multiparous patient for preconception counseling. She is extremely worried about her risk of having a baby with spina bifida. Five years ago, this patient delivered a baby with anencephaly who died shortly after birth. How would you counsel this woman regarding future pregnancies?

a. She does not have a recurrence risk of a neural tube defect above that of the general population
b. She has an increased risk of having another baby with anencephaly because she is over 35 years old
c. When she becomes pregnant, she should undergo diagnostic testing for fetal neural tube defects with a first-trimester chorionic villus sampling
d. When she becomes pregnant, she should avoid hyperthermia in the first trimester because both maternal fevers and the use of hot tubs have been associated with an increased risk of neural tube defects
e. She has a recurrence risk of having another baby with a neural tube defect of less than 1%

1-6. A 29-year-old G1P0 patient at 15 weeks gestational age presents to your office complaining of some shortness of breath that is more intense with exertion. She has no significant past medical history and is not on any medication. The patient denies any chest pain but sometimes feels as though her heart is pounding. She is concerned because she has always been very athletic and cannot maintain the same degree of exercise that she was accustomed to prior to becoming pregnant. On physical exam, her pulse is 90/min. Her blood pressure is 90/50. On cardiac exam, a systolic ejection mummer is identified. The lungs are clear to auscultation and percussion. Which of the following is the most appropriate next step to pursue in the workup of this patient?

a. Refer the patient for a ventilation-perfusion scan to rule out a pulmonary embolism
b. Perform an arterial blood gas
c. Refer the patient to a cardiologist
d. Reassure the patient
e. Order an ECG

I-7. While you are on duty in the emergency room, a 12-year-old boy arrives with pain and inflammation over the ball of his left foot and red streaks extending up the inner aspect of his leg. He remembers removing a wood splinter from the sole of his foot on the previous day. The most likely infecting organism is

a. *Clostridium perfringens*
b. *Clostridium tetani*
c. *Staphylococcus*
d. *Escherichia coli*
e. *Streptococcus*

I-8. A 25-year-old Hispanic male PhD candidate recently traveled to rural Mexico for 1 month to gain further information for his dissertation regarding socioeconomics. While there, he took ciprofloxacin for diarrhea. However, over the 2 to 3 weeks since coming home, he has continued to have occasional loose stools plus vague abdominal discomfort and bloating. There has been no rectal bleeding. The most likely cause of this traveler's diarrhea is

a. *Campylobacter jejuni*
b. Toxigenic *Escherichia coli*
c. *Giardia lamblia*
d. *Cryptosporidium*
e. *Salmonella*
f. *Shigella*

I-9. A 43-year-old woman comes to the emergency room with a temperature of 101°F and a large suppurating ulcer on her left shoulder. This is the third such episode for this woman. Her physical exam is otherwise normal, other than the presence of multiple scars on her abdomen. The woman is admitted to the hospital and is observed to be holding her thermometer next to the light bulb to heat it up. When confronted, she angrily denies any such behavior and signs out of the hospital against medical advice. The patient most likely has which of the following diagnoses?

a. Malingering
b. Somatoform disorder
c. Borderline personality disorder
d. Factitious disorder
e. Body dysmorphic disorder

1-10. A 39-year-old woman has diplopia several times a day for 6 weeks. She consults a physician when the double vision becomes unremitting, and also complains of dull pain behind her right eye. When a red glass is placed over her right eye and she is asked to look at a flashlight off to her left, she reports seeing a white light and a red light. The red light appears to her to be more to the left than the white light. Her right pupil is more dilated than her left pupil and responds less briskly to a bright light directed at it than does the left pupil.

Before any further investigations can be performed, the woman develops the worst headache of her life and becomes stuporous. Her physician discovers that she has marked neck stiffness and photophobia. The physician performs a transfemoral angiogram. This radiologic study is expected to reveal that the woman has

a. An arteriovenous malformation
b. An occipital astrocytoma
c. A sphenoidal meningioma
d. A pituitary adenoma
e. A saccular aneurysm

I-II. A 55-year-old obese woman develops pressurelike substernal chest pain 1 h in duration. Her ECG is shown below. The most likely diagnosis is

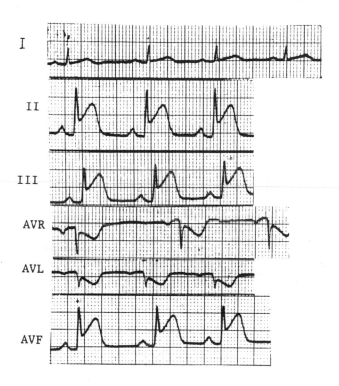

a. Costochondritis
b. Acute anterior myocardial infarction
c. Acute inferior myocardial infarction
d. Pericarditis
e. Esophageal reflux
f. Cholecystitis

1-12. A 55-year-old schizophrenic has been treated with haloperidol for the past 25 years. She presents with constant chewing movements, grimaces, and lip smacking. Her symptoms persist when her haloperidol dose is decreased. Without the neuroleptic, she experiences persecutory delusions and command auditory hallucinations, which tell her to kill her family members. Which of the following antipsychotics should this patient be switched to?

a. Loxitane
b. Molindone
c. Thioridazine
d. Olanzapine
e. Perphenazine

1-13. A healthy 30-year-old G3P2002 presents to the obstetrician's office at 34 weeks for a routine prenatal visit. She has a history of two prior cesarean sections (low-transverse). The first cesarean section was performed secondary to fetal malpresentation (footling breech). The patient then had an elective repeat cesarean section for her second pregnancy. This pregnancy, the patient has had an uncomplicated prenatal course. She tells her physician that she would like to undergo a trial of labor during this pregnancy. However, the patient is interested in permanent sterilization and wonders if it would be better to undergo another scheduled cesarean section so she can have a bilateral tubal ligation performed at the same time. Which of the following statements is true and should be relayed to the patient?

a. A history of two previous cesarean sections is a contraindication to vaginal birth after cesarean section (VBAC)
b. Her risk of uterine rupture with attempted VBAC after two prior cesarean sections is 4 to 9%
c. Her chance of having a successful VBAC is less than 60%
d. The patient should schedule an elective induction if not delivered by 40 weeks
e. If the patient desires a bilateral tubal ligation, it is safer for her to undergo a vaginal delivery followed by a postpartum tubal ligation rather than an elective repeat cesarean section with intrapartum bilateral tubal ligation

1-14. A 70-year-old patient with chronic obstructive lung disease requires 2 L of nasal O_2 to treat his hypoxia, which is sometimes associated with angina. While receiving nasal O_2, the patient develops pleuritic chest pain, fever, and purulent sputum. He becomes stuporous and develops a respiratory acidosis with CO_2 retention and worsening hypoxia. The treatment of choice is

a. Stop oxygen
b. Begin medroxyprogesterone
c. Intubate the trachea and begin mechanical ventilation
d. Observe patient 24 hours before changing therapy
e. Begin sodium bicarbonate

1-15. A 50-year-old man presents to the emergency room with a 6-h history of excruciating abdominal pain and distention. The abdominal film shown below is obtained. The next diagnostic maneuver should be

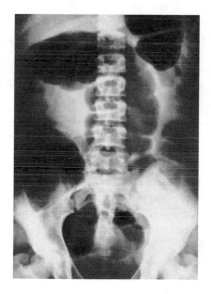

a. Emergency celiotomy
b. Upper gastrointestinal series with small-bowel follow-through
c. CT scan of the abdomen
d. Barium enema
e. Sigmoidoscopy

1-16. A 15-year-old boy has moderate mental retardation, attention deficit disorder, a long face, enlarged ears, and macroorchidism. Development has been steady but always at a delayed pace. The most likely cause for this patient's low intelligence is which of the following?

a. Turner syndrome
b. Klinefelter syndrome
c. Fragile X syndrome
d. Reye syndrome
e. Tuberous sclerosis

1-17. A 60-year-old man with a previous history of appendectomy 30 years ago presents to the emergency room complaining of abdominal pain. He describes the pain as colicky and crampy and feels it builds up, then improves on its own. He has vomited at least 10 times since the pain started this morning. He states that he has not had a bowel movement for 2 days and cannot recall the last time he passed flatus. The abdomen is slightly distended. Abdominal auscultation reveals high-pitched bowel sounds and peristaltic rushes. Percussion reveals a tympanic abdomen. The patient is diffusely tender with palpation but has no rebound tenderness. Rectal examination reveals the absence of stool. Which of the following is the most likely diagnosis?

a. Cholecystitis
b. Diverticulitis
c. Pancreatitis
d. Gastroenteritis
e. Intestinal obstruction

1-18. You are called to the emergency room to see one of your patients. The father of this 3-year-old was spraying the yard with an unknown insecticide. In the emergency room, the child is noted to have bradycardia, muscle fasciculations, meiosis, wheezing, and profound drooling. The most likely agent included in this pesticide is

a. Organophosphate
b. Chlorophenothane (DDT)
c. Sodium cyanide
d. Warfarin
e. Paraquat

1-19. A 35-year-old woman develops an itchy rash over her back, legs, and trunk several hours after swimming in a lake. Erythematous, edematous papules are noted. The wheals vary in size. There are no mucosal lesions and no swelling of the lips (see photo). The most likely diagnosis is

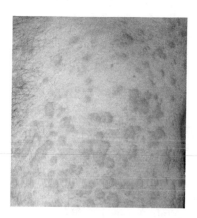

a. Urticaria
b. Folliculitis
c. Erythema multiforme
d. Erythema chronicum migrans

1-20. A 58-year-old woman is seen for evaluation of a swelling in her right vulva. She has also noted pain in this area when walking and during coitus. At the time of pelvic examination, a mildly tender, fluctuant mass is noted just outside the introitus in the right vulva in the region of the Bartholin's gland. What is the most appropriate treatment?

a. Marsupialization
b. Administration of antibiotics
c. Surgical excision
d. Incision and drainage
e. Observation

1-21. A 41-year-old construction worker complains of the sudden onset of severe back pain after lifting some heavy equipment. He describes the pain as being in his right lower back and radiating down the posterior aspect of his right buttock to the knee area. He has no bladder or bowel dysfunction. The pain has improved with bed rest. On physical examination, the patient has tenderness in his lumbar area with palpation. The straight-leg maneuver with the right leg increases the back pain at 80°. The straight-leg maneuver with the left leg also causes thigh pain. Sensation, strength, and reflexes are normal. Which of the following is the most likely diagnosis?

a. Nerve root compression
b. Paravertebral abscess
c. Lumbosacral strain
d. Osteoporosis compression fracture
e. Paget's disease

1-22. A previously healthy 18-month-old has been in a separate room from his family. The family notices the sudden onset of coughing, which resolves over a few minutes. Subsequently, the patient appears to be normal except for increased amounts of drooling and refusal to take foods orally. The most likely explanation for this toddler's condition is

a. Severe gastroesophageal reflux
b. Foreign body in the airway
c. Croup
d. Epiglottitis
e. Foreign body in the esophagus

1-23. A 60-year-old female complains of dry mouth and a gritty sensation in her eyes. She states it is sometimes difficult to speak for more than a few minutes. There is no history of diabetes mellitus or neurologic disease. The patient is on no medications. On exam, the buccal mucosa appears dry and the salivary glands are enlarged bilaterally. The next step in evaluation is

a. Lip biopsy
b. Schirmer test and measurement of autoantibodies
c. IgG antibody to mumps virus
d. Use of corticosteroids

1-24. A 30-year-old man takes a can of beer out of his refrigerator at the end of the day and rapidly swallows a mouthful of its contents before he realizes it is not beer. Within a few minutes he develops severe abdominal cramps, blurred vision, twitching, and loss of consciousness. His wife notifies emergency medical personnel that she had placed some roach spray in the beer can for storage and had left it in the refrigerator to deal with roaches that were nesting there. She claims that she forgot to advise her husband of this. Emergency personnel check the insecticide brand and determine that it is an organophosphate. To counteract the cholinesterase-inhibiting activity of the organophosphate poison, the man should receive

a. Methacholine
b. Pyridostigmine
c. Physostigmine
d. Edrophonium
e. Atropine

1-25. An 18-year-old male is admitted to the emergency room following a motorcycle accident. He is alert and fully oriented, but witnesses to the accident report an interval of unresponsiveness following the injury. Skull films disclose a fracture of the left temporal bone. Following x-ray, the patient suddenly loses consciousness and dilation of the left pupil is noted. This patient should be considered to have

a. A ruptured berry aneurysm
b. An acute subdural hematoma
c. An epidural hematoma
d. An intraabdominal hemorrhage
e. A ruptured arteriovenous malformation

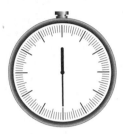

YOU SHOULD HAVE COMPLETED APPROXIMATELY
25 QUESTIONS AND HAVE 30 MINUTES REMAINING.

1-26. An 18-year-old boy is brought into the emergency room after a diving accident. He is awake and alert, has intact cranial nerves, and is able to move his shoulders, but he cannot move his arms or legs. He is flaccid and has a sensory level at C5. Appropriate management includes

a. Naloxone hydrochloride
b. Intravenous methylprednisolone
c. Oral dexamethasone
d. Phenytoin 100 mg tid
e. Hyperbaric oxygen therapy

1-27. A 38-year-old G3P1011 comes to see you for her first prenatal visit at 10 weeks gestational age. She had a previous term vaginal delivery without any complications. You detect fetal heart tones at this visit, and her uterine size is consistent with dates. You also draw her prenatal labs at this visit and tell her to follow up in 4 weeks for a return OB visit. Two weeks later, the results of the patient's prenatal labs come back. Her blood type is A−, with an anti-D antibody titer of 1:4. What is the most appropriate next step in the management of this patient?

a. Schedule an amniocentesis for amniotic fluid bilirubin at 16 weeks
b. Repeat the titer in 4 weeks
c. Repeat the titer at 28 weeks
d. Schedule PUBS to determine fetal hematocrit at 20 weeks
e. Schedule PUBS as soon as possible to determine fetal blood type

1-28. A 41-year-old intravenous drug abuser presents with shortness of breath and pleuritic chest pain. He is febrile with a temperature of 103.5°F. He has no skin lesions, and funduscopic exam is negative. He has jugular venous distension that increases with compression of the liver. The liver is pulsatile. The jugular venous pulse shows a prominent v wave. The patient has splenomegaly. Heart auscultation reveals a holosystolic murmur heard best at the left lower sternal border. The murmur increases with inspiration (Müller maneuver). Which of the following is the most likely diagnosis?

a. Bacterial endocarditis
b. Pericarditis
c. Rheumatic fever
d. Mitral valve prolapse
e. Pericardial effusion

1-29. A 25-year-old woman presents to the emergency room complaining of redness and pain in her right foot up to the level of the midcalf. She reports that her right leg has been swollen for at least 15 years, but her left leg has been normal. On physical examination, she has a temperature of 39°C (102.2°F). The left leg is normal. The right leg is not tender, but it is swollen from the inguinal ligament down and there is an obvious cellulitis of the right foot. The patient's underlying problem is

a. Popliteal entrapment syndrome
b. Acute arterial insufficiency
c. Primary lymphedema
d. Deep venous thrombosis
e. None of the above

1-30. A 33-year-old man presents with diarrhea and weight loss. He denies chills and night sweats but has low-grade fevers. He has no recent travel history. He has no lymphadenopathy; abdominal examination is normal. His stool is negative for blood but positive for leukocytes. Which of the following is the most likely pathogen?

a. *Vibrio cholerae*
b. *Giardia lamblia*
c. *Campylobacter jejuni*
d. *Clostridium perfringens*
e. *Aeromonas hydrophila*
f. *Cryptosporidium*
g. Rotovirus
h. Norwalk virus

1-31. A 29-year-old man contracted HIV-1 through homosexual activity 5 years ago. He had been doing well on HAART, but stopped taking his medications 8 months ago because he thought that he would be better off. Two months ago he was successfully treated for *Pneumocystis carinii* pneumonia. A papovavirus infection of the central nervous system (CNS) in this person would be most likely to produce

a. Adrenoleukodystrophy
b. Multiple sclerosis
c. Subacute sclerosing panencephalitis (SSPE)
d. Progressive multifocal leukoencephalopathy (PML)
e. Metachromatic leukodystrophy

1-32. About 12 days after a mild upper respiratory infection, a 12-year-old boy complains of weakness in his lower extremities. Over several days, the weakness progresses to include his trunk. On physical examination, he has the weakness described and no lower extremity deep tendon reflexes, muscle atrophy, or pain. Spinal fluid studies are notable for elevated protein only. The most likely diagnosis in this patient is

a. Bell palsy
b. Muscular dystrophy
c. Guillain-Barré syndrome
d. Charcot-Marie-Tooth disease
e. Werdnig-Hoffmann disease

1-33. A 70-year-old woman has nausea, vomiting, abdominal distension, and episodic crampy midabdominal pain. She has no history of previous surgery but has a long history of cholelithiasis for which she has refused surgery. Her abdominal radiograph reveals a spherical density in the right lower quadrant. Correct treatment should consist of

a. Ileocolectomy
b. Cholecystectomy
c. Ileotomy and extraction
d. Nasogastric tube decompression
e. Intravenous antibiotics

1-34. You are called in to evaluate the heart of a 19-year-old primigravida at term. Listening carefully to the heart, you determine that there is a split S_1, normal S_2, S_3 easily audible with a 2/6 systolic ejection murmur greater during inspiration, and a soft diastolic murmur. You immediately recognize that

a. The presence of the S_3 is abnormal
b. The systolic ejection murmur is unusual in a pregnant woman at term
c. Diastolic murmurs are rare in pregnant women
d. The combination of a prominent S_3 and soft diastolic murmur is a significant abnormality
e. All findings recorded are normal changes in pregnancy

1-35. A 1-day-old infant who was born by a difficult forceps delivery is alert and active. She does not move her left arm, however, which she keeps internally rotated by her side with the forearm extended and pronated; she also does not move it during a Moro reflex. The rest of her physical examination is normal. This clinical picture most likely indicates

a. Fracture of the left clavicle
b. Fracture of the left humerus
c. Left-sided Erb-Duchenne paralysis
d. Left-sided Klumpke paralysis
e. Spinal injury with left hemiparesis

1-36. A 69-year-old woman slips on the ice and hits her head on the pavement. During the following 3 weeks, she develops a persistent headache, is increasingly distractible and forgetful, and becomes fearful and disoriented at night. Which of the following is the most likely cause of these changes?

a. Subdural hematoma
b. Frontal lobe meningioma
c. Korsakoff's disease
d. Epidural hematoma
e. Multi-infarct dementia

1-37. A 17-year-old male presents with 10 days of progressive tingling paresthesias of the hands and feet followed by evolution of weakness of the legs two evenings before admission. He complains of back pain. He has a history of a diarrheal illness 2 weeks prior. On examination, he has moderate leg and mild arm weakness, but respiratory function is normal. There is mild sensory loss in the feet. He is areflexic. Mental status is normal. Spinal fluid analysis in this case is most likely to show

a. No abnormalities
b. Elevated protein level
c. Elevated white blood cell (WBC) count
d. Elevated pressure
e. Oligoclonal bands

1-38. Two weeks after a viral syndrome, a 9-year-old girl presents to your clinic with a complaint of several days of drooping of her mouth. In addition to the drooping of the left side of her mouth, you note that she is unable to completely shut her left eye. Her smile is asymmetric, but her examination is otherwise normal. This girl likely has

a. Guillain-Barré syndrome
b. Botulism
c. Cerebral vascular accident
d. Brainstem tumor
e. Bell palsy

1-39. A 30-year-old female complains of fatigue, constipation, and weight gain. There is no prior history of neck surgery or radiation. Her voice is hoarse and her skin is dry. Serum TSH is elevated and T₄ is low. The most likely cause of these findings is

a. Autoimmune disease
b. Postablative hypothyroidism
c. Pituitary hypofunction
d. Thyroid carcinoma

1-40. A 30-year-old nursing student presents with confusion, sweating, hunger, and fatigue. Blood sugar is noted to be 40 mg/dL. The patient has no history of diabetes mellitus, although her sister is an insulin-dependent diabetic. The patient has had several similar episodes over the past year, all occurring just prior to reporting for work in the early morning. On this evaluation, the patient is found to have high insulin levels and a low C peptide level. The most likely diagnosis is

a. Reactive hypoglycemia
b. Early diabetes mellitus
c. Factitious hypoglycemia
d. Insulinoma

1-41. A 27-year-old woman has been feeling blue for the past 2 weeks. She has little energy and has trouble concentrating. She states that 6 weeks ago she had been feeling very good, with lots of energy and no need for sleep. She states this pattern has been occurring for at least the past 3 years, though the episodes have never been so severe that she couldn't work. Which of the following diagnoses is most likely?

a. Borderline personality disorder
b. Seasonal affective disorder
c. Cyclothymic disorder
d. Major depression, recurrent
e. Bipolar disorder, depressed

1-42. A 61-year-old right-handed man presents with involuntary twitches of his left hand. He first noticed between 6 months and 1 year ago that when he is at rest, his left hand shakes. He can stop the shaking by looking at his hand and concentrating. The shaking does not impair his activities in any way. He has no trouble holding a glass of water. There is no tremor in his right hand, and his lower extremities are not affected. He has had no trouble walking, and there have been no falls. There have been no behavioral or language changes. On examination, a left hand tremor is evident when the man is distracted. His handwriting is mildly tremulous. He has bilateral cogwheel rigidity with contralateral activation, which is worse on the left. His rapid alternating movements are bradykinetic on the left. The most likely diagnosis in this case is which of the following?

a. Epilepsy
b. Guillain-Barré syndrome
c. Multiple sclerosis
d. Parkinson's disease
e. Stroke

I-43. Three days ago you delivered a 40-year-old G1P1 by cesarean section. The indication for operative delivery was failure to descend after 2 h of pushing. Labor was also significant for prolonged rupture of membranes. The patient had an epidural, which was removed the day following delivery. The nurse pages you to come see the patient on the postpartum floor because she has a fever of 102°F and is experiencing shaking chills. Her BP is 120/70 and her pulse is 120. She has been eating a regular diet without difficulty and had a normal bowel movement this morning. She is attempting to breast-feed, but says her milk has not come in yet. On physical exam, her breasts are mildly engorged and tender bilaterally. Her lungs are clear. Her abdomen is tender over the fundus, but no rebound is present. Her incision has some serous drainage at the right apex, but no erythema is noted. What is the patient's most likely diagnosis?

a. Pelvic abscess
b. Septic pelvic thrombophlebitis
c. Wound infection
d. Metritis
e. Atelectasis

I-44. A 21-year-old man presents with a sore throat. He also complains of dysphagia, odynophagia, and otalgia. His temperature is 102.5°F. The patient speaks with a hot potato voice and is drooling. Examination of the throat reveals a hypertrophied right tonsil that appears to be displaced inferiorly and medially. There is contralateral deflection of the uvula. The patient has trismus and cervical lymphadenopathy. Which of the following is the most likely diagnosis?

a. Retropharyngeal abscess
b. Peritonsillar abscess
c. Exudative pharyngitis
d. Cancer of the right tonsil
e. Mononucleosis

1-45. A 24-year-old woman presents with lethargy, anorexia, tachypnea, and weakness. Laboratory studies reveal a BUN of 150 mg/dL, serum creatinine of 16 mg/dL, and potassium of 6.2 meq/L. Chest x-ray shows increased pulmonary vascularity and a dilated heart. Management of this patient should include

a. Emergency kidney transplantation
b. Creation and immediate use of a forearm arteriovenous fistula
c. Sodium polystyrene sulfonate (Kayexalate) enemas
d. A 100-g protein diet
e. Cardiac biopsy via femoral vein catheterization

1-46. A 30-year-old male patient complains of fever and sore throat for several days. The patient presents to you today with additional complaints of hoarseness, difficulty breathing, and drooling. On examination, the patient is febrile and has inspiratory stridor. Which of the following is the best course of action?

a. Begin outpatient treatment with ampicillin
b. Culture throat for β-hemolytic streptococci
c. Admit to intensive care unit and obtain otolaryngology consultation
d. Schedule for chest x-ray

1-47. A 3-day-old infant with a single second heart sound has had progressively deepening cyanosis since birth but no respiratory distress. Chest radiography demonstrates no cardiomegaly and normal pulmonary vasculature. An electrocardiogram shows an axis of 120° and right ventricular prominence. The congenital cardiac malformation most likely responsible for the cyanosis is

a. Tetralogy of Fallot
b. Transposition of the great vessels
c. Tricuspid atresia
d. Pulmonary atresia with intact ventricular septum
e. Total anomalous pulmonary venous return below the diaphragm

A 34-year-old patient who delivered her first baby 5 weeks ago calls your office and asks to speak with you. She tells you that she is feeling very overwhelmed and anxious. She feels that she cannot do anything right and feels sad throughout the day. She tells you that she finds herself crying all the time and is unable to sleep at night.

I-48. What is the most likely diagnosis?

a. Postpartum depression
b. Maternity blues
c. Postpartum psychosis
d. Bipolar disease
e. Postpartum blues

I-49. A 16-year-old girl presents with lower abdominal pain and fever. On physical examination, a tender adnexal mass is felt. Further questioning in private reveals the following: she has a new sexual partner; her periods are irregular; she has a vaginal discharge. The most likely diagnosis is

a. Appendiceal abscess
b. Pelvic inflammatory disease
c. Ovarian cyst
d. Renal cyst
e. Ectopic pregnancy

I-50. A 1-year-old girl is brought to the physician by her mother. The child had been developing normally until about 6 to 9 months of age. At 9 months, her mother noticed that the girl's head growth had begun to decelerate, she seemed "floppy," and she had lost interest in playing. She had recently been noted to have episodes of crying, screaming, and intense hyperactivity. Which of the following diagnoses is most likely?

a. Asperger's disorder
b. Down syndrome
c. Congenital rubella
d. Rett's disorder
e. Childhood disintegrative disorder

BLOCK 2

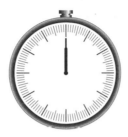

YOU HAVE 60 MINUTES
TO COMPLETE 50 QUESTIONS.

Questions

2-1. A 4-year-old girl is noticed by her grandmother to have a limp and a somewhat swollen left knee. The parents report that the patient occasionally complains of pain in that knee. An ophthalmologic examination reveals findings as depicted in the photograph. The condition most likely to be associated with these findings is

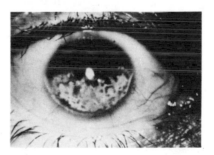

a. Juvenile rheumatoid arthritis
b. Slipped capital femoral epiphysis
c. Henoch-Schönlein purpura
d. Legg-Calvé-Perthes disease
e. Osgood-Schlatter disease

2-2. Two weeks after hospital discharge for documented myocardial infarction, a 65-year-old returns to your office very concerned about low-grade fever and pleuritic chest pain. There is no associated shortness of breath. Lungs are clear to auscultation and heart exam is free of significant murmurs, gallops, or rubs. ECG is unchanged from the last one in the hospital. The most effective therapy is likely

a. Antibiotics
b. Anticoagulation with warfarin (Coumadin)
c. An anti-inflammatory agent
d. An increase in antianginal medication
e. An antianxiety agent

2-3. A 20-year-old G2P1 patient comes to see you at 17 weeks gestational age to review the results of her triple test done 1 week ago. You tell the patient that her MSAFP level is 2.0 MOM. The patient's obstetrical history consists of a term vaginal delivery 2 years ago without complications. What do you tell your patient regarding how to proceed next?

a. Explain to the patient that the blood test is diagnostic of a neural tube defect and she should consult with a pediatric neurosurgeon as soon as possible
b. Tell the patient that the blood test result is most likely a false-positive result and she should repeat the test at 20 weeks
c. Refer the patient for an ultrasound to confirm dates
d. Offer the patient immediate chorionic villus sampling to obtain a fetal karyotype
e. Recommend to the patient that she undergo a cordocentesis to measure fetal serum AFP levels

2-4. A 62-year-old right-handed man has "involuntary twitches" of his left hand. He first noticed between 6 months and 1 year ago that when he is at rest, his left hand shakes. He can stop the shaking by looking at his hand and concentrating. The shaking does not impair his activities in any way. He has no trouble holding a glass of water. There is no tremor in his right hand and the lower extremities are not affected. He has had no trouble walking. There have been no behavioral or language changes. On examination, a left hand tremor is evident when he is distracted. Handwriting is mildly tremulous. He is very mildly bradykinetic on the left. The most likely exam finding would be which of the following?

a. Upper motor neuron pattern of weakness on the left
b. Lower motor neuron pattern of weakness on the left
c. Bilateral upper motor neuron pattern of weakness
d. Mild cogwheel rigidity on the left only with distraction
e. Bilateral severe cogwheel rigidity

2-5. A 40-year-old male complains of exquisite pain and tenderness over the left ankle. There is no history of trauma. The patient is taking a mild diuretic for hypertension. On exam, the ankle is very swollen and tender. There are no other physical exam abnormalities. The next step in management is

a. Begin colchicine and broad-spectrum antibiotics
b. Obtain uric acid level and perform arthrocentesis
c. Begin allopurinol if uric acid level is elevated
d. Obtain ankle x-ray to rule out fracture

2-6. A healthy 31-year-old G3P2002 patient presents to the obstetrician's office at 34 weeks gestational age for a routine return visit. She has had an uneventful pregnancy to date. Her baseline blood pressures were 100–110/60–70, and she has gained a total of 20 lb so far. During the visit, the patient complains of bilateral pedal edema that sometimes causes her feet to ache at the end of the day. Her urine dip indicates trace protein, and her blood pressure in the office is currently 115/75. She denies any other symptoms or complaints. On physical exam, there is pitting edema of both legs without any calf tenderness. How should the obstetrician respond to the patient's concern?

a. Prescribe Lasix to relieve the painful swelling
b. Immediately send the patient to the radiology department to have venous Doppler studies done to rule out deep vein thromboses
c. Admit the patient to L and D to rule out preeclampsia
d. Reassure the patient that this is a normal finding of pregnancy, and no treatment is needed
e. Tell the patient that her leg swelling is due to too much salt intake and instruct her to go on a low-sodium diet

2-7. A 27-year-old man sustains a single gunshot wound to the left thigh. In the emergency room, he is noted to have a large hematoma of his medial thigh. He complains of paresthesias in his foot. On examination, there are weak pulses palpable distal to the injury and the patient is unable to move his foot. The appropriate initial management of this patient is

a. Angiography
b. Immediate exploration and repair
c. Fasciotomy of the anterior compartment
d. Observation for resolution of spasm
e. Local wound exploration

2-8. You are called by a general practitioner to consult on a patient admitted to the hospital 4 days ago. The patient is a 7-month-old white boy with poor weight gain for the past 3 months, who has not gained weight in the hospital despite seemingly adequate nutrition. His guardian is his maternal aunt, as his mother is in jail for unknown reasons. You take a detailed diet history from the guardian, and the amounts of formula and baby food intake seem appropriate for age. Physical examination reveals an active, alert infant with a strong suck reflex who appears wasted. You note generalized lymphadenopathy with hepatomegaly. In addition, you find a severe case of oral candidiasis that apparently has been resistant to treatment. Which of the following is the most appropriate next step in the evaluation or treatment of this child?

a. Increase caloric intake because this is probably a case of underfeeding
b. Order HIV PCR testing because this is likely the presentation of congenitally acquired HIV
c. Draw blood cultures because this could be sepsis
d. Perform a sweat chloride test because this is probably cystic fibrosis
e. Send stool for fecal fat because this is probably a malabsorption syndrome

2-9. A 67-year-old woman with a history of type II diabetes mellitus and atrial fibrillation presents to the emergency room with right body weakness and slurred speech. The onset was sudden while she was brushing her teeth 1 h ago, and she was brought immediately to the emergency room. She has no complaints of word-finding difficulties, no dysesthesia, and no headache. She is taking warfarin. Physical exam findings include blood pressure of 205/90 and irregularly irregular heart beat. There is left side neglect with slurred speech. There is a corticospinal pattern of weakness of the right body, with the face and upper extremity worse than the lower extremity. Routine chemistries and cell counts are normal. Her INR is 1.8. Which of the following should be done next?

a. Administer tissue plasminogen activator
b. Call a vascular surgery consult for possible endarterectomy
c. Order a brain CT
d. Order a cerebral angiogram
e. Start heparin

2-10. A 52-year-old man is sent to see a psychiatrist after he is disciplined at his job because he consistently turns in his assignments late. He states he is not about to turn in anything until it is "perfect, unlike all of my colleagues." He has few friends, because he annoys them with his demands for "precise timeliness" and because of his lack of emotional warmth. This has been a lifelong pattern of behavior for the patient, though he refuses to believe the problems have anything to do with his personal behavior. Which of the following is this patient's most likely diagnosis?

a. Obsessive-compulsive disorder
b. Obsessive-compulsive personality disorder
c. Borderline personality disorder
d. Bipolar disorder, mixed state
e. Anxiety disorder not otherwise specified

2-11. A 19-year-old student presents for a precollege screening visit. On physical examination, the patient has a scant beard (he states he needs to shave only every other month) and gynecomastia. His testes are firm and measure <2 cm each. The patient states that he functions as a normal man sexually although he feels his libido is diminished compared to that of his friends. Which of the following is the most likely diagnosis?

a. Turner syndrome
b. Klinefelter syndrome
c. Ambiguous genitalia
d. Late puberty
e. Normal male

2-12. A 27-year-old G3P2002 who is 34 weeks gestational age calls the on-call obstetrician on a Saturday night at 10:00 P.M. complaining of decreased fetal movement. She says that for the past several hours, her baby has moved only once per hour. She is healthy, has had regular prenatal care, and denies any complications so far during the pregnancy. How should the on-call physician counsel the patient?

a. Instruct the patient to go to labor and delivery for a contraction stress test
b. Reassure the patient that one fetal movement per hour is within normal limits and she does not need to worry
c. Recommend the patient be admitted to the hospital for delivery
d. Counsel the patient that the baby is probably sleeping and that she should continue to monitor fetal kicks. If she continues to experience less than five kicks per hour by morning, she should call you back for further instructions
e. Instruct the patient to go to labor and delivery for a nonstress test

2-13. A 25-year-old female with blonde hair and fair complexion complains of a mole on her upper back. The lesion is 6 mm in diameter, darkly pigmented, and asymmetric, with a very irregular border (see photo). The next step in management is

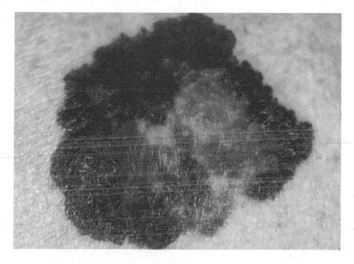

a. Tell the patient to avoid sunlight
b. Follow the lesion for any evidence of growth
c. Obtain metastatic workup
d. Obtain full-thickness excisional biopsy
e. Obtain shave biopsy

2-14. A 21-year-old right-handed female student was working in the photography lab 1 week ago, which required standing all day. After that, she experienced a cold sensation in the left foot and her entire left leg fell asleep. The feeling lasted 4 to 5 days and then slowly went away. Her right lower extremity was fine. Coughing, sneezing, and the Valsalva maneuver did not worsen her symptoms. She had a slight back pain, which she thought was due to using a poor mattress. Past history includes an episode of optic neuritis in the left eye 2 years ago. At that time, she was reportedly depressed and was sleeping constantly. One day, her left eye became blurred and her vision went out. In 1 week, her vision returned to normal. Her vision now is 20/20. She has not had a repeat episode since then. She had an MRI of her brain, which was normal at that time. She drinks alcohol occasionally and does not use any illicit drugs. Her only medication is birth control pills. Examination is significant for brisk reflexes and sustained clonus at the right ankle. Babinski sign is present on the right. Testing is positive for oligoclonal bands. The most likely diagnosis in this case is

a.   Seizure
b.   Transient ischemic attack
c.   Anaplastic astrocytoma
d.   Multiple sclerosis
e.   Parkinson's disease

2-15. A 32-year-old G2P0101 presents to labor and delivery at 34 weeks of gestation, complaining of regular uterine contractions about every 5 min for the past several hours. She has also noticed the passage of a clear fluid per vagina. A nurse places the patient on an external fetal monitor and calls you to evaluate her status. The external fetal monitor demonstrates a reactive fetal heart rate tracing, with regular uterine contractions occurring about every 3 to 4 min. On sterile speculum exam, the cervix is visually closed. A sample of pooled amniotic fluid seen in the vaginal vault is fern- and nitrazine-positive. The patient has a temperature of 102°F, P = 102, and her fundus is tender to deep palpation. Her admission blood work comes back indicating a WBC of 19,000. The patient is very concerned because she had previously delivered a baby at 35 weeks who suffered from respiratory distress syndrome. You perform a bedside sonogram, which indicates oligohydramnios and a fetus whose size is appropriate for gestational age and with a cephalic presentation. What is the next appropriate step in the management of this patient?

a. Administer betamethasone
b. Administer tocolytics
c. Place a cervical cerclage
d. Administer antibiotics
e. Perform emergent cesarean section

2-16. A fully immunized 2-year-old presents to the emergency room with several days of low-grade fever, barking cough, and noisy breathing. Over the last few hours he has developed a fever to 40°C (104°F) and looks toxic. He has inspiratory and expiratory stridor. The family has not noticed drooling, and he seems to be drinking without pain. Direct laryngoscopy reveals a normal epiglottis. The management of this disease process includes

a. Intubation and intravenous antibiotics
b. Inhaled epinephrine and oral steroids
c. Inhaled steroids
d. Observation only
e. Oral antibiotics and outpatient follow-up

2-17. A 14-year-old girl awakens with a mild sore throat, low-grade fever, and a diffuse maculopapular rash. During the next 24 h, she develops tender swelling of her wrists and redness of her eyes. In addition, her physician notes mild tenderness and marked swelling of her posterior cervical and occipital lymph nodes. Four days after the onset of her illness, the rash has vanished. The most likely diagnosis of this girl's condition is

a. Rubella
b. Rubeola
c. Roseola
d. Erythema infectiosum
e. Erythema multiforme

2-18. A 3-year-old child is brought to the emergency room by his parents after they found him having a generalized seizure at home. The child's breath smells of garlic, and he has bloody diarrhea, vomiting, and muscle twitching. Which of the following poisons is it likely that this child has encountered?

a. Thallium
b. Lead
c. Arsenic
d. Carbon monoxide
e. Aluminum

2-19. Following a boating injury in an industrial use river, a patient begins to display fever, tachycardia, and a rapidly expanding area of erythema, blistering, and drainage from a flank wound. An x-ray shows gas in the soft tissues. Which of the following measures is most appropriate?

a. Administration of an antifungal agent
b. Administration of antitoxin
c. Wide debridement
d. Administration of hyperbaric oxygen
e. Early closure of tissue defects

2-20. A 40-year-old male complains of hematuria and an aching pain in his flank. Laboratory data show normal BUN, creatinine, and electrolytes. Hemoglobin is elevated at 18 g/dL and serum calcium is 11 mg/dL. A solid renal mass is found by ultrasound. The most likely diagnosis is

a. Polycystic kidney disease
b. Renal carcinoma
c. Adrenal adenoma
d. Urolithiasis

2-21. A patient is receiving a blood transfusion after a reoperative laparotomy for small bowel obstruction. The nurse notes that the blood has clotted in the tubing. What is the most likely cause?

a. ABO incompatibility
b. Minor blood group incompatibility
c. Rh incompatibility
d. Transfusion through Ringer's lactate
e. Transfusion through 5% dextrose and water

2-22. A 5-year old boy has mental retardation, homonymous hemianopsia, and hemiparesis. He had infantile spasm and still has epilepsy. Head CT reveals calcifications in the cerebral cortex in a railroad track pattern Which of the following does this child most likely have?

a. Glioblastoma multiforme
b. Oligodendroglioma
c. Acoustic schwannoma
d. Craniopharyngioma
e. Sturge-Weber syndrome

2-23. A 16-year-old G1P0 at 38 weeks gestation comes to the labor and delivery suite for the second time during the same weekend that you are on call. She initially presented to L and D at 2:00 P.M. Saturday afternoon complaining of regular uterine contractions. Her cervix was 50/1/−1 vertex, and she was sent home after walking for 2 h in the hospital without any cervical change. It is now Sunday night at 8:00 P.M., and the patient returns to L and D with increasing pain. She is exhausted because she did not sleep the night before because her contractions kept waking her up. The patient is placed on the external fetal monitor. Her contractions are occurring every 2 to 3 min. You reexamine the patient and determine that her cervix is unchanged. What is the best next step in the management of this patient?

a. Perform artificial rupture of membranes to initiate labor
b. Administer an epidural
c. Administer Pitocin to augment labor
d. Achieve cervical ripening with prostaglandin gel
e. Administer 10 mg intramuscular morphine
f. Perform a cesarean section

2-24. Two weeks after a viral syndrome, a 2-year-old child develops bruising and generalized petechiae, more prominent over the legs. No hepatosplenomegaly or lymph node enlargement is noted. The examination is otherwise unremarkable. Laboratory testing shows the patient to have a normal hemoglobin, hematocrit, and white blood count and differential. The platelet count is 15,000/μL. The most likely diagnosis is

a. von Willebrand disease
b. Acute leukemia
c. Idiopathic (immune) thrombocytopenic purpura
d. Aplastic anemia
e. Thrombotic thrombocytopenic purpura

2-25. A 50-year-old construction worker continues to have an elevated blood pressure of 160/95 even after a third agent is added to his antihypertensive regimen. Physical exam is normal, electrolytes are normal, and the patient is taking no over-the-counter medications. The next helpful step for this patient is to

a. Check pill count
b. Evaluate for Cushing syndrome
c. Check chest x-ray for coarctation of the aorta
d. Obtain a renal angiogram
e. Obtain an adrenal CT scan

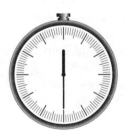

YOU SHOULD HAVE COMPLETED APPROXIMATELY
25 QUESTIONS AND HAVE 30 MINUTES REMAINING.

2-26. A 64-year-old woman is found to have a left-sided pleural effusion on chest x-ray. Analysis of the pleural fluid reveals a ratio of concentration of total protein in pleural fluid to serum of 0.38, a lactate dehydrogenase (LDH) level of 125 IU, and a ratio of LDH concentration in pleural fluid to serum of 0.46. Which of the following disorders is most likely in this patient?

a. Uremia
b. Congestive heart failure
c. Pulmonary embolism
d. Sarcoidosis
e. Systemic lupus erythematosus

2-27. A 56-year-old right-handed woman who had breast cancer 1 year ago began having neurological problems about 1 week ago. She began experiencing nausea, vomiting, and numbness in the right hand and foot. Today she is experiencing crescendo pain in the left retroorbital area. Her headache is throbbing and positional, particularly when she tries to bend forward. The headache was intense in the morning, and at times it woke her up last night. On examination, the only deficits are loss of double simultaneous tactile stimulation and right lower facial droop when smiling. The most appropriate next action would be to

a. Administer intravenous prochlorperazine
b. Give the patient a prescription for zolmitriptan
c. Make a follow-up appointment for next month
d. Order an electroencephalogram to rule out seizures
e. Get a brain MRI

2-28. A 70-year-old man with aortic and mitral valvular regurgitation undergoes an emergency sigmoid colectomy and end colostomy for perforated diverticulitis. His postoperative course is complicated by a myocardial infarction and atrial fibrillation. Four weeks later, he has improved and requests elective colostomy closure. You would recommend

a. Discontinuation of antiarrhythmic and antihypertensive medications on the morning of surgery
b. Discontinuation of beta-blocking medications on the day prior to surgery
c. Control of congestive heart failure with diuretics and digitalis
d. Administration of prophylactic antibiotics other than ampicillin and gentamicin
e. Postponement of elective surgery for 6 to 8 weeks

2-29. A previously well 1-year-old infant has had a runny nose and has been sneezing and coughing for 2 days. Two other members of the family had similar symptoms. Four hours ago, his cough became much worse. On physical examination, he is in moderate respiratory distress with nasal flaring, hyperexpansion of the chest, and easily audible wheezing without rales. The most likely diagnosis is

a. Bronchiolitis
b. Viral croup
c. Asthma
d. Epiglottitis
e. Diphtheria

2-30. An elderly male develops fever 3 days after cholecystectomy. He becomes short of breath, and chest x-ray shows a new right lower lobe infiltrate. Sputum Gram stain shows gram-positive cocci in clumps, and preliminary culture results suggest staphylococci. The initial antibiotic of choice is

a. Penicillinase-resistant penicillin such as nafcillin
b. Vancomycin
c. Antibiotic therapy should be based on the incidence of methicillin-resistant staphylococci in that hospital
d. Quinolones have become the drug of choice for pneumonia

2-31. A 42-year-old man sustains a gunshot wound to the abdomen and is in shock. Multiple units of PRBCs are transfused in an effort to resuscitate him. He complains of numbness around his mouth and displays carpopedal spasm and a positive Chvostek sign. An electrocardiogram demonstrates a prolonged QT interval. The indicated treatment is

a. Intravenous bicarbonate
b. Intravenous potassium
c. Intravenous calcium
d. Intravenous digoxin
e. Intravenous parathyroid hormone

2-32. A 45-year-old man has noticed over the past 6 months that his sense of smell is not as sensitive as it used to be. On examination he has unilateral anosmia, ipsilateral optic atrophy, and contralateral papilledema. He most likely has which of the following?

a.   Pseudotumor cerebri
b.   Multiple sclerosis (MS)
c.   Olfactory groove meningioma
d.   Craniopharyngioma
e.   Nasopharyngeal carcinoma

2-33. A 25-year-old G1P1 comes to see you 6 weeks after an uncomplicated vaginal delivery for a routine postpartum exam. She denies any problems and has been breast-feeding her newborn without any difficulties since leaving the hospital. During the bimanual exam, you note that her uterus is irregular, firm, nontender, and about a 15-week size. Which of the following is the most likely etiology for this enlarged uterus?

a.   Subinvolution of the uterus
b.   The uterus is appropriate size for 6 weeks postpartum
c.   Fibroid uterus
d.   Adenomyosis
e.   Endometritis

2-34. A 50-year-old female is evaluated for hypertension. Her blood pressure is 130/98. She complains of polyuria and of mild muscle weakness. She is on no diuretics or other blood pressure medication. On physical exam, the PMI is displaced to the sixth intercostal space. There is no sign of congestive heart failure and no edema. Laboratory values are as follows:

Na^-: 147 meq/dL
K : 2.3 meq/dL
Cl^-: 112 meq/dL
HCO_3: 27 meq/dL

The patient is on no other medication. She does not eat licorice. The first step in diagnosis is

a.   24-h urine for cortisol
b.   Urinary metanephrine
c.   Plasma renin and aldosterone
d.   Renal angiogram

2-35. A 45-year-old woman presents to her physician with an 8-month history of gradually increasing limb weakness. She first noticed difficulty climbing stairs, then problems rising from chairs, walking more than half a block, and, finally, lifting her arms above shoulder level. Aside from some difficulty swallowing, she has no ocular, bulbar, or sphincter problems and no sensory complaints. Family history is negative for neurological disease. Examination reveals significant proximal limb and neck muscle weakness with minimal atrophy, normal sensory findings, and intact deep tendon reflexes. The most likely diagnosis in this patient is

a. Polymyositis
b. Cervical myelopathy
c. Myasthenia gravis
d. Mononeuropathy multiplex
e. Limb-girdle muscular dystrophy

2-36. A 27-year-old woman comes to a psychiatrist with the chief complaint of feeling depressed her entire life. While she states she has never been so depressed that she has been unable to function, she never feels really good for more than a week or two at a time. She has never been suicidal or psychotic, though her self-esteem is chronically low. Which of the following diagnoses is most likely?

a. Major depression
b. Adjustment disorder
c. Cyclothymia
d. Bipolar disorder
e. Dysthymia

2-37. A 55-year-old man who is extremely obese reports weakness, sweating, tachycardia, confusion, and headache whenever he fasts for more than a few hours. He has prompt relief of symptoms when he eats. These symptoms are most suggestive of which of the following disorders?

a. Diabetes mellitus
b. Insulinoma
c. Zollinger-Ellison syndrome
d. Carcinoid syndrome
e. Multiple endocrine neoplasia, type II

2-38. A 32-year-old G1P0 reports to your office for a routine OB visit at 14 weeks gestational age. Labs drawn at her first prenatal visit 4 weeks ago reveal a platelet count of 60,000. All her other labs were within normal limits. During the present visit, the patient has a blood pressure of 120/70. Her urine dip reveals the presence of trace protein. The patient denies any complaints. The only medication she is currently taking is a prenatal vitamin. On taking a more in-depth history you learn that, prior to pregnancy, your patient had a history of occasional nose and gum bleeds, but no serious bleeding episodes. She has considered herself to be a person who just bruises easily. What is this patient's most likely diagnosis?

a. Alloimmune thrombocytopenia
b. Gestational thrombocytopenia
c. Immune thrombocytopenic purpura
d. HELLP syndrome
e. Pregnancy-induced hypertension

2-39. A 34-year-old woman presents with left-sided chest pain for 8 months. She describes the pain as sharp, intermittent, and associated with palpitations, dizziness, trembling, nausea, paresthesias, and diaphoresis. She experiences three episodes per week. The episodes last 15 min each and may occur at rest or with exertion. The episodes are unpredictable, and the patient often feels as if she is going to die because of the chest pain. The patient does not smoke cigarettes, drink alcohol, or use drugs. She has no family history of heart disease. Her blood pressure and pulse are normal. Physical examination is normal. Electrocardiogram is normal. Which of the following is the most likely diagnosis?

a. Acute myocardial infarction (AMI)
b. Unstable angina
c. Mitral valve prolapse (MVP)
d. Panic disorder
e. Malingering
f. Hyperthyroidism
g. Posttraumatic stress disorder (PTSD)

2-40. The newborn pictured was born at home and has puffy, tense eyelids; red conjunctivae; a copious amount of purulent ocular discharge; and chemosis 2 days after birth. The most likely diagnosis is

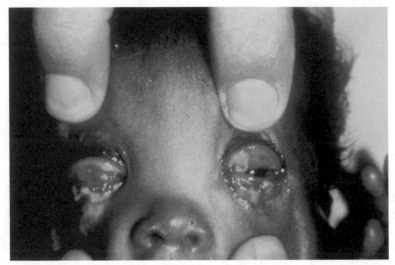

(Courtesy Kathryn Musgrove, M.D.)

a. Dacryocystitis
b. Chemical conjunctivitis
c. Pneumococcal ophthalmia
d. Gonococcal ophthalmia
e. Chlamydial conjunctivitis

2-41. A 65-year-old woman lives alone in a dilapidated house, although her family members have tried in vain to move her to a better dwelling. She wears odd and out-of-fashion clothes and rummages in the garbage cans of her neighbors to look for redeemable cans and bottles. She is very suspicious of her neighbors. She was convinced that her neighbors were plotting against her life for a brief time after she was mugged and thrown onto the pavement by a teenager, but now thinks that this is not the case. She believes in the "power of crystals to protect me" and has them strewn haphazardly throughout her house. What is the most likely diagnosis?

a. Autism
b. Schizophrenia, paranoid type
c. Schizotypal personality disorder
d Avoidant personality disorder
e. Schizoid personality disorder

2-42. A 36-year-old woman has tunnel vision in which she reports the same size area of perception regardless of how far from the testing screen the examination is performed. This history often indicates which of the following?

a. Retinitis pigmentosa
b. Neurosyphilis
c. Sarcoidosis
d. Chorioretinitis
e. Conversion disorder

2-43. A 2-year-old boy is brought into the emergency room with a complaint of fever for 6 days and development of a limp. On examination, he is found to have an erythematous macular exanthem over his body, ocular conjunctivitis, dry and cracked lips, a red throat, and cervical lymphadenopathy. There is a grade II/VI vibratory systolic ejection murmur at the lower left sternal border. A white blood cell count and differential show predominant neutrophils with increased platelets on smear. The most likely diagnosis is

a. Scarlet fever
b. Rheumatic fever
c. Kawasaki disease
d. Juvenile rheumatoid arthritis
e. Infectious mononucleosis

2-44. A 78-year-old female presents to your office for follow-up. She has a history of paroxysmal atrial fibrillation and takes warfarin and digoxin for this problem. Her complaints today are a recent 5-lb weight loss, daily fatigue, and loss of interest in her usual activities. She states she doesn't feel like getting up in the morning. Her spouse adds that she has started taking some alternative therapies from the health food store in an attempt to boost her energy level. On exam, the patient is less animated than usual, and her pulse is irregular at 120/min. She has clear lungs and 1+ edema of the lower extremities. You examine the bag of pills the spouse has brought from the medicine cabinet at home. Which medication is most likely contributing to patient's problem with rapid heart rate?

a. Ginkgo biloba
b. Multivitamin with minerals
c. St. John's wort
d. Soy estrogen
e. Ginseng

2-45. An 8-month-old boy is seen by a pediatrician for the first time. The physician notes that there are no testes in the scrotum. Optimal management of bilateral undescended testicles in an infant is

a. Immediate surgical placement into the scrotum
b. Chorionic gonadotropin therapy for 1 month; operative placement into the scrotum before age 1 if descent has not occurred
c. Observation until the child is 2 years old because delayed descent is common
d. Observation until age 5; if no descent by then, plastic surgical scrotal prostheses before the child enters school
e. No therapy; reassurance of the parent that full masculinization and normal spermatogenesis are likely even if the testicle does not fully descend

2-46. A 72-year-old retired English professor with a long history of hypertension has been having difficulties with tasks he used to find easy and enjoyable, such as crossword puzzles and letter writing, because he cannot remember the correct words and his handwriting has deteriorated. He has also been having difficulties remembering the events of previous days and he moves and thinks at a slower pace. Subsequently, he develops slurred speech. Which of the following diagnoses is most likely in this patient?

a.   Multi-infarct dementia
b.   German-Strausser syndrome
c.   Rett's disorder
d.   Wernicke-Korsakoff syndrome
e.   Alzheimer's disease

2-47. A 32-year-old woman has a 3-year history of oligomenorrhea that has progressed to amenorrhea during the past year. She has observed loss of breast fullness, reduced hip measurements, acne, increased body hair, and deepening of her voice. Physical examination reveals frontal balding, clitoral hypertrophy, and a male escutcheon. Urinary free cortisol and dehydroepiandrosterone sulfate (DHEAS) are normal. Her plasma testosterone level is 6 ng/mL (normal is 0.2 to 0.8). The most likely diagnosis of this patient's disorder is

a.   Cushing syndrome
b.   Arrhenoblastoma
c.   Polycystic ovary syndrome
d.   Granulosa-theca cell tumor

2-48. A 20-year-old ataxic woman with a family history of Friedreich's disease develops polyuria and excessive thirst over the course of a few weeks. She notices that she becomes fatigued easily and has intermittently blurred vision. The most likely explanation for her symptoms is

a.   Inappropriate antidiuretic hormone
b.   Diabetes mellitus
c.   Panhypopituitarism
d.   Progressive adrenal insufficiency
e.   Hypothyroidism

2-49. Physical examination of a baby boy shortly after birth reveals a large bladder and palpable kidneys. A voiding cystourethrogram performed on the baby demonstrates an area of obstruction and proximal dilatation of the urethra, ureters, and kidney. He appears to be otherwise normal. Which of the following is the likely diagnosis?

a. Ureteropelvic junction obstruction
b. Posterior urethral valve
c. Prune belly syndrome
d. Duplication of the collecting system
e. Horseshoe kidney

2-50. A 27-year-old woman (gravida 3, para 2) comes to the delivery floor at 37 weeks gestation. She has had no prenatal care. She complains that, on bending down to pick up her 2-year-old child, she experienced sudden, severe back pain that now has persisted for 2 h. Approximately 30 min ago she noted bright red blood coming from her vagina. By the time she arrives at the delivery floor, she is contracting strongly every 3 min; the uterus is quite firm even between contractions. By abdominal palpation, the fetus is vertex with the head deeply engaged. Fetal heart rate is 130/min. The fundus is 38 cm above the symphysis. Blood for clotting is drawn, and a clot forms in 4 min. Clotting studies are sent to the laboratory. Which of the following actions can wait until the patient is stabilized?

a. Stabilizing maternal circulation
b. Attaching a fetal electronic monitor
c. Inserting an intrauterine pressure catheter
d. Administering oxytocin
e. Preparing for cesarean section

BLOCK 3

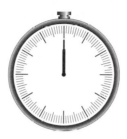

YOU HAVE **60 MINUTES**
TO COMPLETE **50 QUESTIONS.**

Questions

3-1. A 19-year-old woman presents to the emergency room with the chief complaint of a depressed mood for 2 weeks. She states that since her therapist went on vacation she has noted suicidal ideation, crying spells, and an increased appetite. She states that she has left 40 messages on the therapist's answering machine, telling him she is going to kill herself, and that it would serve him right for leaving her. On physical exam, multiple well-healed scars and cigarette burns are noted on the anterior aspect of both forearms. Which of the following diagnoses best fits this patient's clinical presentation?

a. Dysthymic disorder
b. Bipolar disorder
c. Panic disorder
d. Borderline personality disorder
e. Schizoaffective disorder

3-2. A 17-year-old boy is brought to the emergency room by his friends after he "took a few pills" at a party and developed physical symptoms including his neck twisting to one side, his eyes rolling upward, and his tongue hanging out of his mouth. The patient responds immediately to 50 mg of diphenhydramine intramuscularly with the resolution of all physical symptoms. Which of the following substances is most likely to have caused the symptoms?

a. Methamphetamine
b. Meperidine
c. Alprazolam
d. Methylphenidate
e. Haloperidol

3-3. A 35-year-old woman who had been camping in Wisconsin 2 weeks ago develops an erythematous rash on her inner thigh. The macular lesion is 10 cm in diameter and has a distinct red border with central clearing. Two days ago, a second, similar lesion developed. The patient reports no fever, chills, or other symptoms. She has no medical problems or allergies and takes no medications. She does not recall any spider or tick bites. The rest of the physical examination is normal. Which of the following is the most likely diagnosis?

a. Brown recluse spider bite
b. *Borrelia burgdorferi* infection
c. *Bartonella henselae* infection
d. *Mycobacterium marinum* infection
e. *Rickettsia rickettsii* infection

3-4. While you are on call at the hospital covering labor and delivery, a 32-year-old G3P2002 who is 35 weeks calls you complaining of lower back pain. The patient informs you that she had been lifting some heavy boxes while fixing up the baby's nursery. The patient's pregnancy has been complicated by diet-controlled gestational diabetes. The patient denies any regular uterine contractions, rupture of membranes, vaginal bleeding, or dysuria. She denies any fever, chills, nausea, or emesis. She reports that the baby has been moving normally. On physical exam, you note that the patient is obese; her cervix is long and closed. Her abdomen is soft and nontender with no palpable uterine contractions. No flank pain can be elicited. She is afebrile. The external monitor indicates a reactive fetal heart rate strip; there are rare irregular uterine contractions demonstrated on toco. The patient's urinalysis comes back with trace glucose and protein, and is otherwise negative. The patient's most likely diagnosis is which of the following?

a. Labor
b. Musculoskeletal pain
c. Urinary tract infection
d. Chorioamnionitis
e. Round ligament pain

3-5. A 33-year-old operating room nurse accidentally has blood splashed in her eyes during a procedure. The surgical resident who examines her immediately afterward notices that she has 2-mm anisocoria and sends her to the emergency room. She feels well, is alert and talkative, and has no motor dysfunction. On examination, the emergency room physician recognizes that the iris of the eye with the smaller pupil is pale blue, while that of the other eye is brown. The etiology of the woman's anisocoria is probably

a. Conjunctivitis
b. Traumatic third-nerve palsy
c. Carotid artery dissection
d. Pupillary sphincter injury
e. Congenital

3-6. A 43-year-old woman develops acute renal failure following an emergency resection of a leaking abdominal aortic aneurysm. Three days after surgery, the following laboratory values are obtained:

Serum electrolytes (meq/L): Na^+ 127; K^+ 5.9; Cl^- 92; HCO_3- 15
Blood urea nitrogen: 82 mg/dL
Serum creatinine: 6.7 mg/dL

The patient has gained 4 kg since surgery and is mildly dyspneic at rest. Eight hours after these values are reported, the electrocardiogram shown below is obtained. The initial treatment for this patient should be

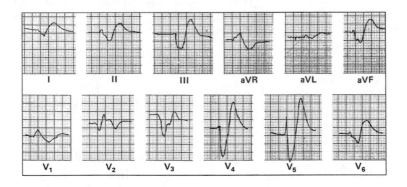

a. 10% calcium gluconate, 10 mL
b. 0.25 mg digoxin every 3 h for three doses
c. Oral Kayexalate
d. 100 mg lidocaine
e. Emergent hemodialysis

3-7. A 15-year-old girl is brought to the pediatric emergency room by the lunchroom teacher, who observed her sitting alone and crying. On questioning, the teacher learned that the girl had taken five tablets after having had an argument with her mother about a boyfriend of whom the mother disapproved. Toxicology studies are negative, and physical examination is normal. The most appropriate course of action would be to

a. Hospitalize the teenager on the adolescent ward
b. Get a psychiatry consultation
c. Get a social service consultation
d. Arrange a family conference that includes the boyfriend
e. Prescribe an antidepressant and arrange for a prompt clinic appointment

3-8. A 66-year-old woman presents for her annual eye examination. She has been seeing floaters recently but has no other complaints. Intraocular pressure measurement by Schiotz tonometry is 21 mmHg. Red reflex is visible and normal. Pupils are equal and reactive to light; extraocular muscles are intact. Examination of the fundi reveals the presence of white, indistinct opaque areas in the superficial retina. They occasionally obscure nearby vessels. There is a positive and normal light reflex. There are no hard exudates, hemorrhages, bony spicule formation, or microaneurysms. The optic cup constitutes 30% of the optic disc, and there is no papilledema. Which of the following is the most likely diagnosis?

a. Glaucoma
b. Early cataract
c. Macular degeneration
d. Hypertensive retinopathy
e. Retinitis pigmentosa
f. Early retinal detachment

3-9. A 73-year-old woman with a long history of heavy smoking undergoes femoral artery–popliteal artery bypass for resting pain in her left leg. Because of serious underlying respiratory insufficiency, she continues to require ventilatory support for 4 days after her operation. As soon as her endotracheal tube is removed, she begins complaining of vague upper abdominal pain. She has daily fever spikes to 39°C (102.2°F) and a leukocyte count of 18,000/mL. An upper abdominal ultrasonogram reveals a dilated gallbladder, but no stones are seen. A presumptive diagnosis of acalculous cholecystitis is made. You recommend

a. Nasogastric suction and broad-spectrum antibiotics
b. Immediate cholecystectomy with operative cholangiogram
c. Percutaneous drainage of the gallbladder
d. Endoscopic retrograde cholangiopancreatography (ERCP) to visualize and drain the common bile duct
e. Provocation of cholecystokinin release by cautious feeding of the patient

3-10. A 13-year-old girl grunts and clears her throat several times in an hour, and her conversation is often interrupted by random shouting. She also performs idiosyncratic, complex motor activities such as turning her head to the right while she shuts her eyes and opens her mouth. She can prevent these movements for brief periods of time, with effort. Which of the following is the most appropriate treatment for this disorder?

a. Individual psychodynamic psychotherapy
b. Lorazepam
c. Methylphenidate
d. Haloperidol
e. Imipramine

3-11. A 35-year-old man injured his thoracic spine in a motor vehicle accident 2 years ago. Initially he had a bilateral spastic paraparesis and urinary urgency, but this has improved. He still has pain and thermal sensation loss on part of his left body and proprioception loss in his right foot. There is still a paralysis of the right lower extremity as well. This patient has which spinal cord condition?

a. Brown-Séquard (hemisection) syndrome
b. Complete transection
c. Posterior column syndrome
d. Syringomyelic syndrome
e. Tabetic syndrome

3-12. A 32-year-old white woman complains of abdominal pain off and on since the age of 17. She notices abdominal bloating relieved by defecation as well as alternating diarrhea and constipation. She has no weight loss, GI bleeding, or nocturnal diarrhea. On examination, she has slight LLQ tenderness and gaseous abdominal distension. Laboratory studies, including CBC, are normal. Your initial approach should be

a. Recommend increased dietary fiber, prn antispasmodics, and follow-up exam in 2 months
b. Refer to gastroenterologist for colonoscopy
c. Obtain antiendomysial antibodies
d. Order UGI series with small bowel follow-through

3-13. A 70-year-old man with a dementing disorder dies in a car accident. During the previous 5 years, his personality had dramatically changed and he had caused much embarrassment to his family due to his intrusive and inappropriate behavior. Pathological examination of his brain shows frontotemporal atrophy, gliosis of the frontal lobes' white matter, characteristic intracellular inclusions, and swollen neurons. Amyloid plaques and neurofibrillary tangles are absent. Which of the following is the correct diagnosis?

a. Alzheimer's disease
b. Pick's disease
c. Creutzfeldt-Jakob disease
d. B_{12} deficiency dementia
e. HIV dementia

3-14. A teenage boy falls from his bicycle and is run over by a truck. On arrival in the emergency room, he is awake and alert and appears frightened but in no distress. The chest radiograph suggests an air-fluid level in the left lower lung field and the nasogastric tube seems to coil upward into the left chest. The best next step in management is

a. Placement of a left chest tube
b. Immediate thoracotomy
c. Immediate celiotomy
d. Esophagogastroscopy
e. Removal and replacement of the nasogastric tube; diagnostic peritoneal lavage

3-15. A 45-year-old woman presents with a 2-year history of nonproductive cough. The cough is not associated with time of day or year, and the patient denies any occupational or environmental exposures. She has never smoked cigarettes. She finds herself clearing her throat frequently during the day and night. She has no nasal discharge, heartburn, or cardiac symptoms. She denies fever, chest pain, or shortness of breath. She takes no medications. On physical examination, her nasopharynx reveals mucopurulent secretions and a cobblestone-appearing mucosa. Lung examination is normal. Chest radiograph is normal. Which of the following is the most likely diagnosis?

a. Reflux disease
b. Asthma
c. Bronchitis
d. Postnasal drip
e. Use of ACE inhibitors
f. Congestive heart failure

3-16. The parents of a 14-year-old boy are concerned about his short stature and lack of sexual development. By history, you learn that his birth weight and length were 3 kg and 50 cm, respectively, and that he had a normal growth pattern, although he was always shorter than children his age. The physical examination is normal. His upper-to-lower segment ratio is 0.98. A small amount of fine axillary and pubic hair is present. There is no scrotal pigmentation; his testes measure 4.0 cm^3 and his penis is 6 cm in length. In this situation you should

a. Measure pituitary gonadotropin
b. Obtain a CT scan of the pituitary area
c. Biopsy his testes
d. Measure serum testosterone levels
e. Reassure the parents that the boy is normal

3-17. You are called to evaluate a 57-year-old man with pressure-like chest pain that occurred while he was shoveling snow. The pain radiates to the jaw and medial aspect of the left arm. The patient denies dizziness, nausea, vomiting, or palpitations. He has a past medical history of hypertension and he smokes two packs of cigarettes per day. He has a brother who had a myocardial infarction that required balloon angioplasty when he was in his forties. The patient has recently been told to modify his diet because of high glucose and cholesterol levels. On physical examination the patient appears pale and diaphoretic. Blood pressure is 160/100 mmHg and pulse is 108/min. His extremities are cool. Heart examination reveals an S_4 gallop. Lungs are normal. Peripheral pulses are palpable and bilaterally equal. He has no peripheral edema. Which of the following is the most likely diagnosis?

a. Right ventricular infarction
b. Cardiogenic shock
c. Acute myocardial infarction
d. Congestive heart failure (CHF)
e. Prinzmetal's angina

3-18. A young man with multiple sclerosis (MS) exhibits paradoxical dilation of the right pupil when a flashlight is redirected from the left eye into the right eye. Swinging the flashlight back to the left eye produces constriction of the right pupil. This patient apparently has

a. Early cataract formation in the right eye
b. Occipital lobe damage on the left
c. Oscillopsia
d. Hippus
e. Optic atrophy

3-19. A 65-year-old male develops the sudden onset of severe knee pain. The knee is red, swollen, and tender. He has a history of diabetes mellitus and cardiomyopathy. An x-ray of the knee shows linear calcification. Definitive diagnosis is best made by

a. Serum uric acid
b. Serum calcium
c. Arthrocentesis and identification of positively birefringent rhomboid crystals
d. Rheumatoid factor

3-20. A 28-year-old G0, LMP 1 week ago, presents to your gynecology clinic complaining of a mass in her left breast that she discovered on a routine breast self-exam in the shower. When you perform a breast exam on her, you palpate a 2-cm firm, nontender mass in the upper inner quadrant of the left breast that is well circumscribed and mobile. You do not detect any skin changes, nipple discharge, or lymphadenopathy. What is this patient's most likely diagnosis?

a. Fibrocystic breast change
b. Fibroadenoma
c. Breast carcinoma
d. Fat necrosis
e. Cystosarcoma phyllodes

3-21. A 37-year-old mildly retarded man with trisomy 21 syndrome has been increasingly forgetful. He makes frequent mistakes when counting change at the grocery store where he has worked for several years. In the past, he used to perform this task without difficulties. He often cannot recall the names of common objects, and he has started annoying customers with his intrusive questions. Which of the following diagnoses is most likely in this patient?

a. Pseudodementia
b. Hypothalamic tumor
c. Alzheimer's disease
d. Wilson's disease
e. Thiamine deficiency

3-22. A 31-year-old man is brought to the emergency room following an automobile accident in which his chest struck the steering wheel. Examination reveals stable vital signs, but the patient exhibits multiple palpable rib fractures and paradoxical movement of the right side of the chest. Chest x-ray shows no evidence of pneumothorax or hemothorax, but a large pulmonary contusion is developing. Proper treatment consists of which of the following?

a. Tracheostomy, mechanical ventilation, and positive end-expiratory pressure
b. Stabilization of the chest wall with sandbags
c. Stabilization with towel clips
d. Immediate operative stabilization
e. No treatment unless signs of respiratory distress develop

3-23. A very concerned mother brings a 2-year-old child to your office because of multiple episodes of a brief, shrill cry followed by a prolonged expiration and apnea. You have been following this child in your practice since birth and know that the child is a product of a normal pregnancy and delivery, has been growing and developing normally, and has no acute medical problems. The mother relates that the first episode in question occurred immediately after the mother refused to give the child some juice. The child became cyanotic and unconscious and had generalized clonic jerks. A few moments later the child awakened and had no residual effects. A second episode of identical nature occurred at the grocery store when the father of the child refused to purchase a toy for the child. Your physical examination reveals a totally delightful and normal child. The most likely diagnosis in this case is

a. Seizure disorder
b. Drug ingestion
c. Hyperactivity with attention deficit
d. Pervasive development disorder
e. Breath-holding spell

3-24. A 47-year-old man with hypertensive nephropathy develops fever, graft tenderness, and oliguria 4 weeks following cadaveric renal transplantation. Serum creatinine is 3.1 mg/dL. A renal ultrasound reveals mild edema of the renal papillae but normal flow in both the renal artery and renal vein. Nuclear scan demonstrates sluggish uptake and excretion. The most appropriate next step is

a. Performing an angiogram
b. Decreasing steroid and cyclosporine dose
c. Beginning intravenous antibiotics
d. Performing renal biopsy, steroid boost, and immunoglobulin therapy
e. Beginning FK 506

3-25. A 43-year-old man comes to the physician with the chief complaint of nervousness and excitability for 3 months. He states that he feels this way constantly, and this is a dramatic change for his normally relaxed personality. He notes that on occasion he becomes extremely afraid of his own impending death, even when there is no objective evidence that this would occur. He notes that he has lost 20 lb and frequently has diarrhea. On mental status examination, he is noted to have pressured speech. On physical examination, he is noted to have a fine tremor and tachycardia. Which of the following disorders is this patient most likely to have?

a. Hyperthyroidism
b. Hypothyroidism
c. Hepatic encephalopathy
d. Hyperparathyroidism
e. Hypoparathyroidism

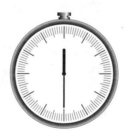

**YOU SHOULD HAVE COMPLETED APPROXIMATELY
25 QUESTIONS AND HAVE 30 MINUTES REMAINING.**

3-26. A 40-year-old man presents to the emergency room complaining of severe abdominal pain that radiates to his back accompanied by several episodes of vomiting. He drinks alcohol daily. On physical examination, the patient is found on the stretcher lying in the fetal position. He is febrile and appears ill. The skin of his abdomen has an area of bluish periumbilical discoloration. There is no flank discoloration. Abdominal examination reveals decreased bowel sounds. The patient has severe midepigastric tenderness on palpation and complains of exquisite pain when your hands are abruptly withdrawn from his abdomen. Rectal examination is normal. Which of the following is the most likely diagnosis?

a. Acute cholecystitis
b. Pyelonephritis
c. Necrotizing pancreatitis
d. Chronic pancreatitis
e. Diverticulitis
f. Appendicitis

3-27. A mentally retarded male adolescent who has been increasingly aggressive and agitated receives several consecutive IM doses of haloperidol, totaling 30 mg in 24 h, as a chemical restraint. The next day, he is rigid, confused, and unresponsive. His blood pressure is 150/95, his pulse is 110/min, and his temperature is 102°F. His white blood cell (WBC) count is 25,000, and CPK level is 1,200 μ/L. What is the most likely diagnosis?

a. Acute dystonic reaction
b. Neuroleptic-induced Parkinson's disease
c. Malignant hyperthermia
d. Neuroleptic malignant syndrome
e. Catatonia

3-28. A patient comes to your office with LMP 4 weeks ago. She denies any symptoms such as nausea, fatigue, urinary frequency, or breast tenderness. She thinks that she may be pregnant because she has not gotten her period yet and is very anxious to find out because she has a history of a previous ectopic pregnancy and wants to be sure to get early prenatal care. Which of the following evaluation methods is most sensitive in diagnosing pregnancy?

a. No evaluation to determine pregnancy is needed because the patient is asymptomatic and therefore cannot be pregnant
b. Serum pregnancy test
c. Detection of fetal heart tones by Doppler equipment
d. Abdominal ultrasound
e. Bimanual exam to assess uterine size

3-29. A 52-year-old woman presents to her private physician with the chief complaint of hoarseness. She sings in her church choir, and her friends noticed a voice change. Her past medical history is significant for heart arrhythmias, which are well controlled for 3 years with amiodarone. Physical examination reveals a woman with coarse hair and skin. Her fingernails are thick, and her eyes appear puffy. The thyroid gland is normal and nontender. Her muscle strength is excellent, but the relaxation phase of her ankle reflex is prolonged. Which of the following is the most likely diagnosis?

a. Cushing's disease
b. Acromegaly
c. de Quervain's disease
d. Amiodarone-induced hypothyroidism
e. Cretinism

3-30. A 22-year-old college student calls his psychiatrist because he notes that for the past week, after cramming hard for finals, that his thoughts have been racing and he is irritable. The psychiatrist notes that the patient's speech is pressured as well. The patient has been stable for the past 6 months on 500 milligrams of valproate twice a day. What is the first step the psychiatrist should take in the management of this patient's symptoms?

a. Hospitalize the patient
b. Increase the valproate by 500 mg/d
c. Prescribe clonazepam 1 mg qhs
d. Start haloperidol 5 mg qd
e. Tell the patient to begin psychotherapy one time per week

3-31. A 65-year-old man undergoes a technically difficult abdominoperineal resection for a rectal cancer during which he receives three units of packed red blood cells. Four hours later in the intensive care unit he is bleeding heavily from his perineal wound. Emergency coagulation studies reveal normal prothrombin, partial thromboplastin, and bleeding times. The fibrin degradation products are not elevated, but the serum fibrinogen content is depressed and the platelet count is 70,000/μL. The most likely cause of the bleeding is

a. Delayed blood transfusion reaction
b. Autoimmune fibrinolysis
c. A bleeding blood vessel in the surgical field
d. Factor VIII deficiency
e. Hypothermic coagulopathy

3-32. A 44-year-old man presents with left arm shaking. Two days ago, the patient noted left arm paresthesias along the lateral aspect of his left arm and left fourth and fifth fingers while he was reading. He thinks he may have been leaning on his left arm at the time; the symptoms resolved after 30 s. This morning, he noted the same feelings, lasting a few seconds, but then his 4th and 5th fingers started shaking rhythmically, and the shaking then migrated to all his fingers, his hand, and then his arm up to his elbow. This episode lasted a total of 30 s. He denies any strange smells or tastes, visual changes, or weakness. Afterward, his fingers felt locked in position for a few seconds. Then he felt as if he did not have control of his hand and had difficulty donning his socks. He and his wife decided to drive to emergency room, and in the car he had trouble putting his seat belt latch into its socket. Examination and routine labs are normal. The next most appropriate action would be to

a. Discharge the patient to follow up in clinic in 2 weeks
b. Obtain a brain MRI
c. Obtain an electroencephalogram
d. Obtain an orthopedic consult
e. Order electromyography and nerve conduction studies

3-33. A 32-year-old G3P3 presents with abdominal pain. Her last menstrual period was 6 weeks ago, and a pregnancy test is positive. The specimen shown below is obtained at laparotomy. The most likely diagnosis is

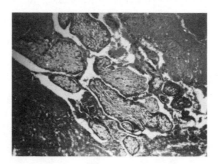

a. Incomplete abortion
b. Missed abortion
c. Hydatidiform mole
d. Tubal ectopic pregnancy
e. Ovarian pregnancy

3-34. A 36-year-old G1P0 at 35 weeks gestation presents to your office complaining of a several-day history of generalized malaise, anorexia, nausea, and emesis. She has also been experiencing abdominal discomfort, which she attributes to indigestion. She has had a poor appetite and has lost several pounds since her last office visit 1 week ago. She denies any headache or visual changes. Her fetal movement has been good, and she denies any regular uterine contractions, vaginal bleeding, or rupture of membranes. This patient is on no medications except for a prenatal vitamin, and has no history of any medical problems. On physical exam, you notice that she is mildly jaundiced and appears to be a little confused. Her vital signs indicate a temperature of 100°F, pulse of 70, and BP of 100/62. She has no significant edema, and in fact appears very dehydrated. You send her to labor and delivery for IV hydration and additional evaluation. Once in labor and delivery, the patient is hooked up to an external fetal monitor, which indicates a fetal heart rate in the 160s that is nonreactive, but with good variability. Blood is drawn and the following results are obtained: WBC = 25,000, Hct = 42.0, platelets = 51,000, SGOT/PT = 287/350, glucose = 43, creatinine = 2.0, fibrinogen = 135, PT/PTT = 16/50 s, serum ammonia level = 90 μmol/L (nl = 11–35). Urinalysis is positive for 3+ protein and large ketones. Which of the following is the patient's most likely diagnosis?

a. Hepatitis B
b. Acute fatty liver of pregnancy
c. Intrahepatic cholestasis of pregnancy
d. Severe preeclampsia
e. Hyperemesis gravidarum

3-35. A 23-year-old woman arrives at the emergency room complaining that, out of the blue, she had been seized by an overwhelming fear, associated with shortness of breath and a pounding heart. These symptoms lasted for approximately 20 min, and, while she was experiencing them, she feared that she was dying or going crazy. The patient has had four similar episodes during the past month, and she has been worrying that they will continue recurring. Which of the following diagnoses is most likely?

a. Acute psychotic episode
b. Hypochondriasis
c. Panic disorder
d. Generalized anxiety disorder
e. Posttraumatic stress disorder

3-36. A 4-year-old boy is seen 1 h after ingestion of a lye drain cleaner. No oropharyngeal burns are noted, but the patient's voice is hoarse. Chest x-ray is normal. Of the following, which is the most appropriate therapy?

a. Immediate esophagoscopy
b. Parenteral steroids and antibiotics
c. Administration of an oral neutralizing agent
d. Induction of vomiting
e. Rapid administration of a quart of water to clear remaining lye from the esophagus and dilute material in stomach

3-37. A 60-year-old, mildly obese woman presents complaining of bilateral medial right knee pain that occurs with prolonged standing. The pain does not occur with sitting or climbing stairs but seems to be worse with other activity and at the end of the day. The patient denies morning stiffness. Examination of the knees reveals no deformity, but there are small effusions. Some mild pain and crepitus are produced with palpation of the medial aspect of the knees. Which of the following is the most likely diagnosis?

a. Rheumatoid arthritis
b. Gouty arthritis
c. Chondromalacia patellae
d. Osteoarthritis
e. Psoriatic arthritis

3-38. A 6-year-old child is hospitalized for observation because of a short period of unconsciousness after a fall from a playground swing. He has developed unilateral pupillary dilatation, focal seizures, recurrence of depressed consciousness, and hemiplegia. Appropriate management would be

a. Spinal tap
b. CT scan
c. Rapid fluid hydration
d. Naloxone
e. Gastric decontamination with charcoal

3-39. An 8-year-old is accidentally hit in the abdomen by a baseball bat. After several minutes of discomfort, he seems to be fine. Over the ensuing 24 h, however, he develops a fever, abdominal pain radiating to the back, and persistent vomiting. On examination, the child appears quite uncomfortable. The abdomen is tender, with decreased bowel sounds throughout, but especially painful, with guarding in the midepigastric region. The test likely to confirm your suspicions is

a. Serum amylase
b. Complete blood count with differential and platelets
c. Serum total and direct bilirubin levels
d. Abdominal radiograph
e. Electrolyte panel

3-40. A previously healthy 15-year-old boy is brought to the emergency room with complaints of about 12 h of progressive anorexia, nausea, and pain of the right lower quadrant. On physical examination, he is found to have a rectal temperature of 38.18°C (100.58°F) and direct and rebound abdominal tenderness localizing to McBurney's point as well as involuntary guarding in the right lower quadrant. At operation through a McBurney-type incision, the appendix and cecum are found to be normal, but the surgeon is impressed by the marked edema of the terminal ileum, which also has an overlying fibrinopurulent exudate. The correct procedure is to

a. Close the abdomen after culturing the exudate
b. Perform a standard appendectomy
c. Resect the involved terminal ileum
d. Perform an ileocolic resection
e. Perform an ileocolostomy to bypass the involved terminal ileum

3-41. A 22-year-old gravida 1, para 0 has just undergone a spontaneous vaginal delivery. As the placenta is being delivered, an inverted uterus prolapses out of the vagina. The maneuver most likely to exacerbate the situations would be to

a. Immediately finish delivering the placenta by removing it from the inverted uterus
b. Call for immediate assistance from other medical personnel
c. Obtain intravenous access and give lactated Ringer solution
d. Apply pressure to the fundus with the palm of the hand and fingers in the direction of the long axis of the vagina
e. Have the anesthesiologist administer halothane anesthesia for uterine relaxation

3-42. A patient with small cell carcinoma of the lung develops lethargy. Serum electrolytes are drawn and show a serum sodium of 118 mg/L. There is no evidence of edema, orthostatic hypotension, or dehydration. Urine is concentrated with an osmolality of 320 mmol/kg. Serum BUN, creatinine, and glucose are within normal range. Which of the following is the next appropriate step?

a. Normal saline infusion
b. Diuresis
c. Fluid restriction
d. Tetracycline

3-43. A 3-day-old infant born at 32 weeks' gestation and weighing 1700 g (3 lb, 12 oz) has three episodes of apnea, each lasting 20 to 25 s and occurring after a feeding. During these episodes, the heart rate drops from 140 to 100 beats per min, and the child remains motionless; between episodes, however, the child displays normal activity. Blood sugar is 50 mg/dL and serum calcium is normal. The child's apneic periods most likely are

a. Due to an immature respiratory center
b. A part of periodic breathing
c. Secondary to hypoglycemia
d. Manifestations of seizures
e. Evidence of underlying pulmonary disease

3-44. Your patient is a 40-year-old G4P5 who is 39 weeks and has progressed rapidly in labor with a reassuring fetal heart rate pattern. She has had an uncomplicated pregnancy with normal prenatal labs including an amniocentesis for advanced maternal age. The patient begins the second stage of labor and after 15 min of pushing starts to demonstrate deep variable heart rate accelerations. You suspect that she may have a fetus with a nuchal cord. You expediently deliver the baby by low outlet forceps and hand the baby over to the neonatologists called to attend the delivery. As soon as the baby is handed off to the pediatric team, it lets out a strong spontaneous cry. The infant is pink with slightly blue extremities that are actively moving and kicking. The heart rate is noted to be 110 on auscultation. You send a cord gas, which comes back with the following arterial blood values: pH 7.29, P_{CO_2} 50, and P_{O_2} 20. What Apgar score should the pediatricians assign to this baby at 1 min of life?

a. 10
b. 9
c. 8
d. 7
e. 6

3-45. A 23-year-old woman returns home after delivering a healthy baby girl. She notes over the next week that she has become increasingly irritable and is not sleeping very well. She worries that she will not be a good mother and that she will make an error in caring for her baby. What is the most likely diagnosis?

a. Postpartum depression
b. Postpartum psychosis
c. Adjustment disorder
d. Postpartum blues
e. Major depression

3-46. A 14-year-old black girl has her right breast removed because of a large mass. The tumor weighs 1400 g and has a bulging, very firm, lobulated surface with a whorl-like pattern, as illustrated below. This neoplasm is most likely

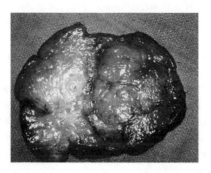

a. Cystosarcoma phyllodes
b. Intraductal carcinoma
c. Malignant lymphoma
d. Fibroadenoma
e. Juvenile hypertrophy

3-47. A 51-year-old woman is diagnosed with invasive cervical carcinoma by cone biopsy. Pelvic examination and rectal-vaginal examination reveal the parametrium to be free of disease, but the upper portion of the vagina is involved with tumor. Intravenous pyelography (IVP) and sigmoidoscopy are negative, but a computed tomography (CT) scan of the abdomen and pelvis shows grossly enlarged pelvic and periaortic nodes. This patient is classified as stage

a. IIa
b. IIb
c. IIIa
d. IIIb
e. IV

3-48. A 28-year-old graduate student presents with confusion and mild right hemiparesis developing over the course of an evening. His girlfriend relates that he has been complaining of severe headaches each morning for the past 2 weeks. While being evaluated in the emergency room, he has a generalized tonic—clonic seizure. When examined 2 h later, he is lethargic and unable to recall recent events, has difficulty naming, and has a right pronator drift. There is mild weakness of abduction of the eyes bilaterally. Funduscopic examination might be expected to show which of the following?

a. Pigmentary degeneration of the retina
b. Hollenhorst plaques
c. Retinal venous pulsations
d. Blurring of the margins of the optic disc
e. Pallor of the optic disc

3-49. A 36-year-old woman is brought to the psychiatrist by her husband because for the past 8 months she refuses to go out of the house because she states that the neighbors are trying to harm her. She is afraid that if they see her they will hurt her, and finds many small bits of evidence supporting this fact. This evidence includes the fact that the neighbors leave their garbage cans out on the street to try to trip her, they park their cars in their driveways so that they can hide behind them and spy on her, and they walk by her house to try to get a look into where she is hiding. She states that her mood is fine, and would be "better if they would leave me alone." She denies hearing the neighbors or anyone else talk to her, but is sure that they are out to "cause her death and mayhem." Which of the following diagnoses is the most likely in this patient?

a. Delusional disorder
b. Schizophreniform disorder
c. Schizoaffective disorder
d. Schizophrenia
e. Major depression with psychotic features

3-50. A 42-year-old nursing student presents to the emergency room with confusion, diaphoresis, and dizziness. She is tremulous and tachycardic. Her serum glucose level is found to be 20 mg/dL, and she responds immediately to intravenous dextrose infusion. The patient states that she has been eating well. After the hypoglycemia is corrected, the physical examination is normal. Bloodwork reveals that insulin levels are high but C-peptide level is low. The rest of the laboratory data are normal. Which of the following is the most likely diagnosis?

a. Insulinoma
b. Surreptitious insulin injection
c. Hypopituitarism
d. Adrenal insufficiency
e. Glucagon deficiency

BLOCK 4

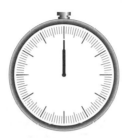

YOU HAVE *60* MINUTES
TO COMPLETE *50* QUESTIONS.

Questions

4-1. A 43-year-old woman with a 1-year history of episodic leg edema and dyspnea is noted to have clubbing of the fingers. Her ECG is shown below. The correct diagnosis is

a. Inferior wall myocardial infarction
b. Right bundle branch block
c. Acute pericarditis
d. Wolff-Parkinson-White syndrome
e. Cor pulmonale

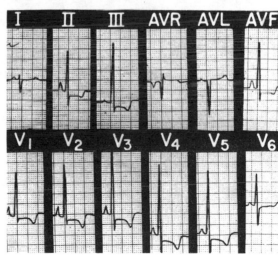

4-2. The previously healthy 4-year-old child pictured presents to the emergency room with a 2-day history of a brightly erythematous rash and temperature of 40°C (104°F). The exquisitely tender, generalized rash is worse in the flexural and perioral areas. The child is admitted and over the next day develops crusting and fissuring around the eyes, mouth, and nose. The desquamation of skin shown occurs with gentle traction. This child most likely has

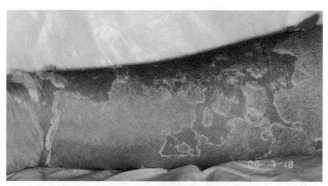

A   *(Courtesy Adelaide Hebert, M.D.)*

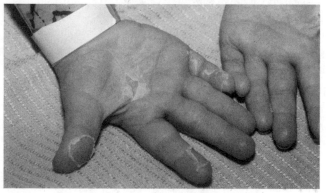

B   *(Courtesy Adelaide Hebert, M.D.)*

a. Epidermolysis bullosa
b. Staphylococcal scalded skin syndrome
c. Erythema multiforme
d. Drug eruption
e. Scarlet fever

4-3. A 4-year-old boy has the onset of episodes of loss of body tone, with associated falls, as well as generalized tonic-clonic seizures. His cognitive function has been deteriorating. EEG shows 1.5- to 2-Hz spike-and-wave discharges. The most likely diagnosis is

a. Landau-Kleffner syndrome
b. Lennox-Gastaut syndrome
c. Juvenile myoclonic epilepsy
d. Mitochondrial encephalomyopathy
e. Febrile seizures

4-4. A 24-year-old patient has returned from a yearlong stay in the tropics. Four weeks ago she noted a small vulvar ulceration that spontaneously healed. Now there is painful inguinal adenopathy with malaise and fever. You are considering the diagnosis of lymphogranuloma venereum (LGV). The diagnosis can be established by

a. Staining for Donovan bodies
b. The presence of antibodies to *Chlamydia trachomatis*
c. Positive Frei skin test
d. Culturing *Haemophilus ducreyi*
e. Culturing *Calymmatobacterium granulomatis*

4-5. A 55-year-old postmenopausal female presents to her gynecologist for a routine exam. She denies any use of hormone replacement therapy and does not report any menopausal symptoms. She denies the occurrence of any abnormal vaginal bleeding. She has no history of any abnormal Pap smears and has been married for 30 years to the same partner. She is currently sexually active with her husband on a regular basis. Two weeks after her exam, her Pap smear comes back as atypical glandular cells of undetermined significance (AGUS). What is the next most appropriate step in the management of this patient?

a. Re-Pap in 4 to 6 months
b. HPV testing
c. Hysterectomy
d. Cone biopsy
e. Colposcopy, endometrial biopsy, endocervical curettage

4-6. A 25-year-old woman is brought to the physician by her boyfriend after he noticed a change in her personality over the preceding 6 months. He states that she often becomes excessively preoccupied with a single theme, often religious in nature. She was not previously a religious person. He notes that she often perseverates on a theme while she is speaking as well, and is overinclusive in her descriptions. Finally, he notes that while previously the two had a satisfying sexual life, now the patient appears to have no sex drive whatsoever. The physician finds the patient to be very emotionally intense as well. Physical examination was normal. Which of the following diagnoses is most likely?

a. Wernicke-Korsakoff syndrome
b. Temporal lobe epilepsy
c. Pick's disease
d. Multiple sclerosis
e. HIV-related dementia

4-7. A 2-year-old child (A) presents with a four-day history of a rash limited to the feet and ankles. The papular rash is both pruritic and erythematous. The 3-month-old sibling of this patient (B) has similar lesions also involving the head and neck. Appropriate treatment for this condition includes

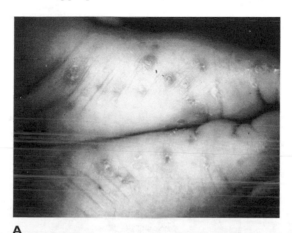

A

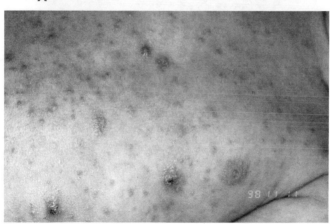

B *(Courtesy Adelaide Hebert, M.D.)*

a. Coal-tar soap
b. Permethrin
c. Hydrocortisone cream
d. Emollients
e. Topical antifungal cream

4-8. A 54-year-old man with a chronic mental illness seems to be constantly chewing. He does not wear dentures. His tongue darts in and out of his mouth, and he occasionally smacks his lips. He also grimaces, frowns, and blinks excessively. Which of the following disorders is most likely in this patient?

a. Tourette's syndrome
b. Akathisia
c. Tardive dyskinesia
d. Parkinson's disease
e. Huntington's disease

4-9. A previously healthy 80-year-old woman presents with early satiety and abdominal fullness. The CT scan shown below is obtained. The lesion is most likely a

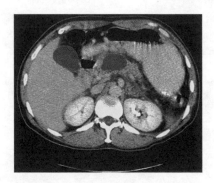

a. Pancreatic pseudocyst
b. Pancreatic adenocarcinoma
c. Pancreatic cystadenocarcinoma
d. Retroperitoneal lymphoma
e. Pancreatic serous cystadenoma

4-10. An 18-year-old male complains of fever and transient pain in both knees and elbows. The right knee was red and swollen for 1 day the week prior to presentation. On physical exam, the patient has a low-grade fever but appears generally well. There is an aortic diastolic murmur heard at the base of the heart. A nodule is palpated over the extensor tendon of the hand. There are pink erythematous lesions over the abdomen, some with central clearing. The following laboratory values are obtained:

Hct: 42
WBC: 12,000/μL
20% polymorphonuclear leukocytes
80% lymphocytes
ESR: 60 mm/h

    The patient's ECG is shown below.

    Which of the following tests is most critical to diagnosis?

a. Blood cultures
b. Antistreptolysin O antibody
c. Echocardiogram
d. Antinuclear antibodies
e. Creatinine phosphokinase

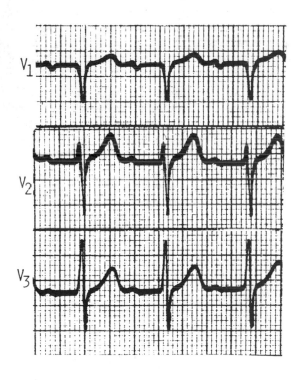

4-11. A 62-year-old woman complains of limb discomfort and trouble getting off the toilet. She is unable to climb stairs and has noticed a rash on her face about her eyes. On examination, she is found to have weakness about the hip and shoulder girdle. Not only does she have a purplish-red discoloration of the skin about the eyes, but she also has erythematous discoloration over the finger joints and purplish nodules over the elbows and knees. Which of the following is the most probable diagnosis?

a. Systemic lupus erythematosus
b. Psoriasis
c. Myasthenia gravis
d. Dermatomyositis
e. Rheumatoid arthritis

4-12. A 41-year-old G1P0 at 39 weeks, who has been completely dilated and pushing for 3 h, has an epidural in place and remains undelivered. She is exhausted and crying and tells you that she can no longer push. Her temperature is 101°F. The fetal heart rate is in the 190s with decreased variability. The patient's membranes have been ruptured for over 24 h, and she has been receiving intravenous ampicillin for a history of colonization with group B strep bacteria. The patient's cervix is completely dilated and effaced and the fetal head is in the direct OA position and is visible at the introitus between pushes. Extensive caput is noted, but the fetal bones are at the +3 station. What is the most appropriate next step in the management of this patient?

a. Deliver the patient by cesarean section
b. Encourage the patient to continue to push after a short rest
c. Attempt operative delivery with forceps
d. Rebolus the patient's epidural
e. Cut a fourth-degree episiotomy

4-13. Five days after going on a nature walk, a 13-year-old boy develops well-demarcated erythematous plaques and vesicles over his arms and face. The plaques are arranged in a linear fashion and are crusting. The boy has some facial edema. He has no history of fever or chills but complains of pruritus. Which of the following is the most likely diagnosis?

a. Rubeola
b. Atopic dermatitis
c. Acute contact dermatitis
d. Impetigo
e. Erythema infectiosum

4-14. A 19-year-old woman presents with severe right-sided flank pain accompanied by fever, shaking, chills, dysuria, and frequency. She is sexually active with one partner and always uses condoms. Her last menstrual period was 5 days ago. On physical examination, her temperature is 103.8°F and her heart rate is 120/min. Blood pressure and respirations are normal. Abdominal examination reveals suprapubic tenderness with palpation. The patient complains of pain when percussion is performed with the ulnar surface of the fist over the right costovertebral angle (CVA). Pelvic examination is normal. Which of the following is the most likely diagnosis?

a. Diverticulitis
b. Acute cystitis
c. Renal calculi
d. Pyelonephritis
e. Appendicitis

4-15. A full-term infant is born after a normal pregnancy; delivery, however, is complicated by marginal placental separation. At 12 h of age, the child, although appearing to be in good health, passes a bloody meconium stool. For determining the cause of the bleeding, which of the following diagnostic procedures should be performed first?

a. A barium enema
b. An Apt test
c. Gastric lavage with normal saline
d. An upper gastrointestinal series
e. A platelet count, prothrombin time, and partial thromboplastin time

4-16. A 60-year-old male has had a chronic cough for over 5 years with clear sputum production. He has smoked one pack of cigarettes per day for 20 years and continues to do so. X-ray of the chest shows hyperinflation without infiltrates. Arterial blood gases show a pH of 7.38, P_{CO_2} of 40 mmHg, and P_{O_2} of 65 mmHg. Spirometry shows an FEV_1/FVC of 65%. The most important treatment modality for this patient is

a. Oral corticosteroids
b. Home oxygen
c. Broad-spectrum antibiotics
d. Smoking cessation program

4-17. A 1-week-old black infant presents to you for the first time with a large, fairly well-defined, purple lesion over the buttocks bilaterally, as shown in the photograph. The lesion is not palpable, and it is not warm or tender. The mother denies trauma and reports that the lesion has been present since birth. This otherwise well-appearing infant is growing and developing normally and appears normal upon physical examination. The most likely diagnosis in this infant is

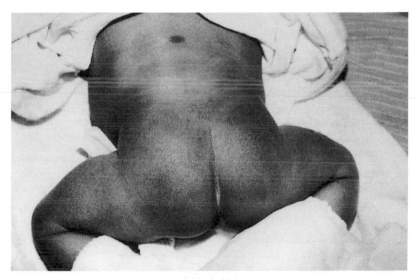

(Courtesy Adelaide Hebert, M.D.)

a. Child abuse
b. Mongolian spot
c. Subcutaneous fat necrosis
d. Vitamin K deficiency
e. Hemophilia

4-18. A 4-year-old boy is brought to the physician by his parents for episodes of waking in the middle of the night screaming. The parents state that when they get to the boy's room during one of these episodes, they find him in his bed, thrashing wildly, his eyes wide open. He pushes them away when they try to comfort him. After 2 min, the boy suddenly falls asleep, and the next day he has no memory of the episode. Which of the following medications is used to treat this disorder?

a. Haloperidol
b. Diazepam
c. Methylphenidate
d. Amitryptiline
e. Valproic acid

4-19. A 39-year-old G1P0 at 39 weeks gestational age is sent to labor and delivery from her obstetrician's office because of a blood pressure reading of 150/100 obtained during a routine OB visit. Her baseline blood pressures during the pregnancy were 100–120/60–70. On arrival to labor and delivery, the patient denies any headache, visual changes, nausea, vomiting, or abdominal pain. The heart rate strip is reactive and the tocodynamometer indicates irregular uterine contractions. The patient's cervix is 50/2–3/0. Her repeat BP is 160/90. Hematocrit is 34.0, platelets are 160,000, SGOT is 22, SGPT is 15, and urinalysis is negative for protein. Which of the following is the most likely diagnosis?

a. Preeclampsia
b. Chronic hypertension
c. Chronic hypertension with superimposed preeclampsia
d. Eclampsia
e. Pregnancy-induced hypertension (gestational hypertension)

4-20. A 35-year-old woman complains of aching all over. She says she sleeps poorly and all her joints hurt. Symptoms have progressed over several years. Physical exam shows multiple points of tenderness over the neck, shoulders, elbows, and wrists. There is no joint swelling or deformity. A complete blood count and erythrocyte sedimentation rate are normal. Rheumatoid factor is negative. There is no tenderness over the median third of the clavicle, the medial malleolus, or the forehead. The best therapeutic option in this patient is

a. Amitriptyline at night
b. Prednisone
c. Aspirin and methotrexate
d. Plaquenil

4-21. For the past year, a 12-year-old boy has had recurrent episodes of swelling of his hands and feet, which has been getting worse recently. These episodes occur following exercise and emotional stress, last for two to three days, and resolve spontaneously. The last episode was accompanied by abdominal pain, vomiting, and diarrhea. The results of routine laboratory workup are normal. An older sister and a maternal uncle have had similar episodes but were not told a diagnosis. The most compatible diagnosis is

a. Systemic lupus erythematosus
b. Focal glomerulosclerosis
c. Congenital nephrotic syndrome
d. Hereditary angioedema
e. Henoch-Schönlein purpura

4-22. A 61-year-old man comes to your office complaining of a popping sensation in his left ear for nearly 2 weeks. He also complains of decreased hearing. Recently, another physician treated him for an acute otitis media with antibiotics. Physical examination reveals a normal right ear canal and tympanic membrane. The left tympanic membrane is gray, retracted, and immobile. Which of the following is the most likely diagnosis?

a. Otitis media with effusion
b. Acute otitis media
c. Mastoiditis
d. Otitis externa
e. Malignant otitis externa

4-23. A 26-year-old heroin addict has been using a street version of artificial heroin. The drug actually contains 1-methyl-4-phenyl-1,2,3,6-tetrahydropyridine (MPTP). The neurological syndrome for which he is at risk is clinically indistinguishable from which of the following?

a. Huntington's disease
b. Friedreich's disease
c. Sydenham's chorea
d. Parkinson's disease
e. Amyotrophic lateral sclerosis

4-24. An elderly diabetic woman with chronic steroid-dependent bronchospasm has an ileocolectomy for a perforated cecum. She is taken to the ICU intubated and is maintained on broad-spectrum antibiotics, renal dose dopamine, and a rapid steroid taper. On postoperative day 2, she develops a fever of 39.2°C (102.5°F), hypotension, lethargy, and laboratory values remarkable for hypoglycemia and hyperkalemia. The most likely diagnosis of this acute event is

a. Sepsis
b. Hypovolemia
c. Adrenal insufficiency
d. Acute tubular necrosis
e. Diabetic ketoacidosis

4-25. A 19-year-old male has a history of athlete's foot but is otherwise healthy when he develops the sudden onset of fever and pain in the right foot and leg. On physical exam, the foot and leg are fiery red with a well-defined indurated margin that appears to be rapidly advancing. There is tender inguinal lymphadenopathy. The most likely organism to cause this infection is

a. *Staphylococcus epidermidis*
b. *Tinea pedis*
c. *Streptococcus pyogenes*
d. Mixed anaerobic infection

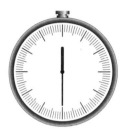

YOU SHOULD HAVE COMPLETED APPROXIMATELY
25 QUESTIONS AND HAVE 30 MINUTES REMAINING.

4-26. A 22-year-old nulliparous woman has recently become sexually active. She consults you because of painful coitus, with the pain located at the vaginal introitus. It is accompanied by painful involuntary contraction of the pelvic muscles. Other than confirmation of these findings, the pelvic examination is normal. Of the following, what is the most common cause of this condition?

a. Endometriosis
b. Psychogenic causes
c. Bartholin's gland abscess
d. Vulvar atrophy
e. Ovarian cyst

4-27. A 78-year-old woman with mild renal insufficiency complains of pain in the right knee on walking that has interfered with her day-to-day activities. Pain is relieved by rest. There are no inflammatory symptoms of redness or swelling. There is minimal joint effusion. An x-ray of the knee shows osteophytes and asymmetric loss of joint space. ESR and white blood cell count are normal. The best initial management of this patient is

a. Nonsteroidal anti-inflammatory agent
b. Intraarticular corticosteroids
c. Acetaminophen
d. Total arthroplasty

4-28. A 3-year-old girl is admitted with the x-ray pictured. The child lives with her parents and a 6-week-old brother. Her grandfather stayed with the family for 2 months before his return to the West Indies 1 month ago. The grandfather had a 3-month history of weight loss, fever, and hemoptysis. Appropriate management of this problem includes

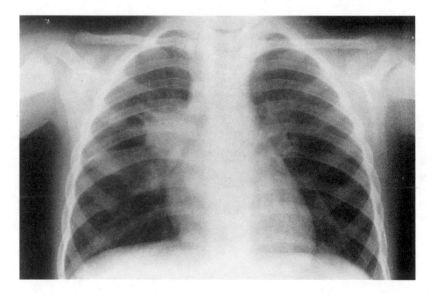

a. Bronchoscopy and culture of washings for all family members
b. Placement of a Mantoux test on the 6-week-old sibling
c. Isolating the 3-year-old patient for 1 month
d. Treating the 3-year-old patient with isoniazid (INH) and rifampin
e. HIV testing for all family members

4-29. A 90-year-old male complains of hip and back pain. He has also developed headaches, hearing loss, and tinnitus. On physical exam the skull appears enlarged, with prominent superficial veins. There is marked kyphosis, and the bones of the leg appear deformed. Plasma alkaline phosphatase is elevated. A skull x-ray shows sharply demarcated lucencies in the frontal, parietal, and occipital bones. X-rays of the hip show thickening of the pelvic brim. The most likely diagnosis is

a. Multiple myeloma
b. Paget's disease
c. Hypercalcemia
d. Metastatic bone disease

4-30. A 25-year-old woman is admitted for hypertensive crisis. In the hospital, blood pressure is labile and responds poorly to antihypertensive therapy. The patient complains of palpitations and apprehension. Her past medical history shows that she developed hypotension during an operation for appendicitis.

Hct: 49% (37–48)
WBC: 11×10^3 mm (4.3–10.8)
Plasma glucose: 160 mg/dL (75–115)
Plasma calcium: 11 mg/dL (9–10.5)

The most likely diagnosis is

a. Pheochromocytoma
b. Renal artery stenosis
c. Essential hypertension
d. Insulin-dependent diabetes mellitus

4-31. A previously healthy 2-year-old black child has developed a chronic cough over the previous 6 weeks. He has been seen in different emergency rooms on two occasions during this period and placed on antibiotics for pneumonia. Upon auscultation, you hear normal breath sounds on the left. On the right side, you hear decreased air movement during inspiration but none upon expiration. The routine chest radiograph shows no infiltrate, but the heart is shifted slightly to the left. The appropriate next step in making the diagnosis in this patient is to

a. Measure the patient's sweat chloride
b. Obtain inspiratory and expiratory chest radiographs
c. Prescribe broad-spectrum oral antibiotics
d. Initiate a trial of inhaled β agonists
e. Prescribe appropriate doses of oral prednisone

4-32. A 54-year-old woman undergoes a laparotomy because of a pelvic mass. At exploratory laparotomy, a unilateral ovarian neoplasm is discovered that is accompanied by a large omental metastasis. Frozen section diagnosis confirms metastatic serous cystadenocarcinoma. The most appropriate intraoperative course of action is

a. Excision of the omental metastasis and ovarian cystectomy
b. Omentectomy and ovarian cystectomy
c. Excision of the omental metastasis and unilateral oophorectomy
d. Omentectomy and bilateral salpingo-oophorectomy
e. Omentectomy, total abdominal hysterectomy, and bilateral salpingo-oophorectomy

4-33. A 64-year-old man with a history of hypertension presents with sharp midsternal chest pain that is intermittent and radiates to his back between his shoulder blades. Blood pressure is 170/110 mmHg in his right arm and 90/60 mmHg in his left arm. Heart auscultation reveals a diastolic murmur. He has a tracheal tug sign. ECG is normal. Chest radiograph reveals a widened mediastinum. Which of the following is the most likely diagnosis?

a. Myocardial infarction
b. Pulmonary embolus
c. Aortic dissection
d. Coarctation of the aorta
e. Aortic stenosis

4-34. An 82-year-old previously healthy woman with a recent upper respiratory infection presents with generalized weakness, headache, and blurry vision. For the past 2 weeks she has had upper respiratory symptoms that started with a sore throat, nasal congestion, and excessive coughing. She went to her primary care doctor 4 days ago and was diagnosed with sinusitis. She was given a prescription for an antibiotic and took it for 2 days, then stopped. She thereafter had chills, lightheadedness, vomiting, blurry vision, general achiness, and a headache that started abruptly and has not gotten better since. Other than blurry vision, she has not had any other visual symptoms. The blurry vision remains when she closes either eye. She also has eye tenderness with movement and mild photosensitivity. She has no drug allergies. Exam findings include temperature of 102.5°F, nuchal rigidity, and sleepiness. The next most appropriate action in this case is which of the following?

a. Get a brain MRI, then perform a lumbar puncture
b. Give the patient a prescription for oral azithromycin and let her go home
c. Immediately give intravenous ceftriaxone plus ampicillin
d. Immediately start intravenous acyclovir
e. Obtain cerebrospinal fluid and blood cultures and observe the patient until the results come back

4-35. A 62-year-old man with chronic schizophrenia is brought to the emergency room after he is found wandering around his halfway house confused and disoriented. His serum sodium concentration is 123 mEq/L. Urine sodium concentration is 5 mEq/L. The patient has been treated with risperidone 4 mg/d for the past 3 years with good symptom control. His roommate reports that the patient often complains of feeling thirsty. Which of the following is the most likely cause of this patient's symptoms?

a. Renal failure
b. Inappropriate antidiuretic hormone (ADH) secretion
c. Addison's disease
d. Psychogenic polydipsia
e. Nephrotic syndrome

4-36. A patient was induced for being postterm at 42⅗ weeks. Immediately following the delivery, you examine the baby with the pediatricians and note the following on physical exam: a small amount of cartilage in the earlobe, occasional creases over the anterior two-thirds of the soles of the feet, 4-mm breast nodule diameter, fine and fuzzy scalp hair, and a scrotum with some but not extensive rugae. Based on this physical exam, what is the approximate gestational age of this male infant?

a. 33 weeks
b. 36 weeks
c. 38 weeks
d. 42 weeks

4-37. A 46-year-old male with HIV and severe penicillin allergy receiving zidovudine, indinavir, and stavudine presents with fever, nonproductive cough, and severe hypoxia. Chest x-ray reveals diffuse increased interstitial markings and a possible lobar consolidation in the left lower lobe. After appropriate evaluation, the patient receives levofloxacin, trimethoprim-sulfamethoxazole, and acyclovir. Initial serum creatinine is 1.6 mg/dL. On day 4, it has risen to 3.8 mg/dL and a normal serum potassium has risen to 7.1 mg/dL. Urinalysis reveals no casts, 10 to 20 WBC/HPF, and rare RBCs. Which drug is the most likely cause of renal failure?

a. Levofloxacin
b. Trimethoprim-sulfamethoxazole
c. Acyclovir
d. Indinavir

4-38. Following blunt abdominal trauma, a 12-year-old girl develops upper abdominal pain, nausea, and vomiting. An upper gastrointestinal series reveals a total obstruction of the duodenum with a coiled spring appearance in the second and third portions. Appropriate management is

a. Gastrojejunostomy
b. Nasogastric suction and observation
c. Duodenal resection
d. TPN to increase the size of the retroperitoneal fat pad
e. Duodenojejunostomy

4-39. A 70-year-old male complains of 2 months of low back pain and fatigue. He has developed fever with purulent sputum production. On physical exam, he has pain over several vertebrae and rales at the left base. Laboratory results are as follows:

Hemoglobin: 7 g/dL
MCV: 86 fL (normal 86 to 98)
WBC: 12,000/µL
BUN: 44 mg/dL
Creatinine: 3.2 mg/dL
Ca: 11.5 mg/dL
Chest x-ray: LLL infiltrate
Reticulocyte count: 1%

The most likely diagnosis is

a. Multiple myeloma
b. Lymphoma
c. Metastatic bronchogenic carcinoma
d. Primary hyperparathyroidism

4-40. A 32-year-old woman presents with the recent onset of petechiae of her lower extremities. She denies menorrhagia and gastrointestinal bleeding. She has no family history of a bleeding disorder and has been in excellent health her entire life. Physical examination is remarkable for petechiae of both legs. There is no hepatosplenomegaly. The rest of the physical examination is normal. Platelet count is 8000/µL. Hemoglobin and white blood cell count are normal. Peripheral smear reveals reduced platelets and an occasional megathrombocyte. Which of the following is the most likely diagnosis?

a. Thrombocytopenic thrombotic purpura (TTP)
b. Hemolytic-uremic syndrome (HUS)
c. Evans syndrome
d. Disseminated intravascular coagulopathy (DIC)
e. Idiopathic thrombocytopenic purpura (ITP)
f. Henoch-Schönlein purpura (HSP)

4-41. A 38-year-old G1P0 presents to the obstetrician's office at 37 weeks gestational age complaining of a rash on her abdomen that is becoming increasingly pruritic. The rash started on her abdomen, and the patient notes that it is starting to spread downward to her thighs. The patient reports no previous history of any skin disorders or problems. She denies any malaise or fever. On physical exam, her physician notes that her abdomen, and most notably her stretch marks, are covered with red papules and plaques. No excoriations or bullae are present. The patient's face, arms, and legs are unaffected by the rash. What is this patient's most likely diagnosis?

a. Herpes gestationis
b. PUPPP
c. Prurigo gravidarum
d. Intrahepatic cholestasis of pregnancy
e. Impetigo herpetiformis

4-42. A 42-year-old man has had a rocky course for the 3 days following a bowel resection of intestinal perforation due to inflammatory bowel disease. His CVP had been 12 to 14 but is now 6 in the face of diminished blood pressure and oliguria. The cause is most likely

a. Pulmonary embolism
b. Hypervolemia
c. Positive-pressure ventilation
d. Pneumothorax
e. Gram-negative sepsis

4-43. A 50-year-old male complains of slowly progressive weakness over several months. Walking has become more difficult, as has using his hands. There are no sensory, bowel, or bladder complaints, or any problems in thinking, speech, or vision. Examination shows distal muscle weakness with muscle wasting and fasciculations. There are also upper motor neuron signs, including extensor plantar reflexes and hyperreflexia in wasted muscle groups. The most likely diagnosis is

a. Polymyositis
b. Duchenne muscular dystrophy
c. Amyotrophic lateral sclerosis
d. Myasthenia gravis

4-44. The family of a 4-year-old boy has recently moved into your area. The child was recently brought to the emergency department for an evaluation of abdominal pain. Although appendicitis was ruled out in the ED and the child's abdominal pain has resolved, the ED physician requested that the family follow up in your office to evaluate an incidental finding of an elevated creatine kinase. The family notes that he was a late walker (began walking independently about 18 months of age), that he is more clumsy than their daughter was at the same age, and that he seems to be somewhat sluggish when he runs, climbs stairs, rises from the ground after he sits, and rides his tricycle. A thorough history and physical examination are likely to reveal which of the following?

a. Hirsutism
b. Past seizure activity
c. Severe proximal muscle weakness
d. Cataracts
e. Enlarged gonads

4-45. An 80-year-old man is admitted to the hospital complaining of nausea, abdominal pain, distention, and diarrhea. A cautiously performed transanal contrast study reveals an apple core configuration in the rectosigmoid area. Appropriate management at this time would include

a. Colonoscopic decompression and rectal tube placement
b. Saline enemas and digital disimpaction of fecal matter from the rectum
c. Colon resection and proximal colostomy
d. Oral administration of metronidazole and checking a *Clostridium difficile* titer
e. Evaluation of an electrocardiogram and obtaining an angiogram to evaluate for colonic mesenteric ischemia

4-46. A 65-year-old man, who was hospitalized for an acute pneumonia 3 days previously, begins screaming for his nurse, stating that "there are people in the room out to get me." He then gets out of bed and begins pulling out his intravenous line. On exam, he alternates between agitation and somnolence. He is not oriented to time or place. His vital signs are: pulse, 126/min; respiration, 32/min; blood pressure, 80/58; temperature, 102.5°F. Which of the following diagnoses best fits this patient's clinical picture?

a. Dementia
b. Schizophreniform disorder
c. Fugue state
d. Delirium
e. Brief psychotic episode

4-47. A 40-year-old cigarette smoker is found on routine physical exam to have a 1-cm white patch on his oral mucosa that does not rub off. There are no other lesions in the mouth. The patient has no risk factors for HIV infection. The lesion is nontender. The next step in management is

a. Culture for *Candida albicans*
b. Follow lesion with annual physical exam
c. Refer to oral surgeon for biopsy of lesion
d. Reassure patient that this is a normal variant

4-48. A 20-year-old female develops urticaria that lasts for 6 weeks and then resolves spontaneously. She gives no history of weight loss, fever, rash, or tremulousness. Physical exam shows no abnormalities. The most likely cause of the urticaria is

a. Connective tissue disease
b. Hyperthyroidism
c. Chronic infection
d. Not likely to be determined

4-49. A 19-year-old primigravida is expecting her first child; she is 12 weeks pregnant by dates. She has vaginal bleeding and an enlarged-for-dates uterus. In addition, no fetal heart sounds are heard. The ultrasound shown below is obtained. The most likely diagnosis of this woman's condition is

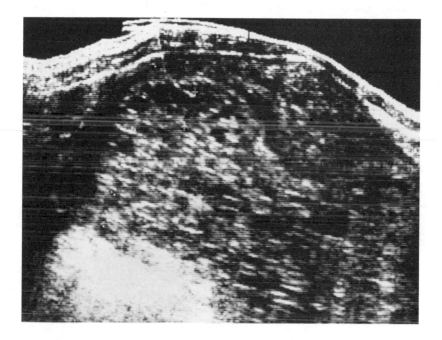

a. Sarcoma botryoides
b. Tuberculous endometritis
c. Adenocarcinoma of the uterus
d. Hydatidiform mole
e. Normal pregnancy

4-50. A 19-year-old male college student returns from spring break in Fort Lauderdale, Florida, with complaints of acute pain and swelling of the scrotum. Physical examination reveals an exquisitely tender, swollen right testis that is rather hard to examine. The cremasteric reflex is absent, but there is no swelling in the inguinal area. The rest of his genitourinary examination appears to be normal. A urine dip is negative for red and white blood cells. Which of the following is the appropriate next step in this man?

a. Administration of antibiotics after culture of urethra for chlamydia and gonorrhea
b. Reassurance
c. Intravenous fluid administration, pain medications, and straining of all voids
d. Ultrasound of the scrotum
e. Laproscopic exploration of both inguinal regions

BLOCK 5

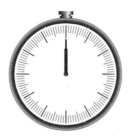

YOU HAVE 60 MINUTES
TO COMPLETE 50 QUESTIONS.

Questions

5-1. A 79-year-old woman presents to the emergency room with a 1-week history of fever, myalgias, nausea, vomiting, and diarrhea. Her symptoms started shortly after she ate at a Mexican restaurant with her daughter and son-in-law. She did not eat raw foods, and her family members did not become ill. She has no past medical history and takes no medications. She has a temperature of 103.2°F and appears extremely ill. She is awake and oriented to person and place but not to time. Heart and lung examinations are normal, and she has no focal neurologic deficits. CT scan of the head is normal. Lumbar puncture reveals pleocytosis, increased protein concentration, and normal glucose. Blood and cerebrospinal fluid cultures identify a gram-positive rod organism. Which of the following is the most likely diagnosis?

a. *Actinomyces* infection
b. *Bacillus cereus* infection
c. Invasive *Listeria* infection
d. Inhalation anthrax infection
e. *Clostridium* botulism infection

5-2. A 25-year-old woman with a history of epilepsy presents to the emergency room with impaired attention and unsteadiness of gait. Her phenytoin level is 37. She has white blood cells in her urine and has a mildly elevated TSH. Examination of the eyes would be most likely to show which of the following?

a. Weakness of abduction of the left eye
b. Lateral beating movements of the eyes
c. Impaired convergence
d. Papilledema
e. Impaired upward gaze

5-3. An 88-year-old man with a history of end-stage renal failure, severe coronary artery disease, and brain metastases from lung cancer presents with acute cholecystitis. His family wants "everything done." The best management option in this patient would be

a. Tube cholecystostomy
b. Open cholecystectomy
c. Laparoscopic cholecystectomy
d. Intravenous antibiotics followed by elective cholecystectomy
e. Lithotripsy followed by long-term bile acid therapy

5-4. A 24-year-old male comes to the physician with the chief complaint that his nose is too big to the point of being hideous. The patient states his nose is a constant embarrassment to him and he would like it surgically reduced. He tells the physician that three previous surgeons had all refused to operate on him because they said his nose was fine, but the patient states that "they just didn't want such a difficult case." The physician observes that the patient's nose is of normal size and shape. Which of the following diagnoses best fits this patient's clinical picture?

a. Schizophrenia
b. Narcissistic personality disorder
c. Body dysmorphic disorder
d. Anxiety disorder not otherwise specified
e. Schizoaffective disorder

5-5. A 28-year-old nulligravid patient complains of bleeding between her periods and increasingly heavy menses. Over the past 9 months she has had two dilation and curettages (D&Cs), which have failed to resolve her symptoms, and oral contraceptives and antiprostaglandins have not decreased the abnormal bleeding. Of the following options, which is most appropriate at this time?

a. Perform a hysterectomy
b. Perform hysteroscopy
c. Perform endometrial ablation
d. Treat with a GnRH agonist
e. Start the patient on a high-dose progestational agent

5-6. A 50-year-old obese female is taking oral hypoglycemic agents. While being treated for an upper respiratory infection, she develops lethargy and is brought to the emergency room. On physical exam, there is no focal neurologic finding or neck rigidity. Laboratory results are as follows.

Na$^-$: 134 meq/L
K$^-$: 4.0 meq/L
HCO$_3$: 25 meq/L
Glucose: 900 mg/dL
BUN: 84 mg/dL
Creatinine: 3.0 mg/dL
BP: 120/80 sitting, 105/65 lying down

The most likely cause of this patient's coma is

a. Diabetic ketoacidosis
b. Hyperosmolar coma
c. Inappropriate ADH
d. Bacterial meningitis

5-7. A 60-year-old white male just moved to town and needs to establish care for coronary artery disease. He had a heart attack last year, but gradually eliminated several prescription medications (he does not recall the names) that he was on at the time of hospital discharge. However, he has been very conscientious about low-fat, low-cholesterol eating habits. Past history is negative for hypertension, diabetes, or smoking. The lipid profile you obtain shows the following:

Total cholesterol: 210 mg/dL
Triglycerides: 190
HDL: 52
LDL (calculated): 120

To optimally treat his lipid status, you suggest which of the following?
a. Continue dietary efforts
b. Add an HMG-CoA reductase inhibitor (statin drug)
c. Add a fibric acid derivative such as gemfibrozil
d. Review his previous medications and resume an angiotensin converting enzyme inhibitor

5-8. A 33-year-old married man who suffers from chronic anxiety presents for a psychiatric consultation. He reports that his marriage is very happy and gives a sexual history that includes daily and satisfying sexual intercourse with his wife. He also masturbates three to four times weekly. He states that his sexual drive has been high ever since he was a teenager. His sexual fantasies are predominantly heterosexual, but occasionally he fantasizes about homosexual encounters while masturbating. During his adult years, while traveling alone, he has had both heterosexual and homosexual experiences on several occasions. He remembers these experiences as pleasurable. The patient admits to some transient guilt about "stepping out" on his wife, but he is not excessively anxious or troubled about his sexual life. On the basis of the patient's sexual history, one could reasonably infer a diagnosis of which of the following?
a. Schizotypal personality disorder
b. Antisocial personality disorder
c. Narcissistic personality disorder
d. Borderline personality disorder
e. No personality disorder

5-9. A 1-year-old child has repeated episodes of vomiting and abdominal distention. An x-ray shows obstruction at the second portion of the duodenum. Laparotomy is performed and an annular pancreas is discovered. For a symptomatic partial duodenal obstruction secondary to an annular pancreas, the operative treatment of choice is

a. A Whipple procedure
b. Gastrojejunostomy
c. Vagotomy and gastrojejunostomy
d. Partial resection of the annular pancreas
e. Duodenojejunostomy

5-10. A 39-year-old woman presents with the sudden onset of pleuritic chest pain and shortness of breath. She has been in good health until 3 days ago, when she noticed some swelling of her left lower extremity. She is not a smoker and denies any recent trauma. On physical examination, she is afebrile but has a respiratory rate of 32/min. Her heart rate is 120/min and her blood pressure is normal. An accentuated (loud) S_2 is heard on heart auscultation. The left lower extremity is swollen, tender to palpation, and erythematous. Dorsiflexion of the left foot (Homan's sign) causes severe calf discomfort. Lung examination and chest radiograph are normal. Arterial blood analysis on room air shows a P_{CO_2} of 30 mmHg and a P_{O_2} of 58 mmHg. Which of the following is the most appropriate next diagnostic step?

a. Transesophageal echocardiogram
b. Transthoracic echocardiogram
c. Cardiac catheterization
d. Ventilation-perfusion scan
e. D-dimer assay

5-11. An 18-year-old college student who has recently become sexually active is seen for severe primary dysmenorrhea. She does not want to get pregnant, and has failed to obtain resolution with heating pads and mild analgesics. Which of the following medications is most appropriate for this patient?

a. Prostaglandin inhibitors
b. Narcotic analgesics
c. Oxytocin
d. Oral contraceptives
e. Luteal progesterone

5-12. A 59-year-old G4P4 presents to your GYN office complaining of losing urine when she coughs, sneezes, or engages in certain types of strenuous physical activity. The problem has gotten increasingly worse over the past few years, to the point where the patient finds her activities of daily living compromised secondary to fear of embarrassment. She denies any other urinary symptoms such as urgency, frequency, or hematuria. In addition, she denies any problems with her bowel movements. Her prior surgeries include a tonsillectomy and appendectomy. She has adult-onset diabetes and her blood sugars are well controlled with oral glucophage. The patient has no history of any gynecologic problems in the past. She has four children that were delivered via spontaneous vaginal deliveries; their weights ranged between 8 and 9 lb. She is currently sexually active with her partner of 25 years. She has been menopausal for 4 years and has never taken any hormone replacement therapy. Her height is 5 ft, 6 in., and she weighs 190 lb. Her blood pressure is 130/80. Based on the patient's history, what is the most likely diagnosis?

a. Overflow incontinence
b. Stress incontinence
c. Urinary tract infection
d. Detrusor instability
e. Vesicovaginal fistula

5-13. A 47-year-old perimenopausal woman presents for her annual checkup. She denies chest pain, shortness of breath, and palpitations. She has no family history of heart disease and does not smoke cigarettes. She has no past medical history of hypertension or diabetes mellitus. She takes no medications and exercises in a fitness center three times a week. Her blood pressure is 110/75 mmHg and her heart rate is 66/min and regular. Physical examination reveals no jugular venous distension. Lung examination is normal. A split S_1 best heard over the tricuspid area is now audible but was not present 1 year ago. There is no peripheral edema. Which of the following is the most appropriate next step in diagnosis?

a. Transthoracic echocardiogram
b. Transesophageal echocardiogram
c. Cardiac isoenzymes
d. Cardiac catheterization
e. Electrocardiogram
f. Cardiac stress test
g. Holter monitor

5-14. A 52-year-old woman develops progressive dementia, tremors, gait ataxia, and myoclonic jerks over the course of 6 months. Her speech is slow and slurred, and hand movements are clumsy. No members of her immediate family have a history of degenerative neurologic disease. Magnetic resonance imaging (MRI) of the head reveals a subtle increase in signal in the basal ganglia bilaterally. EEG reveals disorganized background activity with periodic sharp-wave discharges that occur repetitively at 1-s intervals and extend over both sides of the head. Arteriogram reveals no vascular abnormalities. The clinical picture is most consistent with

a. Multi-infarct dementia
b. Tabes dorsalis
c. Friedreich's disease (Friedreich's ataxia)
d. Subarachnoid hemorrhage
e. Spongiform encephalopathy

5-15. A 38-year-old woman is involved in a motor vehicle accident in which she collides with a bridge abutment head-on. She was wearing a seatbelt. Exam in the ER demonstrates a bruise coinciding with the seat belt straps. Her abdomen is tender. CT scan with contrast is most likely to demonstrate

a. Renal vascular injury
b. Superior mesenteric thrombosis
c. Mesenteric vascular injury
d. Avulsion of the splenic pedicle
e. Diaphragmatic hernia

5-16. A 5-year-old boy who was previously healthy has a 1-day history of low-grade fever, colicky abdominal pain, and a skin rash. He is alert but irritable; temperature is 38.6°C (101.5°F). A diffuse, erythematous, maculopapular, and petechial rash is present on his buttocks and lower extremities, as shown in the following figure. There is no localized abdominal tenderness or rebound; bowel sounds are active. Laboratory data demonstrate

Urinalysis:	30 red blood cells per high-powered field, 2+ protein
Stool:	guaiac positive
Platelet count:	135,000/µL

These findings are most consistent with

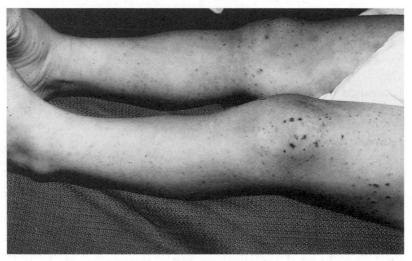

(Courtesy Adelaide Hebert, M.D.)

a. Anaphylactoid purpura
b. Meningococcemia
c. Child abuse
d. Leukemia
e. Hemophilia B

5-17. A 25-year-old man with major depression discusses the potential benefits and side effects of various antidepressants with his psychiatrist. He clearly indicates that he does not want a medication that could decrease his libido or interfere with his ability to obtain and maintain an erection. Which of the listed antidepressants would be appropriate for this patient?

a. Bupropion
b. Clomipramine
c. Amitriptyline
d. Sertraline
e. Paroxetine

5-18. A 76-year-old male presents to the emergency room. He had influenza and now presents with diffuse muscle pain and weakness. His past medical history is remarkable for osteoarthritis, for which he takes ibuprofen. Physical examination reveals a blood pressure of 130/90 with no orthostatic change. The only other finding is diffuse muscle tenderness. Laboratory data includes:

BUN: 30 mg/dL
Creatinine: 6 mg/dL
K: 6.0 meq/L
Uric acid: 18 mg/dL
Ca: 6.5 mg/dL
Po_4: 7.5 mg/dL
CPK: 28,000 IU/L
Urine output: 40 mL/h

Which is the most likely diagnosis?

a. Nonsteroidal anti-inflammatory drug–induced acute renal failure (ARF)
b. Volume depletion
c. Rhabdomyolysis-induced ARF
d. Urinary tract obstruction

5-19. A patient with low-grade fever and weight loss has poor excursion on the right side of the chest with decreased fremitus, flatness to percussion, and decreased breath sounds all on the right. The trachea is deviated to the left. The most likely diagnosis is

a. Pneumothorax
b. Pleural effusion
c. Consolidated pneumonia
d. Atelectasis

5-20. A 45-year-old woman who has been on chronic steroid treatment for her asthma has thin arms and legs but has a large amount of fat deposited on her abdomen, chest, and shoulders. Her skin is thin and atrophic, and she bruises easily. She has purple striae on her abdomen. Physical examination shows an elevated blood pressure, and lab tests show a decreased glucose tolerance. Which of the following psychiatric diagnoses is most likely?

a. Major depression
b. Bipolar-mania
c. Substance-induced mood disorder
d. Delirium
e. Schizoaffective disorder

5-21. On the night after complex lower extremity vascular surgery, a 72-year-old man is seen to vomit, and immediately he appears to be in severe respiratory distress. The nurse calls and tells you that he appears to have aspirated gastric contents into the tracheobronchial tree. Your initial treatment should be

a. Tracheal intubation and suctioning
b. Steroids
c. Intravenous fluid bolus
d. Cricothyroidotomy
e. High positive end-expiratory pressure

5-22. A 75-year-old African American female is admitted with acute myocardial infarction and congestive heart failure, then has an episode of ventricular tachycardia. She is prescribed multiple medications and soon develops confusion and slurred speech. The most likely cause of this confusion is

a. Captopril
b. Digoxin
c. Furosemide
d. Lidocaine
e. Nitroglycerin

5-23. A 57-year-old woman began having weakness and trouble walking 1 year ago. Current exam findings include weak, wasted muscles with spasticity, fasciculations, extensor plantar responses, and hyperreflexia. This case is most suggestive of

a. Dorsal spinal root disease
b. Ventral spinal root disease
c. Arcuate fasciculus damage
d. Motor neuron disease
e. Purkinje cell damage

5-24. A 21-year-old man is brought to the emergency room by his parents because he has not slept, bathed, or eaten in the past 3 days. The parents state that for the past 6 months their son has been acting strangely and "not himself." They state that he has been locking himself in his room, talking to himself, and writing on the walls. Six weeks prior to the emergency room visit, their son became convinced that a fellow student was stealing his thoughts and making him unable to learn his school material. In the past 2 weeks, they have noticed that the patient has become depressed and has stopped taking care of himself, including bathing, eating, and getting dressed. On exam, the patient is dirty, disheveled, and crying. He complains of not being able to concentrate, a low energy level, and feeling suicidal. Which of the following diagnoses is the most likely in this patient?

a. Schizoaffective disorder
b. Schizophrenia
c. Bipolar I disorder
d. Schizoid personality disorder
e. Delusional disorder

5-25. A 28-year-old woman presents with her third episode of left lower extremity deep venous thrombosis. She has a history of two second-trimester miscarriages in the past. Laboratory data reveal an elevated activated partial thromboplastin time (PTT) that is not corrected by dilution with normal plasma and an abnormal dilute Russell's viper venom. Which of the following is the most likely diagnosis?

a. Libman-Sacks disease
b. Livedo reticularis
c. Antiphospholipid syndrome
d. Takayasu's arteritis
e. Sjögren syndrome

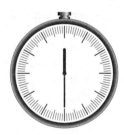

YOU SHOULD HAVE COMPLETED APPROXIMATELY
25 QUESTIONS AND HAVE 30 MINUTES REMAINING.

5-26. A 35-week term infant presents with cyanosis shortly after birth. His arterial oxygen saturation is only 30%. What is the most likely diagnosis?

a. Patent ductus arteriosus
b. Coarctation of the aorta
c. Atrial septal defect
d. Ventricular septal defect
e. Transposition of the great vessels

5-27. A 76-year-old woman is admitted with back pain and hypotension. A CT scan (shown below) is obtained, and the patient is taken to the operating room. Three days after resection of a ruptured abdominal aortic aneurysm, she complains of severe, dull left flank pain and passes bloody mucus per rectum. The diagnosis that must be immediately considered is

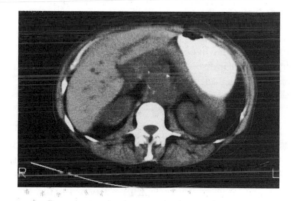

a. Staphylococcal enterocolitis
b. Diverticulitis
c. Bleeding AV malformation
d. Ischemia of the left colon
e. Bleeding colonic carcinoma

5-28. A 5-year-old boy is brought to the psychiatrist because he has difficulty paying attention in school. He fidgets and squirms and will not stay seated in class. At home he is noted to talk excessively and has difficulty waiting for his turn. His language and motor skills are appropriate for his age. Which of the following is the most likely diagnosis?

a. Oppositional defiant disorder (ODD)
b. Attention-deficit/hyperactivity disorder (ADHD)
c. Pervasive developmental disorder
d. Separation anxiety disorder
e. Mild mental retardation

5-29. As you are about to step out of a newly delivered mother's room, she mentions that she wants to breast-feed her healthy infant, but that her obstetrician was concerned about one of the medicines she was taking. Which of the woman's medicines, listed below, is clearly contraindicated in breast-feeding?

a. Ibuprofen as needed for pain or fever
b. Labetolol for her chronic hypertension
c. Lithium for her bipolar disorder
d. Carbamazepine for her seizure disorder
e. Acyclovir for her HSV outbreak

5-30. A 29-year-old G0 comes to your office complaining of a heavy vaginal discharge for the past 2 weeks. The patient describes the discharge as thin in consistency and of a grayish white color. She has also noticed a slight fishy vaginal odor that seems to have started with the appearance of the discharge. She denies any vaginal or vulvar prutitus or burning. She admits to being sexually active in the past, but has not had intercourse during the past year. She denies a history of any sexually transmitted diseases. She is currently on no medications with the exception of her birth control pills. Last month she took a course of amoxicillin for treatment of a sinusitis. On physical exam, the vulva appears normal and the cervix is not inflamed. There is a copious thin whitish discharge in the vaginal vault that is also adherent to the vaginal walls. Wet smear indicates the presence of clue cells. What is the most likely diagnosis?

a. Candidiasis
b. Bacterial vaginosis
c. Trichomoniasis
d. Physiologic discharge
e. Chlamydia

5-31. A 37-year-old woman with progressive multiple sclerosis is being admitted for intravenous glucocorticoid therapy. She was diagnosed with multiple sclerosis 10 years ago after presenting with bilateral decreased visual acuity. She had an abnormal MRI at that time. She has been hospitalized approximately nine times since presentation, with her flares commonly consisting of increasing bilateral lower extremity weakness and decreased sensation manifested as a heavy feeling, waxing and waning generalized fatigue, bilateral hand tingling, and occasional nondescript speech changes that make her sound as though she has a slight accent. She has also had bilateral optic neuritis and one transient episode of aphasia in the past. She was last hospitalized 3 years ago. For the past 2 years she has been on cyclophosphamide and methylprednisolone, originally every 4 weeks, and now every 6 weeks, with the last treatment 1 month ago. She has tried and failed interferon β therapy. For the 2 months prior to admission, the patient has had worsening bilateral lower extremity weakness/heaviness, increased fatigue, and mild low back numbness, as well as intermittent and alternating decreased hearing in both ears at work. She has also noticed mild unsteadiness walking. Included among her admission orders should be

a. Heart-healthy diet
b. Ranitidine 150 mg bid
c. Neurological checks every hour for the first 48 h
d. Placement of central venous line
e. Stat head CT for change in mental status

5-32. A 74-year-old man with a history of previous myocardial infarction and stroke presents with the sudden onset of left-sided vision loss. Blood pressure is 135/85 mmHg. Heart rate is 80/min and regular. Heart and lungs are normal. Funduscopic examination of the left eye reveals a bright yellow refractile deposit wedged at the bifurcation of a peripheral arteriole. The deposit appears to be migrating down the vessel. Which of the following is the most appropriate next step in diagnosis?

a. Holter monitor
b. Cardiac isoenzymes
c. Carotid dopplers
d. Echocardiogram
e. Electrocardiogram
f. CT scan of the head

5-33. An 8-year-old boy is brought to your office with the complaint of abdominal pain. The pain is worse during the week and seems to be less prominent during the weekends and during the summer. The patient's growth and development are normal. The physical examination is unremarkable. Laboratory screening, including stool for guaiac, complete blood count, urinalysis, and chemistry panel, yields normal results. The next step in the care of this patient should be to

a. Perform an upper GI series
b. Perform CT of the abdomen
c. Administer a trial of H_2 blockers
d. Observe the patient and reassure the patient and family
e. Recommend a lactose-free diet

5-34. A 37-year-old woman who recently emigrated from Central America presents with a 20-lb weight loss over the last month. She also complains of generalized weakness and occasional nausea. She has no past medical history and was in previous good health. On physical examination, the patient has increased skin pigmentation. She is afebrile. Her blood pressure is 90/60 mmHg supine and 70/50 mmHg standing. The rest of her physical examination is normal. Laboratory data reveal hyponatremia, hyperkalemia, and a metabolic acidosis. Which of the following is the most likely diagnosis?

a. Sheehan syndrome
b. Craniopharyngioma
c. Addison's disease
d. Empty sella syndrome
e. Insulinoma
f. Schmidt syndrome
g. Pituitary apoplexy

5-35. A 15-month-old boy is brought to the emergency room because of fever and a rash. Six hours earlier he was fine, except for tugging on his ears; another physician diagnosed otitis media and prescribed amoxicillin. During the interim period, the child has developed an erythematous rash on his face, trunk, and extremities. Some of the lesions, which are of variable size, do not blanch on pressure. The child is now very irritable, and he does not interact well with the examiner. Temperature is 39.5°C (103.1°F). He continues to have injected, immobile tympanic membranes, but you are concerned about his change in mental status. The most appropriate next step in the management of this infant is to

a. Begin administration of intravenous ampicillin
b. Begin diphenhydramine
c. Discontinue administration of ampicillin and begin trimethoprim with sulfamethoxazole
d. Perform bilateral myringotomies
e. Perform a lumbar puncture

5-36. A 4-year-old girl is brought to the pediatrician's office. Her father reports that she suddenly became pale and stopped running while he had been playfully chasing her. After 30 min, she was no longer pale and wanted to resume the game. She has never had a previous episode or ever been cyanotic. Her physical examination was normal, as were her chest x-ray and echocardiogram. An electrocardiogram showed the pattern seen below, which indicates

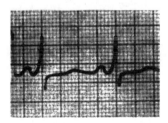

a. Paroxysmal ventricular tachycardia
b. Paroxysmal supraventricular tachycardia
c. Wolff-Parkinson-White syndrome
d. Stokes-Adams pattern
e. Excessive stress during play

5-37. An 80-year-old man has a history of 2 years of progressive gait disturbance and incontinence, which had been attributed to old age and prostatism. Within the past 3 months, he has been forgetful, confused, and withdrawn. His gait is short-stepped, and he turns very slowly, almost toppling over. He has a history of head trauma from 30 years ago. His CT scan is shown below. The most likely diagnosis is

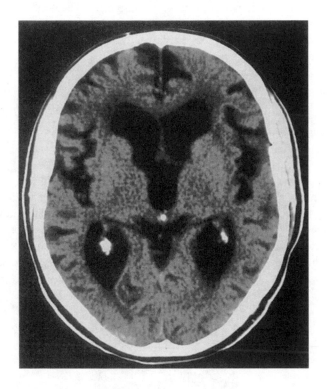

a. Alzheimer's disease
b. Creutzfeldt-Jakob disease
c. Progressive multifocal leukoencephalopathy (PML)
d. Normal-pressure hydrocephalus
e. Chiari malformation

5-38. A 19-year-old woman comes to the emergency room and reports that she fainted at work earlier in the day. She has mild vaginal bleeding. Her abdomen is diffusely tender and distended. In addition, she complains of shoulder and abdominal pain. Her temperature is 97.6°F, pulse rate is 120/min, and blood pressure is 96/50 mmHg. To confirm the diagnosis suggested by the available clinical data, the best diagnostic procedure is

a. Pregnancy test
b. Posterior colpotomy
c. Dilation and curettage
d. Culdocentesis
e. Laparoscopy

5-39. A 53-year-old woman presents with complaints of weakness, anorexia, malaise, constipation, and back pain. While being evaluated, she becomes somewhat lethargic. Laboratory studies include a normal chest x ray; serum albumin 3.2 mg/dL; serum calcium 14 mg/dL; serum phosphorus 2.6 mg/dL; serum chloride 108 mg/dL; BUN 32 mg/dL; and creatinine 2.0 mg/dL. Appropriate initial management includes

a. Intravenous normal saline infusion
b. Administration of thiazide diuretics
c. Administration of intravenous phosphorus
d. Use of mithramycin
e. Neck exploration and parathyroidectomy

5-40. A 20-year-old woman presents with a hematoma of the pinna of her right ear following a fall and injury to the ear. Which of the following is appropriate therapy?

a. Ice packs and prophylactic antibiotics
b. Excision of the hematoma
c. Needle aspiration
d. Incision, drainage, and pressure bandage
e. Observation alone

5-41. A 67-year-old musician presents with a long history of low back pain. Pain is worsened with prolonged standing and with exercise. For the last several months, the patient has noticed that the back pain comes on with walking less than one block and radiates to the buttocks. The pain is relieved by sitting for several minutes. On physical examination, there are no neurologic deficits and bilateral straight-leg raising maneuvers are normal. Peripheral pulses are strong and bilaterally equal. Which of the following is the most likely diagnosis?

a. Lumbar spinal stenosis
b. Peripheral vascular disease
c. Lumbosacral sprain
d. Disk herniation
e. Diffuse idiopathic skeletal hyperostosis

5-42. A 5-year-old girl sustains a cut on her face from broken glass. Initially, the injury appears superficial except for a small area of deeper penetration just above the right eyebrow. Within 4 days, the child complains of periorbital pain and double vision. The tissues about the eye are erythematous, and the eye appears to bulge slightly. The optic disc is sharp, and no afferent pupillary defect is apparent. Visual acuity in the affected eye is preserved. This child probably has

a. Orbital cellulitis
b. Cavernous sinus thrombosis
c. Transverse sinus thrombosis
d. Optic neuritis
e. Diphtheritic polyneuropathy

5-43. A 15-year-old boy is arrested for shooting the owner of the convenience store he tried to rob. He has been in Department of Youth Services custody several times for a variety of crimes against property, possession of illegal substances, and assault and battery. He is cheerful and unconcerned during the arrest, more worried about not losing his leather jacket than about the fate of the man he has injured. Which of the following is the most appropriate diagnosis in this case?

a. Oppositional defiant disorder
b. Antisocial personality disorder
c. Narcissistic personality disorder
d. Conduct disorder
e. Substance abuse

5-44. A newborn infant develops respiratory distress immediately after birth. His abdomen is scaphoid. No breath sounds are heard on the left side of his chest, but they are audible on the right. Immediate intubation is successful with little or no improvement in clinical status. Emergency chest x-ray is shown (A) along with an x-ray 2 h later (B). The most likely explanation for this infant's condition is

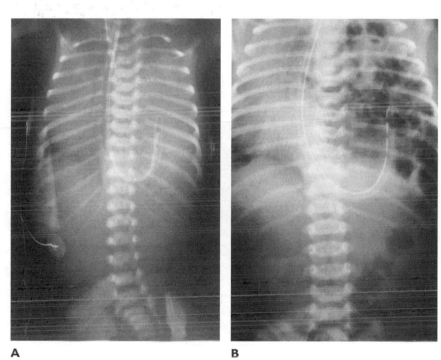

A   B

(Courtesy Susan John, M.D.)

a. Pneumonia
b. Cyanotic heart disease
c. Diaphragmatic hernia
d. Choanal atresia
e. Pneumothorax

5-45. A 62-year-old man presents with a 2-year history of tremors of the right hand that disappear with voluntary movement. He has no past medical history and takes no medications. Review of systems is positive for anhidrosis and a 5-year history of impotence. On physical examination, the patient is alert and oriented. He has a resting tremor of his hands that has a pill-rolling quality. His face is expressionless (masklike), and his movements are slow. He has difficulty getting out of a chair and is unable to complete the get-up-and-go test in under 15 s. There is a decrease in tone and strength of the extremities. Deep tendon reflexes are diminished. The Babinski reflex is normal (flexor). Which of the following is the most likely diagnosis?

a. Benign essential tremor
b. Parkinson's disease
c. Shy-Drager syndrome
d. Creutzfeldt-Jakob disease
e. Cerebellar tremor
f. Progressive supranuclear palsy

5-46. An obese 50-year-old woman undergoes a laparoscopic cholecystectomy. In the recovery room, she is found to be hypotensive and tachycardic. Her arterial blood gases reveal a pH of 7.29, PaO_2 of 60 kPa, and $PaCO_2$ of 54 kPa. The most likely cause of this woman's problem is

a. Acute pulmonary embolism
b. CO_2 absorption from induced pneumoperitoneum
c. Alveolar hypoventilation
d. Pulmonary edema
e. Atelectasis from high diaphragm

5-47. A 32-year-old G2P1001 at 20 weeks gestational age presents to the emergency room complaining of constipation and abdominal pain for the past 24 h. The patient also admits to bouts of nausea and emesis since eating a very spicy meal at a new Thai restaurant the evening before. She denies a history of any medical problems. During her last pregnancy, the patient underwent an elective cesarean section at term to deliver a fetus in the breech presentation. The emergency room doctor who examines her pages you and reports that the patient has a low-grade fever of 100°F, with a normal pulse and blood pressure. She is minimally tender to deep palpation with hypoactive bowel sounds. She has no rebound tenderness. The patient has a WBC of 13,000, and electrolytes are normal. What is the appropriate next step in the management of this patient?

a. The history and physical exam are consistent with constipation, which is commonly associated with pregnancy; the patient should be discharged with reassurance and instructions to give herself a soapsuds enema and follow a high-fiber diet with laxative use as needed
b. The patient should be prepped for the operating room immediately to have an emergent appendectomy
c. The patient should be reassured that her symptoms are due to the spicy meal consumed the evening before and should be given Pepto-Bismol to alleviate the symptoms
d. The patient should be sent to radiology for an upright abdominal x-ray
e. Intravenous antiemetics should be ordered to treat the patient's hyperemesis gravidarum

5-48. A 56-year-old man is brought into the emergency room after having collapsed at work 30 min ago. He has no medical history and takes no medications. He is alert and speaking but has no awareness of any deficit. He has a right gaze preference, dense left face and arm plegia, and mild left leg weakness. When asked to raise his legs, he lifts only the right leg. He has reduced blink to threat from the left side. The most appropriate initial diagnostic step is

a. Head CT
b. Cerebral angiogram
c. C-spine MRI
d. T2-weighted brain MRI
e. Skull x-rays

5-49. A 68-year-old man is admitted to the coronary care unit with an acute myocardial infarction. His postinfarction course is marked by congestive heart failure and intermittent hypotension. On the fourth hospital day, he develops severe midabdominal pain. On physical examination, blood pressure is 90/60 mmHg and pulse is 110/min and regular; the abdomen is soft with mild generalized tenderness and distension. Bowel sounds are hypoactive; stool hematest is positive. The next step in this patient's management should be which of the following?

a. Barium enema
b. Upper gastrointestinal series
c. Angiography
d. Ultrasonography
e. Celiotomy

5-50. A 32-year-old woman who has a chronic psychiatric disorder, multiple medical problems, and alcoholism comes to the physician because her breasts have started leaking a whitish fluid. What is the most likely cause of this symptom?

a. Haloperidol
b. Oral contraceptives
c. Hypothyroidism
d. Cirrhosis
e. Pregnancy

BLOCK 6

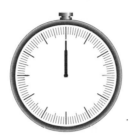

YOU HAVE 60 MINUTES
TO COMPLETE 50 QUESTIONS.

Questions

6-1. A 26-year-old G1P1 comes to see you in your office for preconception counseling because she wants to get pregnant again. She denies a history of any illegal drug use but admits to smoking a few cigarettes each day and occasionally drinking some beer. When you advise her not to smoke or drink at all during this pregnancy, she gets defensive because she smokes and drinks very little, and she did the same during her previous pregnancy 2 years ago and her baby was just fine. Which of the following statements is true regarding the effects of tobacco and alcohol on pregnancy?

a. Small amounts of alcohol, such as a glass of wine or beer a day at dinner time, are safe; only binge drinking of large amounts of alcohol has been associated with fetal alcohol syndrome
b. Fetal alcohol syndrome can be diagnosed prenatally via identifying fetal anomalies on sonogram done antenatally
c. Cigarette smoking is associated with an increased risk of spontaneous abortion
d. In most studies, cigarette smoking has been associated with an increased risk of congenital anomalies
e. Tobacco use in pregnancy is a common cause of mental retardation and developmental delay in neonates

6-2. A five-year-old boy is brought into the emergency room immediately after an unfortunate altercation with a neighbor's immunized Chihuahua that occurred while the child was attempting to dress the dog as a super-hero. The fully immunized child has a small, irregular, superficial lacera-tion on his right forearm that has stopped bleeding. His neuromuscular examination is completely normal, and his perfusion is intact. Management should include

a. Antimicrobial prophylaxis
b. Tetanus booster immunization and tetanus toxoid in the wound
c. Copious irrigation
d. Primary rabies vaccination for the child
e. Destruction of the dog and examination of brain tissue for rabies

6-3. A 26-year-old trauma victim is being resuscitated following an auto accident complicated by hypotension from a fractured pelvis and resultant hemorrhage. The patient becomes hypotensive with a normal CVP, olig-uric, and febrile and complains of flank pain. The most likely diagnosis is

a. Hypovolemic shock
b. Acute adrenal insufficiency
c. Gram-negative bacteremia
d. Transfusion reaction
e. Ureteral obstruction

6-4. A 40-year-old white male complains of weakness, weight loss, and abdominal pain. On examination, the patient has diffuse hyperpigmenta-tion and a palpable liver edge. Polyarthritis of the wrists and hips is also noted. Fasting blood sugar is 185 mg/dL. The most likely diagnosis is

a. Insulin-dependent diabetes mellitus
b. Pancreatic carcinoma
c. Addison's disease
d. Hemochromatosis

6-5. Aunt Mary is helping her family move to a new apartment. During the confusion, 3-year-old Jimmy is noted to be stumbling about, his face flushed and his speech slurred. The contents of Aunt Mary's purse are strewn about on the floor. In the emergency room, Jimmy is found to have a rapid heartbeat, blood pressure of 42/20, and dilated pupils. ECG shows prolonged QRS and QT intervals. Jimmy suddenly starts to convulse. His condition is most likely to be the result of poisoning with

a. Barbiturates
b. Tricyclic antidepressants
c. Diazepam
d. Organophosphates
e. Arsenic

6-6. A 34-year-old woman comes to the physician with the chief complaint of pain in her neck and back. She states that 7 months previously she had been in a car accident in which she was hit from behind by a man who was angry that she wasn't traveling fast enough. Immediately after the accident the man got out of the car and began screaming at the patient. The patient had been taken to the hospital, and an exam showed severe bruising and muscular rigidity of her back and neck, but no other damage. However, the patient states she has been completely disabled by her pain since that time. She states that her life would be perfect without the pain, and pleads with the physician to make it stop. On physical exam, she has mild muscular tension in her neck and back, but otherwise her diagnostic workup is within normal limits. Which of the following diagnoses is most likely?

a. Pain disorder
b. Malingering
c. Factitious disorder
d. Hypochondriasis
e. Conversion disorder

6-7. A 65-year-old man who smokes cigarettes and has chronic obstructive pulmonary disease falls and fractures the seventh, eighth, and ninth ribs in the left anterolateral chest. Chest x-ray is otherwise normal. Appropriate treatment might include

a. Strapping the chest with adhesive tape
b. Immobilization with sandbags
c. Tube thoracostomy
d. Peritoneal lavage
e. Surgical fixation of the fractured ribs

6-8. A 40-year-old male presents to the office with a history of palpitations that last for a few seconds and occur two or three times a week. There are no other symptoms. ECG shows a rare single unifocal premature ventricular contraction (PVC). The most likely cause of this finding is

a. Underlying coronary artery disease
b. Valvular heart disease
c. Hypertension
d. Apathetic hyperthyroidism
e. Idiopathic or unknown

6-9. A little girl who was underweight and hypotonic in infancy is obsessed with food, eats compulsively, and, at age 4, is already grossly overweight. She is argumentative, oppositional, and rigid. She has a narrow face, almond-shaped eyes, and a small mouth. Which of the following is the most likely diagnosis?

a. Down syndrome
b. Fragile X syndrome
c. Fetal alcohol syndrome
d. Hypothyroidism
e. Prader-Willi syndrome

6-10. A healthy 30-year-old G1P0 at 41 weeks gestational age presents to labor and delivery at 11:00 P.M. because she is concerned that her baby has not been moving as much as normal for the past 24 h. She denies any complications during the pregnancy. She denies any rupture of membranes, regular uterine contractions, or vaginal bleeding. On arrival to labor and delivery, her blood pressure is initially 140/90 but decreases with rest to 120/75. Her prenatal chart indicates that her baseline blood pressures are 100–120/60–70. The patient is placed on an external fetal monitor. The fetal heart rate baseline is 180 bpm with absent variability. There are uterine contractions every 3 min accompanied by late fetal heart rate decelerations. Physical exam indicates that the cervix is long/closed/−2. Which of the following is the appropriate plan of management for this patient?

a. Proceed with emergent cesarean section
b. Administer intravenous $MgSO_4$ and induce labor with Pitocin
c. Ripen cervix overnight with prostaglandin F_2 (Cervidil) and proceed with Pitocin induction in the morning
d. Admit the patient and schedule a cesarean section in the morning, after the patient has been NPO for 12 h
e. Induce labor with misoprostil (Cytotec)

6-11. A pregnant woman is discovered to be an asymptomatic carrier of *Neisseria gonorrhoeae*. A year ago, she was treated with penicillin for a gonococcal infection and developed a severe allergic reaction. Treatment of choice at this time is

a. Tetracycline
b. Ampicillin
c. Spectinomycin
d. Chloramphenicol
e. Penicillin

6-12. A 7-year-old boy with sickle cell disease presents with severe left upper quadrant pain that started suddenly 2 h before he arrived at the emergency room. He has no previous history of pain in that area. Physical examination reveals a temperature of 98.6°F and a normal blood pressure. Heart rate is 108/min. Heart and lung examinations are normal. There is fullness and tenderness in the left upper quadrant of the abdomen with palpation, but there is no audible rub. There is no hepatomegaly or rebound tenderness, and FOBT is negative. The rest of the physical examination is normal. Hemoglobin is 6.1 g/dL. Which of the following is the most likely diagnosis?

a. Vasoocclusive crisis
b. Splenic infarction
c. Splenic sequestration crisis
d. Left pleural effusion
e. Pulmonary infarction

6-13. A 35-year-old man is brought to see a psychiatrist by his wife, who states her husband keeps getting lost, even in places he has been familiar with for years. The patient's father was institutionalized and died at age 37. On exam, the patient is oriented to person only. He cannot accurately make change for a dollar, though he used to work as a banker. Which of the following diagnostic tests would be most useful for this patient?

a. EEG
b. Liver function tests
c. Serum amylase
d. Blood toxicology screen
e. MRI

6-14. A 65-year-old man who is hospitalized with pancreatic carcinoma develops abdominal distension and obstipation. The following abdominal radiograph is obtained. Appropriate management is best achieved by

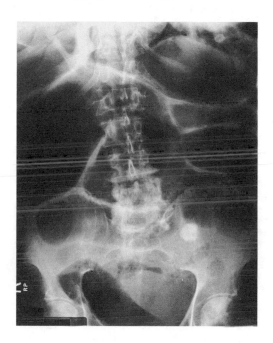

a. Urgent colostomy or cecostomy
b. Discontinuation of anticholinergic medications and narcotics and correction of metabolic disorders
c. Digital disimpaction of fecal mass in the rectum
d. Diagnostic and therapeutic colonoscopy
e. Detorsion of volvulus and colopexy or resection

6-15. A 19-year-old primiparous woman develops toxemia in her last trimester of pregnancy and during the course of her labor is treated with magnesium sulfate. At 38 weeks' gestation, she delivers a 2100-g infant with Apgar scores of 1 at 1 min and at 5 at 5 min. Laboratory studies at 18 h of age reveal a hematocrit of 79%, platelet count of 100,000/μL, glucose 38 mg/dL, magnesium 2.5 meq/L, and calcium 8.7 mg/dL. Soon after, this the infant has a generalized convulsion. The most likely cause of the infant's seizure is

a. Polycythemia
b. Hypoglycemia
c. Hypocalcemia
d. Hypermagnesemia
e. Thrombocytopenia

6-16. A 65-year-old man was diagnosed with lung cancer 6 months ago. Over the last 2 months, he has had worsening severe proximal muscle weakness. He is most likely to have which of the following?

a. Dermatomyositis
b. Trichinosis
c. Multiple sclerosis (MS)
d. Progressive multifocal leukoencephalopathy (PML)
e. Myasthenia gravis

6-17. A 30-year-old male complains of unilateral headaches with rhinorrhea and tearing of the eye on the side of the headache. Episodes are precipitated by alcohol. Headaches may become a problem for weeks to months, after which a headache-free period occurs. The most likely diagnosis is

a. Migraine
b. Cluster headache
c. Sinusitis
d. Tension headache

6-18. You receive a telephone call from the mother of a 4-year-old child with sickle cell anemia. She tells you that the child is breathing fast, coughing, and has a temperature of 40°C (104°F). The most conservative, prudent approach is to

a. Prescribe aspirin and ask her to call back if the fever does not respond
b. Make an office appointment for the next available opening
c. Make an office appointment for the next day
d. Refer the child to the laboratory for an immediate hematocrit, white blood cell count, and differential
e. Admit the child to the hospital as an emergency

6-19. A 54-year-old obese woman presents with the chief complaint of hemoptysis. She states that over the last day she has coughed up approximately 10 mL of blood-streaked sputum. She denies fever, chills, chest pain, or shortness of breath. She does admit to a recent upper respiratory tract infection with cough and a copious amount of sputum production. She remembers similar episodes of cough with bloody sputum occurring after colds for the last several years. She smokes one pack of cigarettes per day since high school. Examinations of the pharynx and lungs are normal. Which of the following is the most likely diagnosis?

a. Chronic bronchitis
b. Tuberculosis
c. Adenocarcinoma of the lung
d. Congestive heart failure
e. Pulmonary infarction

6-20. A 24-year-old woman comes to the emergency room with the chief complaint that "my stomach is rotting out from the inside." She states that for the last 6 months she has been crying on a daily basis and that she has decreased concentration, energy, and interest in her usual hobbies. She has lost 25 lb during that time. She cannot get to sleep, and when she does, she wakes up early in the morning. For the past 3 weeks, she has become convinced that she is dying of cancer and is rotting on the inside of her body. She has also heard a voice calling her name in the past 2 weeks when no one is around. Which of the following is the most appropriate diagnosis for this patient?

a. Delusional disorder
b. Schizoaffective disorder
c. Schizophreniform disorder
d. Schizophrenia
e. Major depression with psychotic features

6-21. One of your obstetric patients presents to the office at 25 weeks complaining of severe left calf pain and swelling. The area of concern is slightly edematous, but no erythema is apparent. The patient demonstrates a positive Homan sign, and you are concerned that she may have a deep vein thrombosis. Which of the following diagnostic modalities do you order?

a. MRI
b. Computed tomographic scanning
c. Venography
d. Real-time ultrasonography

6-22. Three weeks after an upper respiratory illness, a 25-year-old male develops weakness of his arms and legs over several days. On physical exam he is tachypneic, with shallow respirations and symmetric muscle weakness in both arms and legs. There is no obvious sensory deficit, but motor reflexes cannot be elicited. The most likely diagnosis is

a. Myasthenia gravis
b. Multiple sclerosis
c. Guillain-Barré syndrome
d. Dermatomyositis
e. Diabetes mellitus

6-23. A 65-year-old male with diabetes mellitus, bronzed skin, and cirrhosis of the liver is being treated for hemochromatosis previously confirmed by liver biopsy. The patient experiences increasing right upper quadrant pain, and his serum alkaline phosphatase is now elevated. There is a 15-lb weight loss. The next step in management should be to

a. Increase frequency of phlebotomy for worsening hemochromatosis
b. Obtain CT scan to rule out hepatoma
c. Obtain hepatitis B serology
d. Obtain antimitochondrial antibody to rule out primary biliary cirrhosis

6-24. This 30-year-old woman presented with weakness, bone pain, an elevated parathormone level, and a serum calcium level of 15.2 mg/dL. Skeletal survey films were taken, including the hand films and chest x-ray shown. The most likely cause of these findings is

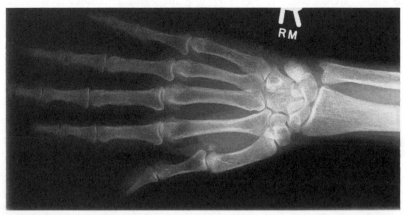

A

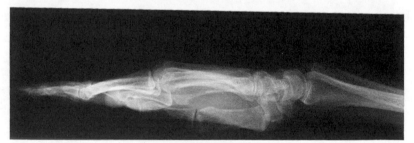

B

 a. Sarcoidosis
 b. Vitamin D intoxication
 c. Paget's disease
 d. Metastatic carcinoma
 e. Primary hyperparathyroidism

6-25. A 10-year-old boy has been having bellyaches for about 2 years. They occur at night as well as during the day. Occasionally, he vomits after the onset of pain. Occult blood has been found in his stool. His father also gets frequent stomachaches. The most likely diagnosis is

a. Peptic ulcer
b. Appendicitis
c. Meckel diverticulum
d. Intussusception
e. Pinworm infestation

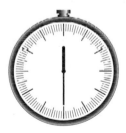

**YOU SHOULD HAVE COMPLETED APPROXIMATELY
25 QUESTIONS AND HAVE 30 MINUTES REMAINING.**

6-26. An anxious young woman who is taking birth control pills presents to the emergency room with shortness of breath. The absence of which of the following would make the diagnosis of pulmonary embolus unlikely?

a. Wheezing
b. Pleuritic chest pain
c. Tachypnea
d. Hemoptysis
e. Right-sided S_3 heart sound

6-27. Within 1 day of admission, the patient's right-sided weakness began to abate, and within 1 week it completely resolved. On the fourth day of hospitalization, the patient abruptly lost consciousness and exhibited clonic movements starting in his right side and generalizing to his left side. The movements stopped within 3 min, but he had residual right-sided weakness for 24 h. CT scan was unchanged from that obtained on admission. The most appropriate treatment to institute involves

a. Heparin
b. Recombinant tissue plasminogen activator (r-TPA)
c. Lamotrigine
d. Phenytoin
e. Warfarin

6-28. A patient delivered a baby boy 2 days ago and is trying to decide whether or not to have you perform a circumcision on her newborn. The boy is in the well baby nursery and is doing very well. The patient had an uncomplicated vaginal delivery, and the baby weighed 6 lb, 10 oz. In counseling this patient, you tell her which of the following recommendations from the American Pediatric Association?

a. Circumcisions should be performed routinely because they decrease the incidence of male urinary tract infections
b. Circumcisions should be performed routinely because they decrease the incidence of penile cancer
c. Circumcisions should be performed routinely because they decrease the incidence of sexually transmitted diseases
d. Circumcisions should not be performed routinely because of insufficient data regarding risks and benefits
e. Circumcisions should not be performed routinely because it is a risky procedure and complications such as bleeding and infection are common

6-29. An 80-year-old with a past history of myocardial infarction is found to have left bundle branch block on ECG. He is asymptomatic with blood pressure 130/80, lungs clear to auscultation, and no leg edema. On cardiac auscultation, the most likely finding is

a. Fixed (wide) split S_2
b. Paradoxical (reversed) split S_2
c. S_3
d. S_4
e. Opening snap
f. Midsystolic click

6-30. A 23-year-old man comes to the physician with the complaint that his memory has worsened over the past 2 months and that he has difficulty concentrating. He has lost interest in his friends and his work. He has difficulty with abstract thoughts and problem solving. He has also felt depressed. MRI scan shows parenchymal abnormalities. Which of the following diagnoses is most likely?

a. Alzheimer's disease
b. Vascular dementia
c. HIV-related dementia
d. Lewy body disease
e. Binswanger's disease

6-31. A 31-year-old right-handed woman has a history of alcohol abuse requiring detox. Currently, she says she is drinking about nine beers 3 days per week. She drank five glasses of wine and 3 beers 5 days ago, and she had 10 beers last night. This morning, she awoke feeling well. She was speaking with her fiancé, went to the bathroom, and got back into bed. She had no headache, fever, chills, nausea, vomiting, or pain. Suddenly her body became stiff with arms flexed for a few seconds, followed by rhythmic jerking of both arms. Her legs were shaking, but less so. Her eyes were open, and she was foaming at the mouth. After 1 min, this stopped, and she initially did not recognize her fiancé or his sister. She slowly returned to a normal level of consciousness over a 10-min period. She remembers events just prior to the episode, and she remembers being in the car on the way to the hospital. Her only medication is a multivitamin. She denies illicit drugs. Her examination is entirely normal. Routine labs and a brain MRI are normal. The most likely underlying cause of her condition is

a. Autoimmune
b. Genetic
c. Infectious
d. Neoplastic
e. Toxic/metabolic

6-32. A 35-year-old construction worker presents with complaints of nocturnal parasthesias of the thumb and the index and middle fingers. There is some atrophy of the thenar eminence. Tinel sign is positive. The most likely diagnosis is

a. Carpal tunnel syndrome
b. De Quervain's tenosynovitis
c. Amyotrophic lateral sclerosis
d. Rheumatoid arthritis of the wrist joint

6-33. A 23-year-old previously healthy man presents to the emergency room after sustaining a single gunshot wound to the left chest. The entrance wound is 3 cm inferior to the nipple and the exit wound is just below the scapula. A chest tube is placed that drains 400 mL of blood and continues to drain 50 to 75 mL/h during the initial resuscitation. Initial blood pressure of 70/0 mmHg has responded to 2 L crystalloid and is now 100/70 mmHg. Abdominal examination is unremarkable. Chest x-ray reveals a reexpanded lung and no free air under the diaphragm. The next management step should be

a. Admission and observation
b. Peritoneal lavage
c. Exploratory thoracotomy
d. Exploratory celiotomy
e. Local wound exploration

6-34. A 24-year-old man with chronic schizophrenia is brought to the emergency room after his parents found him in his bed and were unable to communicate with him. On examination, the man is confused and disoriented. He has severe muscle rigidity and a temperature of 103°F. His blood pressure is elevated, and he has a leucocytosis. Which of the following is the best first step in the pharmacologic treatment of this man?

a. Haloperidol
b. Lorazepam
c. Bromocriptine
d. Benztropine
e. Lithium

6-35. Your 18-year-old college freshman calls to state that he has had fever, muscular pain (especially in the neck), headache, and malaise. He describes the area from the back of his mandible toward the mastoid space as being full and tender and that his earlobe on the affected side appears to be sticking upward and outward. Drinking sour liquids causes much pain in the affected area. You quickly retrieve his immunization card and suddenly realize that he has failed to get vaccinated for

a. Mumps
b. Varicella
c. Rubella
d. Measles
e. Herpangina

6-36. A 50-year-old male complains of low back pain and stiffness, which becomes worse on bending and is relieved by lying down. There are no symptoms of fever, chills, weight loss, or urinary problems. He has had similar pain several years ago. On exam, there is paraspinal tenderness and spasm of the lower lumbar back. There are no sensory deficits, and reflexes are normal. The next step in management is

a. Lumbosacral spine films
b. Stretching exercises
c. Weight training
d. Activity as tolerated, optional 2-day bedrest
e. MRI

6-37. A 40-year-old G3P3 comes to your office for a routine annual GYN exam. She tells you that she gets up several times during the night to void. On further questioning, she admits to you that during the day she sometimes gets the urge to void, but sometimes cannot quite make it to the bathroom. She attributes this to getting older and is not extremely concerned, although she often wears a pad when she goes out in case she loses some urine. This patient is very healthy otherwise and does not take any medication on a regular basis. She has had three normal spontaneous vaginal deliveries of infants weighing between 7 and 8 lb. An office dipstick of her urine does not indicate any blood, bacteria, WBCs, or protein. Based on her office presentation and history, what is this patient's most likely diagnosis?

a. Urinary stress incontinence
b. Urinary tract infection
c. Overflow incontinence
d. Bladder dyssynergia
e. Vesicovaginal fistula

6-38. A 43-year-old woman complains of lancinating pains radiating into the right side of her jaw. This discomfort has been present for more than 3 years and has started occurring more than once a week. The pain is paroxysmal and routinely triggered by cold stimuli, such as ice cream and cold drinks. She has sought relief with multiple dental procedures and has already had two teeth extracted. Multiple neuroimaging studies reveal no structural lesions in her head. Assuming there are no contraindications to the treatment, a reasonable next step would be to prescribe

a. Clonazepam (Klonopin) 1 mg orally three times daily
b. Diazepam (Valium) 5 mg orally two times daily
c. Divalproex sodium (Depakote) 250 mg orally three times daily
d. Indomethacin (Indocin) 10 mg orally three times daily
e. Carbamazepine (Tegretol) 100 mg orally three times daily

6-39. A 26-year-old man comes to the physician with the chief complaint of a depressed mood for the past 5 weeks. He has been feeling down, with decreased concentration, energy, and interest in his usual hobbies. Six weeks prior to this office visit he had been to the emergency room for an acute asthma attack, for which he had been started on prednisone. Which of the following diagnoses is most likely?

a. Mood disorder secondary to a general medical condition
b. Substance-induced mood disorder
c. Major depression
d. Adjustment disorder
e. Dysthymia

6-40. A pedestrian is hit by a speeding car. Radiologic studies obtained in the emergency room, including a retrograde urethrogram, are consistent with a pelvic fracture with a rupture of the urethra superior to the urogenital diaphragm. Management should consist of

a. Immediate percutaneous nephrostomy
b. Immediate placement of a Foley catheter through the urethra into the bladder to align and stent the injured portions
c. Immediate reconstruction of the ruptured urethra after initial stabilization of the patient
d. Immediate exploration of the pelvis for control of hemorrhage from pelvic fracture and drainage of pelvic hematoma
e. Immediate placement of a suprapubic cystostomy tube

6-41. A 19-year-old with insulin-dependent diabetes mellitus is taking 30 units of NPH insulin each morning and 15 units at night. Because of persistent morning glycosuria with some ketonuria, the evening dose is increased to 20 units. This worsens the morning glycosuria, and now moderate ketones are noted in urine. The patient complains of sweats and headaches at night. The next step in management is

a. Increase the evening dose of insulin
b. Increase the morning dose of insulin
c. Switch from human NPH to pork insulin
d. Obtain blood sugar levels between 2:00 and 5:00 A.M.

6-42. A 22-year-old man is being treated with fluoxetine for major depression. Hoping to become less depressed more quickly, he also begins taking a relative's phenelzine, a monoamine oxidase inhibitor (MAOI). Two days later he is brought to the emergency department after becoming confused. He also complains of visual hallucinations and myoclonic jerks. On physical examination, he is flushed and diaphoretic. His temperature is 39.5°C (103°F). Which of the following is the most likely diagnosis?

a. Meningitis
b. Overdose of fluoxetine
c. Neuroleptic malignant syndrome
d. Serotonin syndrome
e. Extrapyramidal side effect

6-43. A 37-year-old woman develops cholecystitis and requires cholecys-tectomy. Her family advises the physicians involved that she has a long history of alcoholism and benzodiazepine use, including diazepam (Valium), lorazepam (Ativan), and clonazepam (Klonopin). Approximately 7 days after the surgery, the patient becomes increasingly agitated, delusional, and suspicious. Routine investigations reveal no evidence of focal or systemic infection. Hepatic, renal, and hematologic parameters are largely normal. Within 24 h of these cognitive and affective changes, the patient has a gen-eralized tonic-clonic seizure. Magnetic resonance imaging (MRI) and computed tomography (CT) studies of the brain are normal, and her CSF is unremarkable. In consideration of the abuse history provided by the family, medication orders prior to the surgery should have included

a. Haloperidol
b. Chlorpromazine
c. Trihexyphenidyl
d. Prochlorperazine
e. Thiamine

6-44. A 40-year-old woman's cognitive functions have progressively dete-riorated for several years, to the point where she needs nursing home–level care. She is depressed, easily irritated, and prone to aggressive outbursts, a dramatic change from her premorbid personality. She also presents with irregular, purposeless, and asymmetrical movements of her face, limbs, and trunk, which worsen when she is upset and disappear in sleep. Her MRI shows atrophy of the caudal nucleus and the putamen. Which of the following diagnoses is most likely in this patient?

a. Creutzfeldt-Jakob disease
b. Wilson's disease
c. Huntington's disease
d. Alzheimer's disease
e. Multi-infarct dementia

6-45. A 39-year-old man with a 12-year history of human immunodeficiency virus (HIV) presents with 3+ pitting edema of the lower extremities. He denies fever, polyuria, frequency, nocturia, and hematuria. He does not drink alcohol, smoke cigarettes, or use illicit drugs. He has no past medical history of hypertension or diabetes mellitus. He is compliant with his HIV medication. Blood pressure is 120/80 mmHg; heart, lung, and abdominal examinations are normal. Serum albumin is 2.8 mg/dL (normal = 3.5 to 5.7 mg/dL), and 24-hour urine protein is 3800 mg/dL (normal < 150 mg/dL). The patient has significantly elevated lipid (predominantly LDL) levels. Which of the following is the most likely cause for the lipid abnormalities?

a. A defect in the LDL receptor resulting in an increase in lipid levels
b. A defect in the VLDL receptor resulting in an increase in lipid levels
c. Increased lipoprotein clearance of lipids from the blood by lipoprotein lipase
d. Decreased lipoprotein clearance of lipids from the blood by lipoprotein lipase
e. Decreased hepatic synthesis of proteins

6-46. The mother of a 2-year-old girl reports that her daughter complains of burning when she urinates and that she has foul-smelling discharge from her vagina. She has noticed that there is some slight staining on the front of her underwear, but she reports no fever, nausea, vomiting, or other constitutional signs. The child does not attend day care, and she has demonstrated no change in behavior. The physical examination is normal with an intact hymen, but the child's vulva is reddened and with a malodorous scent noted. Her urinalysis and culture are normal. The most likely explanation for this child's condition is

a. Sexual abuse
b. Pinworms in the vagina
c. Chemical vulvovaginitis
d. Pediculosis pubis
e. Giardiasis

6-47. A 32-year-old woman with alcoholism and cocaine use dating back at least 10 years comes to the emergency room after 48 h of recurrent vomiting and hematemesis. She reports abdominal discomfort that preceded the vomiting by a few days. For at least 36 h, she has been unable to keep ethanol in her stomach. Intravenous fluid replacement is started while she is being transported to the emergency room, and while in the emergency room she complains of progressive blurring of vision. Over the course of 1 h, she becomes increasingly disoriented, ataxic, and dysarthric. The most likely explanation for her rapid deterioration is

a. Dehydration
b. Hypomagnesemia
c. Wernicke's encephalopathy
d. Hypoglycemia
e. Cocaine overdose

6-48. A 29-year-old G0 who comes to your OB/GYN office complaining of PMS. On taking a more detailed history, you learn that the patient suffers from emotional lability and depression for about 10 days prior to her menses. She reports that once she begins to bleed she feels back to normal. The patient also reports a long history of premenstrual fatigue, breast tenderness, and bloating. Her previous health care provider placed her on oral contraceptives to treat her PMS 6 months ago. She reports that the pills have alleviated all her PMS symptoms except for the depression and emotional symptoms. Which of the following would be the best treatment for this patient's problem?

a. Spironolactone
b. Evening primrose oil
c. Fluoxetine
d. Progesterone supplements
e. Vitamin B_6

6-49. A 63-year-old male alcoholic with a 50-pack-year history of smoking presents to the emergency room with fatigue and confusion. Physical examination reveals a blood pressure of 110/70 with no orthostatic change. Heart, lung, and abdominal examination are normal and there is no pedal edema. Laboratory data is as follows:

Na: 110 meq/L
K: 3.7 meq/L
Cl: 82 meq/L
HCO_3: 20 meq/L
Glucose: 100 mg/dL
BUN: 5 mg/dL
Creatinine: 0.7 mg/dL
Urinalysis: normal

The most likely diagnosis is
a. Volume depletion
b. Inappropriate secretion of antidiuretic hormone
c. Polydipsia
d. Cirrhosis

6-50. The delivery of a newborn boy is remarkable for oligohydramnios. The pictured infant is also noted to have undescended testes and clubfeet, and to be in respiratory distress. The most likely diagnosis to explain these findings is

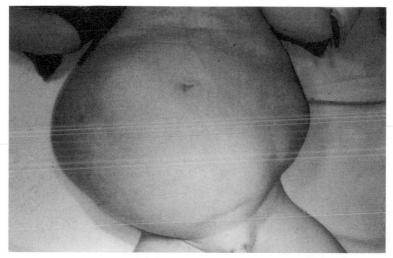

(Courtesy Michael L. Ritchey, M.D.)

a. Surfactant deficiency
b. Turner syndrome
c. Prune belly syndrome
d. Hermaphroditism
e. Congenital adrenal hyperplasia

BLOCK 7

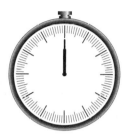

**YOU HAVE 60 MINUTES
TO COMPLETE 50 QUESTIONS.**

Questions

7-1. A 22-year-old college student comes to the physician with the complaint of shortness of breath during anxiety-provoking situations, such as exams. She also notes perioral tingling, carpopedal spasms, and feelings of derealization at the same time. All of the symptoms pass after the anxiety over the situation has faded. The episodes have never occurred "out of the blue." Which of the following is the most likely diagnosis?

a. Panic disorder
b. Generalized anxiety disorder
c. Hyperventilation
d. Anxiety disorder not otherwise specified
e. Anxiety disorder secondary to a general medical condition

7-2. A 65-year-old woman has a life-threatening pulmonary embolus 5 days following removal of a uterine malignancy. She is immediately heparinized and maintained in good therapeutic range for the next 3 days, then passes gross blood from her vagina and develops tachycardia, hypotension, and oliguria. Following resuscitation, an abdominal CT scan reveals a major retroperitoneal hematoma. You should now

a. Immediately reverse heparin by a calculated dose of protamine and place a vena caval filter (e.g., a Greenfield filter)
b. Reverse heparin with protamine, explore and evacuate the hematoma, and ligate the vena cava below the renal veins
c. Switch to low-dose heparin
d. Stop heparin and observe closely
e. Stop heparin, give fresh frozen plasma (FFP), and begin warfarin therapy

7-3. A 35-year-old female has progressive numbness of the right arm and difficulty seeing objects in the left visual field. She is known to be HIV-positive, but has not consistently taken medications in the past. On examination, she appears healthy, but has a right homonymous hemianopsia and decreased sensory perception in her left upper extremity and face. Her CD4 count is 75 cells per μL, and her MRI is consistent with a demyelinating lesion of the left parietooccipital area. CSF PCR for JC virus is positive. Which of the following is the most appropriate treatment in this case?

a. Amphotericin B
b. Cranial radiation
c. Highly active antiretroviral therapy (HAART)
d. Intravenous acyclovir
e. Intravenous ceftriaxone

7-4. A 38-year-old man arrives at the emergency room with the chief complaint of hematemesis for 3 h. He does not drink alcohol and has no previous medical history. He spent the previous night vomiting approximately 10 to 12 times after eating some "bad chicken." The patient is squirming on the stretcher and is retching. He is afebrile with a heart rate of 120/min and a blood pressure of 90/60 mmHg. Abdominal exam is positive for diffuse tenderness, but the patient has no rigidity, guarding, or rebound tenderness. There is no hepatosplenomegaly. Rectal exam is negative for occult blood. A nasogastric tube is inserted and reveals bright red blood. Which of the following is the most likely diagnosis?

a. Esophageal varices
b. Mallory-Weiss tear
c. Gastritis
d. Peptic ulcer disease
e. Boerhaave syndrome
f. Dieulafoy lesion

7-5. A 19-year-old man is brought to the physician by his parents after he called them from college, terrified that the Mafia was after him. He states he has eaten nothing for the past 6 weeks other than canned beans because "they are into everything—I can't be too careful." He is convinced that the Mafia has put cameras in his dormitory room and that they are watching his every move. He occasionally hears the voices of two men talking about him when no one is around. His roommate states that for the past 2 months the patient has been increasingly withdrawn and suspicious. Which of the following is the most likely diagnosis for this patient?

a. Delusional disorder
b. Schizoaffective disorder
c. Schizophreniform disorder
d. Schizophrenia
e. PCP intoxication

7-6. A 29-year-old G3P2 black woman in the thirty-third week of gestation is admitted to the emergency room because of acute abdominal pain that has been increasing during the past 24 h. The pain is severe and is radiating from the epigastrium to the back. The patient has vomited a few times and has not eaten or had a bowel movement since the pain started. On examination, you observe an acutely ill patient lying on the bed with her knees drawn up. Her blood pressure is 150/100 mmHg, her pulse is 110/min, and her temperature is 38.8°C (100.8°F). On palpation, the abdomen is somewhat distended and tender, mainly in the epigastric area, and the uterine fundus reaches 31 cm above the symphysis. Hypotonic bowel sounds are noted. Fetal monitoring reveals a normal pattern of fetal heart rate (FHR) without uterine contractions. On ultrasonography, the fetus is in vertex presentation and appropriate in size for gestational age; fetal breathing and trunk movements are noted, and the volume of amniotic fluid is normal. The placenta is located on the anterior uterine wall and of grade 2 to 3. Laboratory values show mild leukocytosis (12,000 cells per µL); a hematocrit of 43; mildly elevated serum glutamic-oxaloacetic transaminase (SGOT), serum glutamic-pyruvic transaminase (SGPT), and bilirubin; and serum amylase of 180 U/dL. Urinalysis is normal. The most probable diagnosis in this patient is

a. Acute degeneration of uterine leiomyoma
b. Acute cholecystitis
c. Acute pancreatitis
d. Acute appendicitis
e. Severe preeclamptic toxemia

7-7. A 41-year-old patient with a long history of schizophrenia presents with confusion and disorientation. His wife states that he drinks several liters of water daily. His blood pressure is 110/70 mmHg, pulse is 104/min, respirations are 20/min, and temperature is 98.6°F. The patient has no orthostatic changes in blood pressure or pulse. Heart and lung examinations are normal. The neurologic exam reveals a dysarthric man who is oriented only to person. He has no focal neurologic deficits. Laboratory data reveal a serum sodium concentration of 105 meq/L and the diagnosis of primary polydipsia is made. The patient is admitted and the sodium is corrected to normal (135 meq/L) within 12 hours. While awaiting a psychiatry consult, the patient develops flaccid quadriplegia, then becomes comatose. Which of the following is the most likely diagnosis?

a. Relapse into hyponatremia
b. Acute schizophrenia
c. New stroke
d. Myocardial infarction
e. Central pontine myelinolysis

7-8. A 26-year-old woman is brought to the emergency room by her husband after she begins screaming that her children are calling to her and becomes hysterical. The husband states that 2 weeks previously the couple's two children were killed in a car accident, and since that time the patient has been agitated, disorganized, and incoherent. He states that she will not eat because she believes he has been poisoning her food, and she has not slept in the past 2 days. In the emergency room, the patient believes that the nurses are going to cause her harm as well. The patient is sedated and later sent home. One week later all her symptoms remit spontaneously. Which of the following is the most likely diagnosis for this patient?

a. Delirium
b. Schizophreniform disorder
c. Major depression with psychotic features
d. Brief psychotic disorder
e. Posttraumatic stress disorder

7-9. A previously healthy 8-year-old boy has a 3-week history of low-grade fever of unknown source, fatigue, weight loss, myalgia, and headaches. On repeated examinations during this time, he is found to have developed a heart murmur, petechiae, and mild splenomegaly. The most likely diagnosis is

a. Rheumatic fever
b. Kawasaki disease
c. Scarlet fever
d. Endocarditis
e. Tuberculosis

7-10. A 34-year-old secretary climbs 12 flights of stairs every day to reach her office because she is terrified by the thought of being trapped in the elevator. She has never had any traumatic event occur with an elevator, but nonetheless has been terrified of them since childhood. Which of the following diagnoses is most likely?

a. Social phobia
b. Performance anxiety
c. Generalized anxiety disorder
d. Specific phobia
e. Agoraphobia

7-11. A 67-year-old man has a history of progressive memory loss for 2 years. His examination is otherwise normal. A diagnosis of Alzheimer's disease is made. Which of the following medications may retard the progress of this patient's deterioration?

a. Donepezil
b. L-dopa
c. Risperidone
d. Prednisone
e. Vitamin B_{12}

7-12. A 64-year-old man afflicted with severe emphysema, who receives oxygen therapy at home, is admitted to the hospital because of upper gastrointestinal bleeding. The bleeding ceases soon after admission, and the patient becomes agitated and then disoriented; he is given 5 mg of intramuscular diazepam (Valium). Twenty minutes later he is unresponsive. Physical examination reveals a stuporous but arousable man who has papilledema and asterixis. Arterial blood gases are as follows: pH 7.17; PO_2 42 kPa; PCO_2 95 kPa. The best immediate therapy is to

a. Correct hypoxemia with high-flow nasal oxygen
b. Correct acidosis with sodium bicarbonate
c. Administer 10 mg intravenous dexamethasone
d. Intubate the patient
e. Call for neurosurgical consultation

7-13. The nurse from the level II neonatal intensive care nursery calls you to evaluate a baby. The infant, born at 32 weeks' gestation, is now 1 week old and had been doing well on increasing nasogastric feedings. This afternoon, however, the nurse noted that the infant has vomitted the last two feedings and seems less active. Your examination reveals a tense and distended abdomen with decreased bowel sounds. As you are evaluating the child, he has a grossly bloody stool. Your management of this infant should include

a. Surgical consultation for an emergent exploratory laparotomy
b. Continued feeding of the infant, as gastroenteritis is usually self-limited
c. Stool culture to identify the etiology of the bloody diarrhea and an infectious diseases consultation
d. Stopping feeds, beginning intravenous fluids, ordering serial abdominal films, and initiating systemic antibiotics
e. Upper GI series and barium enema to evaluate for obstruction

7-14. An 18-year-old G0 comes to see you complaining of a 3-day history of urinary frequency, urgency, and dysuria. She panicked this morning when she noticed the presence of bright red blood in her urine. She also reports some midline lower abdominal discomfort. She had intercourse for the first time 5 days ago and reports that she used condoms. On physical exam, there is no discharge from the cervix or in the vagina and the cervix appears normal. Bimanual exam is normal except for mild suprapubic tenderness. There is no flank tenderness, and the patient's temperature is normal. What is the most likely diagnosis?

a. *Chlamydia* cervicitis
b. Pyelonephritis
c. Cystitis
d. Bladder dyssynergia
e. Kidney stone

7-15. A 19-year-old previously healthy college student presents with a 5-day history of fever, generalized malaise, and sore throat. He denies cough. He does not use illicit drugs and uses condoms with his one sexual partner. He has been vaccinated against hepatitis B. On physical examination the patient appears jaundiced and has a temperature of 101.7°F. The pharynx is erythematous but has no exudate. There is bilateral tender cervical lymphadenopathy. Liver size is 14 cm in the MCL, and the spleen tip is palpable 2 cm below the left costal margin. The white blood cell count is elevated and many atypical forms are reported. Which of the following is the most likely diagnosis?

a. Drug-induced hepatitis
b. Mononucleosis syndrome
c. Hepatitis B infection
d. Hepatitis C infection
e. *Mycoplasma pneumoniae*

7-16. A 47-year-old nurse presents to your office complaining of a poorly healing ulcer of her left second digit. The ulcer started a week ago and is painless. The patient has tried using over-the-counter antibacterial and hydrocortisone creams without improvement. She denies trauma to the hand. The patient has a temperature of 101.1°F and left-sided epitrochlear and axillary adenopathy. She has a 4-cm ulcer on the dorsal side of the left second digit covered by a black eschar and surrounded by an extensive amount of nonpitting edema. Which of the following is the most likely diagnosis?

a. Smallpox infection
b. Cutaneous anthrax
c. Cat-scratch disease
d. Leprosy infection
e. Brown recluse spider bite

7-17. A 59-year-old woman presents complaining of a cough productive of sputum for nearly 10 years. Her cough occurs during the day, and she produces sputum daily. The woman states that as a child, she had several episodes of pneumonia requiring hospital admissions and antibiotics. Several times a year, her sputum becomes purulent and she requires antibiotic therapy. She denies smoking cigarettes and has worked as a seamstress all of her life. On physical examination, the lungs are clear without wheezes, rhonchi, or crackles. A chest radiograph reveals tram-track markings at the bases. Which of the following is the most likely diagnosis?

a. Asthma
b. Cystic fibrosis
c. Chronic bronchitis
d. Emphysema
e. Bronchiectasis

7-18. A 25-year-old woman is found to have an anterior neck mass. Her thyroid scan, shown below, exhibits findings that are consistent with which of the following disorders?

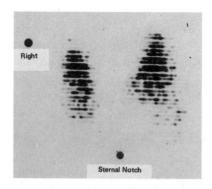

a. Carcinoma
b. Toxic adenoma
c. Toxic multinodular goiter
d. Graves' disease
e. de Quervain's (subacute) thyroiditis

7-19. Parents bring a 5-day-old infant to your office. The mother is O negative and was Coombs positive at delivery. The term child weighed 3055 g at birth and had a baseline hemoglobin (16 gm/dL) and a total serum bilirubin (3 mg/dL). He passed a black tarlike stool within the first 24 h of life. He was discharged at 30 h of life with a stable axillary temperature of 36.5°C (97.7°F). Today the infant's weight is 3000 g, his axillary temperature is 35°C (95°F), and he is jaundiced to the chest. Parents report frequent yellow, seedy stool. You redraw labs and find his hemoglobin is now 14 gm/dL, and his total serum bilirubin is 13 mg/dL. The change in which of the following parameters is of most concern?

a. Hemoglobin
b. Temperature
c. Body weight
d. Bilirubin
e. Stool

7-20. A 35-year-old female complains of slowly progressive dyspnea. Her history is otherwise unremarkable, and there is no cough, sputum production, pleuritic chest pain, or thrombophlebitis. She has taken appetite suppressants at different times. On physical exam, there is jugular venous distention, a palpable right ventricular lift, and a loud P_2 heart sound. Chest x-ray shows clear lung fields. ECG shows right axis deviation. A perfusion lung scan is normal with no segmental deficits. The most likely diagnosis in this patient is

a. Primary pulmonary hypertension
b. Recurrent pulmonary emboli
c. Cardiac shunt
d. Interstitial lung disease

7-21. A 75-year-old man has malaise and slowly progressive weight loss for the better part of 3 months. Laboratory tests reveal a hematocrit of 32%, an erythrocyte sedimentation rate (ESR) of 97 mm/h, and a white blood cell (WBC) count of 10,700 cells per μL. Serum CPK and thyroxine (T_4) levels are normal. Which of the following is the most likely explanation for the patient's complaints?

a. Polymyositis
b. Dermatomyositis
c. Polymyalgia rheumatica
d. Rheumatoid arthritis
e. Hyperthyroid myopathy

7-22. A social worker makes a routine visit on a 3-year-old boy who has just been returned to his biological mother after spending 3 months in foster care for severe neglect. The child initially appears very shy and clings fearfully to his mother. Later on, he starts playing in a very destructive and disorganized way. When the mother tries to stop him from throwing blocks at her, he starts kicking and biting. The mother becomes enraged and starts shouting. Which of the following is most likely to be this child's diagnosis?

a. Oppositional defiant disorder
b. ADHD
c. Reactive attachment disorder
d. PTSD
e. Major depression

7-23. Since you are a new intern, you ordered all of the diagnostic studies you could think of instead of just the ones your senior resident told you were most appropriate. The nurse calls to inform you that the infant's studies are back. Both the mother and baby have O-positive blood. The baby's direct serum bilirubin is 0.2 mg/dL, with a repeat total serum bilirubin of 11.8 mg/dL. Urine bilrubin is positive. The mother's white count is 13,000/µL with a differential of 50% polymorphonuclear cells, 45% lymphocyes, and 5% monocytes. The hemoglobin is 17 g/dL, and the platelet count is 278,000/µL. Reticulocyte count is 1.5%. The peripheral smear does not show fragments or abnormal cell shapes. Blood cultures are pending in the laboratory. Liver enzymes and liver ultrasound are normal. G6PD levels and osmotic fragility testing are normal. The most likely diagnosis in this infant is

a. Rh or ABO hemolytic disease
b. Physiologic jaundice
c. Sepsis
d. Congenital spherocytic anemia
e. Biliary atresia

7-24. A married 41-year-old G5P3114 presents to your office for a routine exam. This patient has been married for 20 years and is very happy being a stay-at-home mom. She is healthy and denies any medical problems except migraine headaches that are sometimes exacerbated by her menses. She reports that all her pregnancies were uncomplicated except for the development of gestational diabetes when she was pregnant with her last child. She drinks alcohol socially, and admits to smoking occasionally. She reports that her menses are regular and denies any dysmenorrhea or PMS. When questioned about her family history, she states that she thinks her grandmother was diagnosed with ovarian cancer when she was in her 50s. She denies a family history of any other cancers or medical diseases. She is tired of using condoms for contraception, and wants to discuss her options for birth control with you. She and her husband are sure that they do not want to have additional children in the future. Her BP is 140/90; height is 5 ft, 5 in.; weight is 150 lb. What is the most common cause of death in women of this patient's age?

a. HIV
b. Cardiac disease
c. Accidents
d. Suicide
e. Cancer

7-25. A 57-year-old woman sees blood on the toilet paper. Her Doctor notes the presence of an excoriated bleeding 2.8-cm mass at the anus. Biopsy confirms the clinical suspicion of anal cancer. In planning the management of a 2.8-cm epidermoid carcinoma of the anus, the first therapeutic approach should be

a. Abdominoperineal resection
b. Wide local resection with bilateral inguinal node dissection
c. Local radiation therapy
d. Systemic chemotherapy
e. Combined radiation therapy and chemotherapy

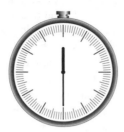

YOU SHOULD HAVE COMPLETED APPROXIMATELY
25 QUESTIONS AND HAVE 30 MINUTES REMAINING.

7-26. A 77-year-old nursing home patient is brought to the emergency room because of low-grade fever. She has no vomiting or diarrhea. She has no cough or foul-smelling urine. Her chest radiograph and urinalysis are normal. A 2.5-cm stage 3 pressure ulcer is visible over her sacrum. Which of the following is the most effective intervention for this patient's skin lesion?

a. Wet to dry dressings
b. Dry to wet dressings
c. Frequent turning
d. Whirlpool therapy
e. Surgical debridement

7-27. A 61-year-old man with a history of hypertension has been in excellent health until he presents with vertigo and unsteadiness lasting for 2 days. He then develops nausea, vomiting, dysphagia, hoarseness, ataxia, left facial pain, and right-sided sensory loss. There is no weakness. On examination, he is alert, with a normal mental status. He vomits with head movement. There is skew deviation of the eyes, left ptosis, clumsiness of the left arm, and titubation. He has loss of pin and temperature sensation on the right arm and leg and decreased joint position sensation in the left foot. He is unable to walk. Magnetic resonance imaging (MRI) in this patient might be expected to show which of the following?

a. Basilar artery tip aneurysm
b. Right lateral medullary infarction
c. Left lateral medullary infarction
d. Left medial medullary infarction
e. Right medial medullary infarction

7-28. An ill appearing 2-week-old girl is brought to the emergency room. She is pale and dyspneic with a respiratory rate of 80 breaths per min. Heart rate is 195 beats per min, heart sounds are distant, and a gallop is heard. There is cardiomegaly by x-ray. An echocardiogram demonstrates poor ventricular function, dilated ventricles, and dilation of the left atrium. An electrocardiogram shows ventricular depolarization complexes that have low voltage. The diagnosis suggested by this clinical picture is

a. Myocarditis
b. Endocardial fibroelastosis
c. Pericarditis
d. Aberrant left coronary artery arising from pulmonary artery
e. Glycogen storage disease of the heart

7-29. A patient presents for her first initial OB visit after performing a home pregnancy test and gives a last menstrual period of about 8 weeks ago. She says she is not entirely sure of her dates, however, because she has a long history of irregular menses. Which of the following is the most accurate way of dating the pregnancy?

a. Determination of uterine size on pelvic examination
b. Quantitative serum HCG level
c. Crown-rump length on abdominal or vaginal ultrasound
d. Determination of progesterone level along with serum HCG level

7-30. A 45-year-old housewife has been drinking in secret for several years. She started with one or two small glasses of Irish cream per night to help her sleep, but, with time, her nightly intake has increased to 4 to 5 hard liquor shots. Now she needs a few glasses of wine in the early afternoon to prevent shakiness and anxiety. During the past year, she could not take part in several important family events, including her son's high school graduation, because she was too ill or she did not want to risk missing her nightly drinking. She is ashamed of her secret and has tried to limit her alcohol intake but without success. Which of the following diagnoses is most likely?

a. Alcohol abuse
b. Alcohol addiction
c. Addictive personality disorder
d. Alcohol dependence
e. Alcohol-induced mood disorder

7-31. A 2-year-old boy develops bloody diarrhea shortly after eating in a fast-food restaurant. A few days later, he develops pallor and lethargy; his face looks swollen and his mother reports that he has been urinating very little. Laboratory evaluation reveals low hematocrit and platelet count and positive blood and protein in the urine. Which of the following diagnoses is likely to explain these symptoms?

a. Henoch-Schönlein purpura
b. IgA nephropathy
c. Intussusception
d. Meckel diverticulum
e. Hemolytic-uremic syndrome

7-32. A 30-year-old male is admitted to the hospital after a motorcycle accident that resulted in a fracture of the right femur. The fracture is managed with traction. Three days later the patient becomes confused and tachypneic. A petechial rash is noted over the chest. Lungs are clear to auscultation. Arterial blood gases show PO_2 of 50, PCO_2 of 28, and pH of 7.49. The most likely diagnosis is

a. Unilateral pulmonary edema
b. Hematoma of the chest
c. Fat embolism
d. Pulmonary embolism
e. Early *Staphylococcus aureus* pneumonia

7-33. A 32-year-old woman is referred to the emergency room for renal failure that was discovered in a pre-employment screening examination. The patient has a blood urea nitrogen (BUN) of 100 mg/dL and a serum creatinine of 8.4 mg/dL. Her only complaint is bilateral flank pain. Family history reveals that her mother and one sibling have renal failure and receive hemodialysis. Her mother has had a recent stroke. The patient's blood pressure is 170/100 mmHg. Heart examination reveals a midsystolic click and murmur that increases with Valsalva maneuver. Kidneys are palpated bilaterally and are each 20 cm. Which of the following is the most likely diagnosis?

a. Horseshoe kidney
b. Polycystic kidney disease
c. Bilateral hydronephrosis
d. Kidney carcinoma
e. Medullary sponge kidney

7-34. A healthy 25-year-old G1P0 at 40 weeks gestational age comes to your office to see you for a routine OB visit. The patient complains to you that on several occasions she has experienced dizziness, light-headedness, and feeling as if she is going to pass out when she lies down on her back to take a nap. What is the appropriate plan of management for this patient?

a. Do an ECG
b. Monitor her for 24 h with a Holter monitor to rule out an arrhythmia
c. Do an arterial blood gas analysis
d. Refer her immediately to a neurologist
e. Reassure her that nothing is wrong with her and encourage her not to lie flat on her back

7-35. A 9-year-old boy is brought to your clinic by his parents because he has begun to have episodes of eye fluttering lasting several seconds. Sometimes he loses track of his thoughts in the middle of a sentence. There was one fall off a bicycle that may have been related to one of these events. There are no other associated symptoms, and the episodes may occur up to 20 or more times per day. The boy's development and health have been normal up until this point. He did have two head injuries as a young child: the first when he fell off a tricycle onto the ground, and the second when he fell off of a playset onto his head. Both episodes resulted in a brief loss of consciousness and he did not think clearly for part of the day afterward, but had no medical intervention. The test most likely to confirm this patient's diagnosis is

a. Brain CT scan
b. Brain MRI
c. Electroencephalogram
d. Lumbar puncture
e. Nerve conduction study

7-36. A 55-year-old woman who has a history of severe depression and who had radical mastectomy for carcinoma of the breast 1 year previously develops polyuria, nocturia, and excessive thirst. Laboratory values are as follows:

Serum electrolytes: Na^- 149 meq/L; K^- 3.6 meq/L
Serum calcium: 9.5 mg/dL
Blood glucose: 110 mg/dL
Blood urea nitrogen: 30 mg/dL
Urine osmolality: 150 mOsm/kg

The most likely diagnosis is

a. Psychogenic polydipsia
b. Renal glycosuria
c. Hypercalciuria
d. Diabetes insipidus
e. Inappropriate antidiuretic hormone syndrome

7-37. A 10-month-old boy, recently arrived from Guyana, has a 5-h history of crying, with intermittent drawing up of his knees to his chest. On the way to the emergency room he passes a loose, bloody stool. He has had no vomiting and has refused his bottle since the crying began. Physical examination is noteworthy for an irritable infant whose abdomen is very difficult to examine because of constant crying. His temperature is 38.8°C (101.8°F). The rectal ampulla is empty, but there is some gross blood on the examining finger. The most helpful study in the immediate management of this patient would be

a. Stool culture
b. Examination of the stool for ova and parasites
c. An air-contrast enema
d. Examination of the blood smear
e. Coagulation studies

7-38. At age 5, a child is noted to have the loss of ankle jerks. At age 10, limb ataxia develops, followed by a peripheral neuropathy. During adolescence, retinitis pigmentosa develops. Acanthocytosis is present. These are all characteristic of which of the following?

a. Multiple sclerosis (MS)
b. Sickle cell disease
c. Abetalipoproteinemia
d. Progressive multifocal leukoencephalopathy (PML)
e. HIV subacute encephalomyelitis

7-39. You are asked to provide a consult on a 13-year-old boy who wishes to join his high school track team. The patient is asymptomatic but carries a diagnosis of having a functional heart murmur. Heart examination reveals a nonradiating systolic ejection murmur heard best at the left sternal border. The murmur does not increase with Valsalva maneuver, hand grip, or inspiration. Which of the following is the most appropriate next step in management?

a. No further management is necessary
b. Transthoracic echocardiogram
c. Transesophageal echocardiogram
d. Electrocardiogram
e. Holter monitor
f. Stress test

7-40. A 70-year-old intensive care unit patient complains of fever and shaking chills. The patient develops hypotension, and blood cultures are positive for gram-negative bacilli. The patient begins bleeding from venipuncture sites and around his Foley catheter. Laboratory studies are as follows:

Hct: 38%
WBC: 15,000/μL
Platelet count: 40,000/μL (normal 130,000 to 400,000)
Peripheral blood smear: fragmented RBCs
PT: elevated
PTT: elevated
Plasma fibrinogen: 70 mg/dL (normal 200 to 400)

The best course of therapy in this patient is

a. Begin heparin
b. Treat underlying disease
c. Begin plasmapheresis
d. Give vitamin K
e. Begin red blood cell transfusion

7-41. A 55-year-old man comes to the physician with the chief complaint of daytime drowsiness. He states that although he goes to bed at 10 P.M. and doesn't get up until 6 A.M., he is chronically tired and must take naps during the day. He wakes up in the morning with a headache and a dry mouth. His wife states he snores loudly. Which of the following is the most likely diagnosis?

a. Obstructive sleep apnea
b. Narcolepsy
c. Central apnea
d. Recurrent hypersomnia
e. Major depression

7-42. An elderly homeless male is evaluated for anemia. On exam, he has purpura and ecchymoses of the legs. Perifollicular papules and perifollicular hemorrhages are also noted. There is swelling and bleeding of gums around the patient's teeth as well as tenderness around a hematoma of the calf. The most likely diagnosis is

a. Elder abuse
b. Scurvy
c. Pellagra
d. Beriberi

7-43. A 25-year-old woman arrives in the emergency room following an automobile accident. She is acutely dyspneic with a respiratory rate of 60/min. Breath sounds are markedly diminished on the right side. The first step in managing the patient should be to

a. Take a chest x-ray
b. Draw arterial blood for blood gas determination
c. Decompress the right pleural space
d. Perform pericardiocentesis
e. Administer intravenous fluids

7-44. A 59-year-old man has fine, scaly plaques over his abdomen that have been recurrent for 15 years. Several skin biopsies have been nondiagnostic (lymphocytic epidermal infiltrate), and the lesions respond poorly to topical steroids. The rest of the physical examination is remarkable for a small axillary lymph node. Which of the following is the most likely diagnosis?

a. Lichen planus
b. Pityriasis rosea
c. Mycosis fungoides
d. Kaposi's sarcoma
e. Seborrheic keratosis

7-45. A 7-year-old child is brought by her mother for a school physical. His growth parameters show his height to be fiftieth percentile and his weight to be significantly higher than ninety-fifth percentile. His mother complains that he always seems sleepy during the day and that he has started complaining of headaches. His second-grade teacher has commented that he has difficulty staying awake in class. His mother complains that he wakes up the whole house with his snoring at night. The next step in evaluating and managing this condition should be to

a. Try steroids to decrease tonsillar and adenoid hypertrophy
b. Refer to an otolaryngologist for tonsillectomy and adenoidectomy
c. Arrange for continuous positive airway pressure (CPAP) at home
d. Arrange for home oxygen therapy for use at night
e. Arrange for polysomnography

7-46. A healthy 42-year-old G2P1001 presents to labor and delivery at 30 weeks gestation complaining of a small amount of bright red blood per vagina earlier in the day. The bleeding occurred shortly after intercourse. It started off as spotting and then progressed to a light menses. By the time the patient arrived at L and D, the bleeding had completely resolved. The patient denies any regular uterine contractions, but admits to occasional abdominal cramping. She reports the presence of good fetal movements. She denies any complications during the pregnancy. She had a normal screening sonogram at 20 weeks as part of her routine prenatal care. Her obstetrical history is significant for a previous low transverse cesarean section at term for a fetus that was footling breech. She wants to have an elective repeat cesarean section with a tubal ligation for delivery of this baby when she gets to term. What is the appropriate next step in the management of this patient?

a. Send her home, since the bleeding has completely resolved and she is experiencing good fetal movements
b. Perform a sterile digital exam
c. Perform an amniocentesis to rule out infection
d. Perform a sterile speculum exam
e. Perform an ultrasound exam

7-47. A 32-year-old woman is brought to the emergency room after she complained of chest pain. She is noted to be hypervigilant and anxious, with a pulse of 120/min and a BP of 140/97. She has widely dilated pupils. Her toxicology screen is positive. Which of the following drugs is most likely the one found?

a. Cocaine
b. Ritalin
c. Heroin
d. PCP
e. LSD

7-48. A 29-year-old male with HIV, on indinavir, zidovudine, and stavu dine, presents with severe edema and a serum creatinine of 2.0 mg/dL. He has had bone pain for 5 years and takes large amounts of acetominophen with codeine, aspirin, and ibuprofen. He is on prophylactic trimethoprim sulfamethoxazole. Blood pressure is 170/110; urinalysis shows 4+ protein, 5 to 10 RBC, 0 WBC; 24-h urine protein is 6.2 g. What is the most likely cause of his renal disease?

a. Indinavir toxicity
b. Analgesic nephropathy
c. Trimethoprim sulfamethoxazole–induced interstitial nephritis
d. Focal sclerosis

7-49. A 65-year-old man is having a neurological exam because of tingling in his feet. During the course of the examination, it is noticed that pupillary constriction occurs with attempted adduction of the globe. This suggests which of the following?

a. Mesencephalic infarction
b. Pontine glioma
c. Acute glaucoma
d. Iridocyclitis
e. Aberrant third-nerve regeneration

7-50. Two days after admission to the hospital for a myocardial infarction, a 65-year-old man complains of severe, unremitting midabdominal pain. His cardiac index is 1.6. Physical examination is remarkable for an absence of peritoneal irritation or distension despite the patient's persistent complaint of severe pain. Serum lactate is 9 (normal is less than 3). In managing this problem, you should

a. Perform computed tomography
b. Perform mesenteric angiography
c. Perform laparoscopy
d. Perform flexible sigmoidoscopy to assess the distal colon and rectum
e. Defer decision to explore the abdomen until the arterial lactate is greater than 10

BLOCK 8

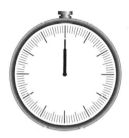

YOU HAVE **60 MINUTES**
TO COMPLETE **50 QUESTIONS.**

Questions

8-1. A 24-year-old primigravid woman, who is intent on breast-feeding, decides on a home delivery. Immediately after the birth of a 4.1-kg (9-lb) infant, the patient bleeds massively from extensive vaginal and cervical lacerations. She is brought to the nearest hospital in shock. Over 2 h, 9 units of blood are transfused, and the patient's blood pressure returns to a reasonable level. A hemoglobin value the next day is 7.5 g/dL, and 3 units of packed red blood cells are given. The most likely late sequela to consider in this woman would be

a. Hemochromatosis
b. Stein-Leventhal syndrome
c. Sheehan syndrome
d. Simmonds syndrome
e. Cushing syndrome

8-2. A 34-year-old black female presents to your office with symptoms of cough, dyspnea, and lymphadenopathy. Physical exam shows cervical adenopathy and hepatomegaly. Her chest radiograph is shown below. How should you pursue diagnosis?

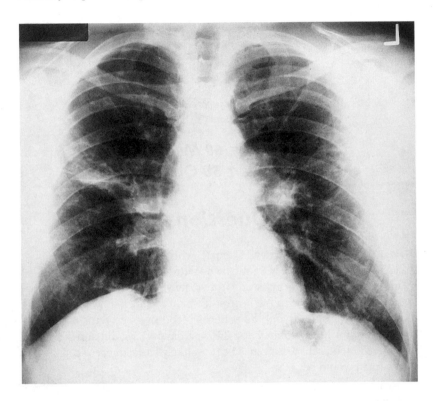

a. Open lung biopsy
b. Liver biopsy
c. Bronchoscopy and transbronchial lung biopsy
d. Scalene node biopsy
e. Serum angiotensin converting enzyme (ACE) level

8-3. A 30-year-old paraplegic male has a long history of urinary tract infection secondary to an indwelling Foley catheter. He develops fever and hypotension requiring hospitalization, fluid therapy, and intravenous antibiotics. He improves, but over 1 week becomes increasingly short of breath and tachypneic. He develops frothy sputum, diffuse rales, and diffuse alveolar infiltrates. There is no fever, jugular venous distention, S$_3$ gallop, or peripheral or sacral edema. The best approach to a definitive diagnosis in this patient is

a. Blood cultures
b. CT scan of the chest
c. Pulmonary capillary wedge pressure
d. Ventilation-perfusion scan

8-4. A 56-year-old man undergoes a left upper lobectomy. An epidural catheter is inserted for postoperative pain relief. Ninety minutes after the first dose of epidural morphine, the patient complains of itching and becomes increasingly somnolent. Blood gas measurement reveals the following: pH 7.24; Paco$_2$ 58; Pao$_2$ 100; HCO$_3^-$ 28. Initial therapy should include

a. Endotracheal intubation
b. Intramuscular diphenhydramine (Benadryl)
c. Epidural naloxone
d. Intravenous naloxone
e. Alternative analgesia

8-5. A demanding 25-year-old woman begins psychotherapy stating she is both desperate and bored. She reports that for the past 5 or 6 years she has experienced periodic anxiety and depression and has made several suicidal gestures. She also reports a variety of impulsive and self-defeating behaviors and sexual promiscuity. She wonders if she might be a lesbian, though most of her sexual experiences have been with men. She has abruptly terminated two previous attempts at psychotherapy. In both cases she was enraged at the therapist because he was unwilling to prescribe anxiolytic medications. Which of the following is the most likely diagnosis?

a. Dysthymia
b. Histrionic personality disorder
c. Antisocial personality disorder
d. Borderline personality disorder
e. Impulse control disorder not otherwise specified

8-6. A 48-year-old male has been unable to have intercourse with his wife of 20 years since she disclosed to him that she was having an affair with his younger and more attractive work partner. He continues having spontaneous nocturnal erections. This patient's sexual dysfunction is most likely due to which of the following?

a. An organic disorder
b. A psychogenic determinant
c. A form of paraphilia
d. An irreversible psychodynamic process
e. A sexual identity disorder

8-7. A 60-year-old right-handed man underwent heart transplantation 2 weeks ago for severe ischemic cardiomyopathy. He had an uneventful postoperative course and went home after 1 week. He is now readmitted from an outside hospital where he was admitted with headaches, increasing confusion, and a generalized seizure. He relates that he has had difficulty seeing for several days. On exam, he has a blood pressure of 180/100. His pupils are equal and reactive, but he has difficulty reading and finding objects presented to him. Motor and sensory function are normal. An MRI shows several areas of T2 signal abnormality in the occipital and parietal lobe white matter bilaterally. A diffusion-weighted MRI sequence, sensitive to the changes of acute infarction, is negative. This patient's history, exam, and laboratory findings are most consistent with which of the following diagnoses?

a. Cyclosporine toxicity
b. Steroid psychosis
c. Occipital lobe infarction
d. Ischemic optic neuropathies
e. Retinal detachment

8-8. A 13-year-old boy has a 3-day history of low-grade fever, upper respiratory symptoms, and a sore throat. A few hours before his presentation to the emergency room, he has an abrupt onset of high fever, difficulty swallowing, and poor handling of his secretions. He indicates that he has a marked worsening in the severity of his sore throat. His pharynx has a fluctuant bulge in the posterior wall. Appropriate initial therapy for this patient would be

a. Narcotic analgesics
b. Trial of oral penicillin V
c. Surgical consultation for incision and drainage under general anesthesia
d. Rapid streptococcal screen
e. Monospot test

8-9. Shortly after the administration of an inhalational anesthetic and succinylcholine for intubation prior to an elective inguinal hernia repair in a 10-year-old boy, he becomes markedly febrile and displays a tachycardia of 160, and his urine changes color to a dark red. The correct approach should be

a. Complete the procedure but pretreat with dantrolene prior to future elective surgery
b. Administer inhalational anesthetic agents
c. Administer succinylcholine
d. Hyperventilate with 100% oxygen
e. Acidify the urine to prevent myoglobin precipitation in the renal tubules

8-10. A 7-year-old girl acutely develops double vision that worsens over the course of a few days. Examination reveals a sixth-nerve (abducens) palsy. She is most likely to have which of the following?

a. Pontine glioma
b. Medullary glioma
c. Mesencephalic infarction
d. Pontine infarction
e. Medullary infarction

8-11. On Monday morning, a septuagenarian man has a moderate-sized abdominal aneurysm resected. On Friday, he is noted to be markedly distended, with an abdominal radiograph on which the cecum is measured as 12 cm across. Proper management at this time would be

a. Decompression of the large bowel via colonoscopy
b. Replacement of the nasogastric tube and administration of low-dose cholinergic drugs
c. Continued nothing-by-mouth orders, administration of a gentle saline enema, and encouragement of ambulation
d. Immediate return to the operating room for operative decompression by transverse colostomy
e. Right hemicolectomy

8-12. A 24-year-old G0 presents to your office complaining of vulvar discomfort. More specifically, she has been experiencing intense burning and pain with intercourse. The discomfort occurs at the vaginal introitus primarily with penile insertion into the vagina. The patient also experiences the same pain with tampon insertion and when the speculum is inserted during a gynecologic exam. The problem has become so bad that she can no longer have sex, which is causing problems in her marriage. She is otherwise healthy and denies any medical problems. She is experiencing regular menses and denies any dysmenorrhea. On physical exam, the region of the vulva around the opening of the vagina appears erythematous and inflamed and is tender to touch with a cotton swab. What is the most likely diagnosis?

a. Vulvar vestibulitis
b. Atrophic vaginitis
c. Contact dermatitis
d. Lichen sclerosus
e. Vulvar intraepithelial neoplasia

8-13. A 22-year-old man sustains a gunshot wound to the abdomen. At exploration, an apparently solitary distal small-bowel injury is treated with resection and primary anastomosis. On postoperative day 7, small-bowel fluid drains through the operative incision. The fascia remains intact. The fistula output is 300 mL/day and there is no evidence of intraabdominal sepsis. Correct treatment includes

a. Early reoperation to close the fistula tract
b. Broad-spectrum antibiotics
c. Total parenteral nutrition
d. Somatostatin to lower fistula output
e. Loperamide to inhibit gut motility

8-14. A 43-year-old man is admitted to the neurology service after he went blind suddenly the morning of admission. The patient does not seem overly concerned with his sudden lack of vision. The only time he gets upset during the interview is when discussing his mother's recent death in Mexico— he was to bring his mother to the USA, but did not because he had been using drugs and did not save the needed money. Physical exam is completely negative. Which of the following diagnoses is most likely?

a. Conversion disorder
b. Hypochondriasis
c. Factitious disorder
d. Malingering
e. Delusional disorder

8-15. A 56-year-old woman who was diagnosed with paranoid schizophrenia in her early twenties has received daily doses of various typical neuroleptics for many years. For the past 2 years, she has had symptoms of tardive dyskinesia. Discontinuation of the neuroleptic is not possible because she becomes aggressive and violent in response to command hallucinations when she is not medicated. Which of the following actions should be taken next?

a. Start the patient on benztropine
b. Start the patient on amantadine
c. Start the patient on propranolol
d. Start the patient on diphenhydramine
e. Switch the patient to clozapine

8-16. A 4-year-old boy presents with a history of constipation since the age of 6 months. His stools, produced every 3 to 4 days, are described as large and hard. Physical examination is normal; rectal examination reveals a large ampulla, poor sphincter tone, and stool in the rectal vault. The plain film of his abdomen is shown. The next step in the management of this child should be

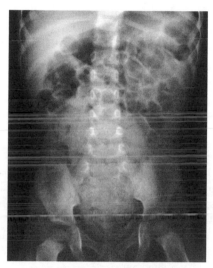

(Courtesy Susan John, M.D.)

a. Lower GI barium study
b. Parental reassurance and dietary counseling
c. Serum electrolyte measurement
d. Upper GI barium study
e. Initiation of synthroid

8-17. A woman with a history of left mastectomy and subsequent radiation therapy for breast cancer 2 years ago presents with a 3-cm mass along the edge of the surgical suture line. She denies fever, chills, night sweats, and weight loss. Physical examination reveals some generalized induration and a tanned appearance of the skin overlying the mastectomy secondary to radiation therapy. There is a nonmobile nontender mass along the suture line that is not warm or fluctuant. She has no axillary lymphadenopathy. A biopsy specimen of the breast mass is most likely to show which of the following?

a. Fibroadenoma
b. Malignancy
c. Benign cyst
d. Abscess
e. Lipoma

8-18. A 56-year-old woman complains of a 10-lb weight loss over a 2-month period. She has generalized malaise and anorexia. She does not smoke cigarettes or drink alcohol. She has no past medical history and takes no medications. Three years ago, her colonoscopy, mammogram, and Papanicolaou smear were negative. Physical examination reveals a temperature of 100.4°F. Heart, lung, and abdominal examinations are normal. A 2-cm fixed hard nontender node is palpable in the right supraclavicular area. Which of the following is the most appropriate next step?

a. Chest radiograph
b. Colonoscopy
c. Mammography
d. CT scan of the chest
e. Papanicolaou smear

8-19. A 30-year-old male complains of leg weakness and paresthesias of the arm and leg. Five years previously he had an episode of transient visual loss. On physical exam, there is hyperreflexia, bilateral Babinski signs, and cerebellar dysmetria with poor finger-to-nose movement. When the patient is asked to look to the right, the left eye does not move normally past the midline. Nystagmus is noted in the abducting eye. A more detailed history suggests the patient has had several episodes of gait difficulty that have resolved spontaneously. He appears to be stable between these episodes. He has no systemic symptoms of fever or weight loss. The most likely diagnosis in this patient is

a. Multiple sclerosis
b. Vitamin B_{12} deficiency
c. Systemic lupus erythematosus
d. Hypochondriasis

8-20. After several years of successful anti-Parkinsonian treatment, a patient abruptly develops acute episodes of profound bradykinesia and rigidity. Remission of these signs occurs as abruptly as the onset. This patient probably suffers from

a. Acute dystonia
b. Absence attacks
c. On-off phenomenon
d. Complex partial seizures
e. Drug toxicity

8-21. A 47-year-old woman is brought to the emergency room after she jumped off an overpass and broke both her legs. In the emergency room she states that she wanted to kill herself because the devil had been tormenting her for many years. She becomes fearful in the emergency room as well, thinking that the devil has possessed the nursing staff working there. After stabilization of her fractures, she is admitted to the psychiatric unit, where she is treated with risperidone and sertraline. After 2 weeks she is no longer suicidal and her mood is euthymic. However, she still believes that the devil is recruiting people to try to persecute her. The patient has had 3 similar episodes prior to this one in the past 10 years. During each of these three episodes, she has been suicidal and anhedonic and has had low energy levels. During these times she also has early morning awakening, is unable to concentrate, and loses 5 to 10 lb because she has no appetite. She has never stopped believing that the devil is persecuting her during all this time. Which of the following is the most appropriate diagnosis for this patient?

a. Delusional disorder
b. Schizoaffective disorder
c. Schizophrenia, paranoid type
d. Schizophreniform disorder
e. Major depression with psychotic features

8-22. A 90-year-old G5P5 with multiple medical problems is brought into your gynecology clinic accompanied by her granddaughter. The patient has hypertension, chronic anemia, coronary artery disease, and osteoporosis. She is mentally alert and oriented and lives in an assisted living facility. She takes numerous medications, but is very functional at the current time. She is a widow and not sexually active. Her chief complaint is a sensation of heaviness and pressure in the vagina. She denies any significant urinary or bowel problems. On performance of a physical exam, you note that the cervix is at the level of the introitus. Based on the physical exam, what is the most likely diagnosis?

a. Normal exam
b. First-degree uterine prolapse
c. Second-degree uterine prolapse
d. Third-degree uterine prolapse
e. Complete procidentia

8-23. A 55-year-old man with recent onset of atrial fibrillation presents with a cold, pulseless left lower extremity. He complains of left leg paresthesia and is unable to dorsiflex his toes. Following a successful popliteal embolectomy, with restoration of palpable pedal pulses, the patient is still unable to dorsiflex his toes. The next step in management should be

a. Electromyography (EMG)
b. Measurement of anterior compartment pressure
c. Elevation of the left leg
d. Immediate fasciotomy
e. Application of a posterior splint

8-24. A 22-year-old woman presents to the emergency room with an episode of acute painful loss of vision in the right eye. On examination, there is right afferent pupillary defect and papillitis on funduscopic examination. She has no history of neurologic symptoms. An MRI shows a few foci of T2 signal increase in a periventricular distribution. Appropriate treatment for presumed optic neuritis in this patient would be

a. Oral prednisone
b. Intravenous methylprednisolone
c. Cyclophosphamide
d. Plasma exchange
e. Intravenous gamma globulin

8-25. At birth, an infant is noted to have an abnormal neurologic examination. Over the next few weeks he develops severe progressive central nervous system degeneration, an enlarged liver and spleen, macroglossia, coarse facial features, and a cherry red spot in the eye. The laboratory finding likely to explain this child's problem is

a. Reduced serum hexosaminidase A activity
b. Deficient activity of acid beta-galactosidase
c. A defective gene on the X chromosome
d. Complete lack of acid beta-galactosidase activity
e. Deficient activity of galactosyl-3-sulfate-ceramide sulfatase (cerebroside sulfatase)

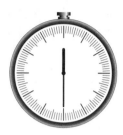

YOU SHOULD HAVE COMPLETED APPROXIMATELY
25 QUESTIONS AND HAVE 30 MINUTES REMAINING.

8-26. An intrauterine pregnancy of approximately 10 weeks gestation is confirmed in a 30-year-old gravida 5, para 4 woman with an IUD in place. The patient expresses a strong desire for the pregnancy to be continued. On examination, the string of the IUD is noted to be protruding from the cervical os. The most appropriate course of action is to

a. Leave the IUD in place without any other treatment
b. Leave the IUD in place and continue prophylactic antibiotics throughout pregnancy
c. Remove the IUD immediately
d. Terminate the pregnancy because of the high risk of infection
e. Perform a laparoscopy to rule out a heterotopic ectopic pregnancy

8-27. A 75-year-old man with a history of recent memory impairment is admitted with headache, confusion, and a left homonymous hemianopsia. He has recently had two episodes of brief unresponsiveness. There is no history of hypertension. Computed tomography (CT) scan shows a right occipital lobe hemorrhage with some subarachnoid extension of the blood. An MRI scan with gradient echo sequences reveals foci of hemosiderin in the right temporal and left frontal cortex. The likely cause of this patient's symptoms and signs is

a. Gliomatosis cerebri
b. Multi-infarct dementia
c. Mycotic aneurysm
d. Amyloid angiopathy
e. Undiagnosed hypertension

8-28. A 48-year-old woman develops pain in the right lower quadrant while playing tennis. The pain progresses and the patient presents to the emergency room later that day with a low-grade fever, a white blood count of 13,000, and complaints of anorexia and nausea as well as persistent, sharp pain of the right lower quadrant. On examination, she is tender in the right lower quadrant with muscular spasm and there is a suggestion of a mass effect. An ultrasound is ordered and shows an apparent mass in the abdominal wall. Which of the following is the most likely diagnosis?

a. Acute appendicitis
b. Cecal carcinoma
c. Hematoma of the rectus sheath
d. Torsion of an ovarian cyst
e. Cholecystitis

8-29. A 32-year-old woman undergoes a cholecystectomy for acute cholecystitis and is discharged home on the sixth postoperative day. She returns
to the clinic 8 months after the operation for a routine visit and is noted by
the surgeon to be jaundiced. Laboratory values on readmission show total
bilirubin 5.6 mg/dL; direct bilirubin 4.8 mg/dL; alkaline phosphatase 250
IU (normal 21 to 91 IU); SGOT 52 kU (normal 10 to 40 kU); SGPT 51 kU
(normal 10 to 40 kU). An ultrasonogram shows dilated intrahepatic ducts.
The patient undergoes the transhepatic cholangiogram seen below. Appropriate management is

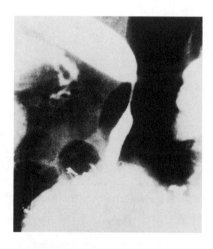

a. Choledochoplasty with insertion of a T tube
b. End-to-end choledochocholedochal anastomosis
c. Roux-en-Y choledochojejunostomy
d. Percutaneous transhepatic dilatation
e. Choledochoduodenostomy

8-30. A 75-year-old patient presents to the ER after a sudden syncopal episode. He is again alert and in retrospect describes occasional substernal chest pressure and shortness of breath on exertion. His lungs have a few bibasilar rales, and his blood pressure is 110/80. On cardiac auscultation, the classic finding you expect to hear is

a. A harsh systolic crescendo-decrescendo murmur heard best at the upper right sternal border
b. A diastolic decrescendo murmur heard at the mid-left sternal border
c. A holosystolic murmur heard best at the apex
d. A midsystolic click

8-31. A 26-year-old graduate student presents to the emergency room with a severe left-sided throbbing headache associated with nausea, vomiting, and photophobia. She has tried taking ibuprofen without relief. On further questioning, she relates that she has been having similar headaches three to four times per month for the past year. Her mother had a similar problem. Her exam is normal. Appropriate therapy for this patient's present headache might include which of the following drugs?

a. Ergotamine tartrate
b. Nitroglycerine
c. Verapamil
d. Amitriptyline hydrochloride
e. Phenobarbital

8-32. For the past 10 years, the memory of a 74-year-old woman has progressively declined. Lately, she has caused several small kitchen fires by forgetting to turn off the stove, she cannot remember how to cook her favorite recipes, and she becomes disoriented and confused at night. She identifies an increasing number of objects as "that thing" because she cannot recall the correct name. Her muscle strength and balance are intact. Which of the following is the most likely diagnosis?

a. Huntington's disease
b. Multi-infarct dementia
c. Creutzfeldt-Jakob disease
d. Alzheimer's disease
e. Wilson's disease

8-33. A 57-year-old woman is involved in a motor vehicle accident in which she strikes the windshield and is briefly unconscious. She makes a full recovery, except that 3 months later she complains she cannot taste the food she is eating. Her complaint is most likely due to

a. Medullary infarction
b. Temporal lobe contusion
c. Sphenoid sinus hemorrhage
d. Phenytoin use to prevent seizures
e. Avulsion of olfactory rootlets

8-34. A 62-year-old man presents for his annual health maintenance visit. The review of systems is positive for occasional fatigue and headache. The patient admits to generalized pruritus following a warm bath or shower. He has plethora and engorgement of the retinal veins. A spleen is palpated on abdominal examination. The patient's hematocrit is 63%, and he has a leukocytosis and thrombocytosis. Peripheral blood smear is normal. The patient does not smoke. Which of the following is the most likely diagnosis?

a. Spurious polycythemia
b. Essential thrombocytosis
c. Myelofibrosis
d. Polycythemia vera
e. Secondary polycythemia
f. Chronic myeloid leukemia
g. Erythropoietin-secreting renal tumor

8-35. Every morning on school days, an 8-year-old girl becomes tearful and distressed and claims she feels sick. Once in school, she often goes to the nurse, complaining of headaches and stomach pains. At least once a week, she misses school or is picked up early by her mother due to her complaints. Her pediatrician has ruled out organic causes for the physical symptoms. The child is usually symptom free on weekends, unless her parents go out and leave her with a baby sitter. Which of the following is the most likely diagnosis?

a. Separation anxiety disorder
b. Major depression
c. Somatization disorder
d. Generalized anxiety disorder
e. Attachment disorder

8-36. You are awakened in the night by your 2-year-old son, who has developed noisy breathing on inspiration, marked retractions of the chest wall, flaring of the nostrils, and a barking cough. He has had a mild upper respiratory infection (URI) for 2 days. The most likely diagnosis is

a. Asthma
b. Epiglottitis
c. Bronchiolitis
d. Viral croup
e. Foreign body in the right mainstem bronchus

8-37. A 2-year-old girl is playing in the garage, only partially supervised by her father, who is mowing the grass. He finds her in the garage, gagging and vomiting. She smells of gasoline. In a few minutes she stops vomiting, but later that day she develops cough, tachypnea, and subcostal retractions. She is brought to your emergency center. The first step in her management is to

a. Administer charcoal
b. Begin nasogastric lavage
c. Administer ipecac
d. Perform pulse oximetry and arterial blood gas
e. Administer gasoline binding agent intravenously

8-38. A 40-year-old alcoholic male is being treated for tuberculosis, but he has not been compliant with his medications. He complains of increasing weakness and fatigue. He appears to have lost weight, and his blood pressure is 80/50 mmHg. There is increased pigmentation over the elbows. Cardiac exam is normal. The next step in evaluation should be

a. CBC with iron and iron-binding capacity
b. Erythrocyte sedimentation rate
c. Early morning serum cortisol and cosyntropin stimulation
d. Blood cultures

8-39. A 56-year-old woman has been treated for 3 years for wheezing on exertion, which was diagnosed as asthma. Chest radiograph, shown below, reveals a midline mass compressing the trachea. The most likely diagnosis is

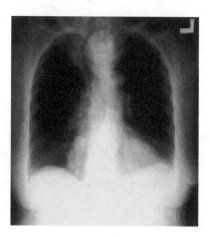

a. Lymphoma
b. Neurogenic tumor
c. Lung carcinoma
d. Goiter
e. Pericardial cyst

8-40. A 66-year-old man presents with a scanty cough and pleuritic chest pain. He also complains of fever and watery diarrhea. He smokes one pack of cigarettes per day and lives in an apartment building that is undergoing renovation. He has no past medical history and takes no medications. Physical examination reveals a toxic-appearing man with a temperature of 103.2°F. His heart rate is 60/min. Chest auscultation reveals bilateral scattered crackles. Abdominal examination reveals diffuse tenderness. Laboratory results reveal hyponatremia, hypophosphatemia, elevated liver function tests, and thrombocytopenia. A chest radiograph reveals bilateral infiltrates. Which of the following is the most likely diagnosis in this patient?

a. Pontiac fever
b. Legionnaires' disease
c. Influenza
d. Tuberculosis
e. Psittacosis

8-41. A 74-year-old man presents with the abrupt onset of pain in the left lower abdomen, which has been progressively worsening over the last 2 days. He states that the pain is unremitting. He has some diarrhea but no nausea or vomiting. He has no dysuria or hematuria. His temperature is 102°F. Bowel sounds are decreased. The patient has involuntary guarding. There is tenderness and rebound tenderness when the left lower quadrant is palpated. The referred rebound test is positive. A fixed sausage-like mass is palpable in the area of tenderness. There is no costovertebral angle (CVA) tenderness. Rectal examination reveals brown stool, which is fecal occult blood test (FOBT) positive. Bloodwork demonstrates a leukocytosis. Which of the following is the most likely diagnosis?

a. Colon cancer
b. Diverticulitis
c. Pancreatitis
d. Pyelonephritis
e. Appendicitis

8-42. An 18-year-old consults you for evaluation of disabling pain with her menstrual periods. The pain has been present since menarche and is accompanied by nausea and headache. History is otherwise unremarkable, and pelvic examination is normal. You diagnose primary dysmenorrhea and recommend initial treatment with which of the following?

a. Ergot derivatives
b. Antiprostaglandins
c. Gonadotropin-releasing hormone (GnRH) analogues
d. Danazol
e. Codeine

8-43. For the past 3 months, a 15-year-old girl has had to turn her light on and off 23 times at exactly 10:30 P.M. before she can go to bed. She can spend from 1 to 2 h on this ritual because she has to start again if she is interrupted or loses count. She is upset if the position of the order of the objects she has on her desk is changed even slightly and cannot stop worrying about her family's safety. In conjunction with pharmacologic treatment, which therapy has been proven effective for this disorder?

a. Play therapy
b. Psychodynamic psychotherapy
c. Group therapy
d. Cognitive-behavioral therapy
e. Family therapy

8-44. A 31-year-old homosexual man has had headache, sleepiness, and poor balance that have worsened over the past week. The patient is known to be HIV-seropositive, but has done well in the past and has not seen a doctor in over 1 year. On examination, his responses are slow and he has some difficulty sustaining attention. He has a right hemiparesis with increased reflexes on the right. Routine cell counts and chemistries are normal. Of the following, which is the most appropriate thing to do next?

a. Get a head CT with contrast
b. Get a noncontrast head CT
c. Perform a lumbar puncture
d. Start antiretroviral therapy
e. Start intravenous heparin

8-45. A 69-year-old man is brought to see his physician by his wife. She notes that over the past year he has had a slow stepwise decline in his cognitive functioning. One year ago she felt his thinking was "as good as it always was," but now he gets lost around the house and can't remember simple directions. The patient states he feels fine, though he is depressed about his loss of memory. He is eating and sleeping well. Which of the following diagnoses is most likely?

a. Multi-infarct dementia
b. Mood disorder secondary to a general medical condition
c. Schizoaffective disorder
d. Delirium
e. Major depression

8-46. A 55-year-old man complains of chronic intermittent epigastric pain, and gastroscopy demonstrates a 2-cm ulcer of the distal lesser curvature. Endoscopic biopsy yields no malignant tissue. After a 6-week trial of H_2 blockade and antacid therapy, the ulcer is unchanged. Proper therapy at this point is

a. Repeat trial of medical therapy
b. Local excision of the ulcer
c. Billroth I partial gastrectomy
d. Billroth I partial gastrectomy with vagotomy
e. Vagotomy and pyloroplasty

8-47. A 22-year-old woman consults you for treatment of hirsutism. She is obese and has facial acne and hirsutism on her face and periareolar regions and a male escutcheon. Serum LH level is 35 mIU/mL and FSH is 9 mIU/mL. Androstenedione and testosterone levels are mildly elevated, but serum DHAS is normal. The patient does not wish to conceive at this time. Which of the following single agents is the most appropriate treatment of her condition?

a. Oral contraceptives
b. Corticosteroids
c. GnRH
d. Parlodel
e. Wedge resection

8-48. A 61-year-old man, who smokes five packs of cigarettes per day and has hypertension, had an abdominal aortic aneurysm repair 8 h ago. The surgery went very well, and there were no reported perioperative complications. Now the patient is unable to move his legs and states that they are "numb." On examination, he has a flaccid paresis of both lower extremities and has impaired pinprick sensation to a T9 level bilaterally. Joint proprioception is normal. The most likely diagnosis in this case is

a. Cerebral stroke
b. Conversion disorder
c. Multiple sclerosis
d. Spinal cord compression
e. Spinal cord infarct

8-49. A term, 4200-g female infant is delivered via cesarean section because of cephalopelvic disproportion. The amniotic fluid was clear, and the infant cried almost immediately after birth. Within the first 15 min of life, however, the infant's respiratory rate increased to 80 breaths per min, and she began to have intermittent grunting respirations. The infant was transferred to the level 2 nursery and was noted to have an oxygen saturation of 94%. The chest radiograph showed fluid in the fissure, overaeration, and prominent pulmonary vascular markings. The most likely diagnosis in this infant is

a. Diaphragmatic hernia
b. Meconium aspiration
c. Pneumonia
d. Idiopathic respiratory distress syndrome
e. Transient tachypnea of the newborn

8-50. A 70-year-old woman complains of insomnia and feeling sad. Her husband died 2 months ago, and she has had these symptoms since the funeral. She feels guilty that she did not care for her husband well enough. She has recently moved to a smaller apartment. She denies weight loss or functional impairment. On occasion, she has thought she heard her husband's voice. The best approach to management is

a. Hospitalization and suicide precautions
b. Antipsychotic medication
c. Bereavement support for at least 1 year
d. Treatment for major depression

BLOCK I

Answers

1-1. The answer is d. *(Tierney, 42/e, pp 1357–1358.)* The postal worker from New Jersey is presenting with symptoms most consistent with **inhalation anthrax.** Sentinel clues include chest pain, shortness of breath, malaise, headache, fever, dry cough, abdominal pain, and nausea. Chest radiograph may show a widened mediastinum (mediastinitis) and pleural effusions (thoracentesis will show these to be hemorrhagic). This presentation rapidly leads to sepsis, shock, and respiratory failure. Although anthrax was previously rare except among high-risk groups such as farmers, tannery workers, wool workers, and veterinarians, bioterroristic use has resulted in cases. Patients with **pneumonic plague** present with mucopurulent sputum, chest pain, and hemoptysis. **Tularemia** is a gram-negative coccobacillus that causes pneumonia accompanied by bilateral hilar adenopathy. Patients with **hemorrhagic fever** present with generalized mucous membrane hemorrhage and evidence of pulmonary, renal, neurologic, and hematopoietic dysfunction. **Hantavirus** is a rodent-borne RNA virus more common in the Southwestern United States; patients present in a shocklike state with thrombocytopenia and leukocytosis.

1-2. The answer is e. *(Kaplan, 8/e, p 94.)* The frontal lobes are associated with the regulation of emotions, the manifestation of behavioral traits usually connected to the personality of an individual, and executive functions (the ability to make appropriate judgments and decisions and to form concepts). They also contain the inhibitory systems for behaviors such as bladder and bowel release. Damage of the frontal lobes causes impairment of these functions but it is not, strictly speaking, a form of dementia, because memory, language, calculation ability, praxis, and IQ are often preserved. Personality changes, disinhibited behavior, and poor judgment are usually seen with lesions of the dorsolateral regions of the frontal lobes. Lesions of the mesial region, which is involved in the regulation of the initiation of movements and emotional responses, cause slowing of motor functions, speech, and emotional reactions. In the most severe cases, patients are mute and akinetic. Lesions of the orbitofrontal area are accompanied by abnormal social behaviors, an excessively good opinion of oneself, jocularity, sexual disinhibition, and lack of concern for others.

1-3. The answer is c. (*Sabiston, 15/e, pp 81–84.*) A ruptured abdominal aneurysm is a surgical emergency often accompanied by serious hypotension and vascular collapse before surgery and massive fluid shifts with renal failure after surgery. In this case, all the hemodynamic parameters indicate inadequate intravascular volume, and the patient is therefore suffering from hypovolemic hypotension. The low urine output indicates poor renal perfusion, while the high urine specific gravity indicates adequate renal function with compensatory free water conservation. The administration of a vasopressor agent would certainly raise the blood pressure, but it would do so by increasing peripheral vascular resistance and thereby further decrease tissue perfusion. The deleterious effects of shock would be increased. A vasodilating agent to lower the systemic vascular resistance would lead to profound hypotension and possibly complete vascular collapse because of pooling of an already depleted vascular volume. This patient's blood pressure is critically dependent on an elevated systemic vascular resistance. To properly treat this patient, rapid fluid infusion and expansion of the intravascular volume must be undertaken. This can be easily done with lactated Ringer's solution or blood (or both) until improvements in such parameters as the pulmonary capillary wedge pressure, urine output, and blood pressure are noted.

1-4. The answer is b. (*Osborn, pp 593–594.*) Calcified masses appear hyperdense without contrast enhancement, whereas highly vascular lesions may appear dense on CT scanning after the patient has received intravenous contrast material. Tumors, granulomas, and other intracranial lesions enhance because of a breakdown in the blood-brain barrier. More cystic lesions may exhibit enhancement limited to the periphery of the cyst.

1-5. The answer is d. (*Cunningham, 21/e, pp 958–960, 977–978.*) The incidence of neural tube defects in the general population is approximately 1.4 to 2.0/1000. It is a multifactorial defect and is not influenced by maternal age. Women who have a previously affected child have a neural tube defect recurrence risk of about 3 to 4%. This patient is at increased risk of having another child with a neural tube defect and therefore should be offered prenatal diagnosis with an amniocentesis and targeted ultrasound. A chorionic villus sampling will determine a fetus's chromosomal makeup but will give no information regarding AFP levels or risk for a neural tube defect. Hyperthermia at the time of neural tube formation in the embryo, as can occur with maternal fever or sauna baths, can increase the relative risk of a neural tube defect up to sixfold.

1-6. The answer is d. (*Cunningham, 21/e, pp 181–182, 185–186, 1236–1237.*) The patient's symptoms and physical exam are most consistent with the physiologic dyspnea, which is common in pregnancy. The increased awareness of breathing that pregnant women experience, which can occur as early as the end of the first trimester, is due to an increase in lung tidal volume. The increase in minute ventilation that occurs during pregnancy may make patients feel as if they are hyperventilating and may also contribute to the feeling of dyspnea. The patient in this case needs to be reassured and counseled regarding these normal changes of pregnancy. She needs to understand that she may have to modify her exercise regimen accordingly. There is no need to refer this patient to a cardiologist or order an ECG. Systolic ejection murmurs are common findings in pregnant women and are due to a normal increased blood flow across the aortic and pulmonic valves. The incidence of pulmonary embolism in pregnancy is about 1 in 6400. In many of these cases there is clinical evidence of a DVT. The most common symptoms of a PE are dyspnea, chest pain, apprehension, cough, hemoptysis, and tachycardia. On physical exam, there may be an accentuated pulmonic closure sound, rales, or a friction rub. A strong suspicion for a PE should be followed up with a ventilation-perfusion scan. Large perfusion defects and ventilation mismatches would suggest the presence of a PE.

1-7. The answer is e. (*Greenfield, 2/e, p 1970.*) The significant observation in this question is the description of lymphangitic inflammatory streaking up the inner aspect of the patient's leg. This is highly suggestive of a streptococcal infection, and the presumptive therapy should be high doses of a bactericidal antibiotic. Penicillin remains the mainstay of therapy against presumed streptococcal infections. Most streptococcal cellulitis is adequately treated by penicillin, elevation of the infected extremity, and attention to the local wound to ascertain adequate local drainage and absence of any persisting foreign body. However, the clinician must be alert to the possibility of a more fulminant and life- or limb-threatening infection by clostridia, microaerophilic streptococci, or other potentially synergistic organisms that can produce rapidly progressive deep infections in fascia of muscle. Smears and cultures of drainage fluid or aspirates should be taken. Close observation of the wound is essential, and aggressive debridement in the operating room is mandatory at the slightest suggestion that fasciitis or myonecrosis may be ensuing.

1-8. The answer is c. *(Braunwald, 15/e, pp 834–838, 1227–1228.)* The bacterial pathogens listed usually cause acute diarrhea, sometimes bloody. They usually respond to fluoroquinolones, although some resistance is emerging, particularly with regard to *Campylobacter. Giardia* gives a more subacute to chronic picture as described in this patient. It responds to metronidazole therapy. *Cryptosporidium* is less common and occurs in immunocompromised patients.

1-9. The answer is d. *(Ebert, pp 378, 383.)* Factitious disorder usually presents with physical or mental symptoms that are induced by the patient to meet the psychological need to be taken care of (primary gain). These patients will often mutilate themselves repeatedly in a frantic effort to be cared for by the hospital system. Moving between hospitals so that they don't get caught is frequent, especially when the patient is directly confronted. Malingering is similar to factitious disorder in that symptoms are faked, but the reason in malingering is for some secondary gain, such as getting out of jail. Somatization disorder is characterized by the recurrent physical complaints that are not explained by physical factors and that cause significant impairment or result in seeking medical attention. Pain of any part of the body and dysfunctions of multiple systems are typical. The *DSM-IV* diagnostic criteria for somatization disorder include at least four pain symptoms, one sexual symptom, and one pseudoneurological symptom. These symptoms can be present at any time in the duration of the disorder. Somatization disorder usually emerges in adolescence or early twenties and follows a chronic course. Somatization disorder is diagnosed predominantly in women, with a prevalence of 0.2 to 0.5%, and rarely in men. Body dysmorphic disorder is characterized by distorted beliefs about the patient's own appearance, often with delusional qualities. Borderline personality disorder patients may mutilate themselves, but the object is generally attention getting or stress relief.

1-10. The answer is e. *(Victor, pp 890–892.)* The clinical picture suggests that a saccular aneurysm has become symptomatic by compressing structures about the base of the brain and subsequently leaking. Aneurysms enlarge with age and usually do not bleed until they are several millimeters across. Persons with intracerebral or subarachnoid hemorrhages before the age of 40 are more likely to have their hemorrhages because of arteriovenous malformations than because of aneurysms. Aneurysms occur with equal frequency in men and women below the age of 40; however, in their forties and fifties, women are more susceptible to symptomatic aneurysms. This is especially true of aneurysms that develop on the internal carotid on that segment of the artery that lies within the cavernous sinus. An angiogram is useful in establishing the site and character of the aneurysm. A CT scan would be more likely to reveal subarachnoid, intraventricular, or intraparenchymal blood, but it would reveal the structure of an aneurysm only if it were several (>5) millimeters across. An MRI will reveal relatively large aneurysms if the system is calibrated and programmed to look at blood vessels. This patient had a transfemoral angiogram, a technique that involves the introduction of a catheter into the femoral artery; the catheter is threaded retrograde in the aorta and up into the carotid or other arteries of interest.

1-11. The answer is c. *(Braunwald, 15/e, pp 1267–1269.)* The ECG shows ST segment elevation in inferior leads II, III, and a VF with reciprocal ST depression in a VL, which is highly consistent with an acute inferior MI. An anterior MI would produce ST segment elevation in the precordial leads. Pericarditis classically produces pleuritic chest pain and diffuse ST segment elevation (except aVR) on ECG. Costochondritis, esophageal reflux, cholecystitis, and duodenal ulcer disease can all cause the symptoms of substernal chest pain, but not these ECG findings.

1-12. The answer is d. *(Kaplan, 8/e, p 1033.)* Tardive dyskinesia often improves when the dosage of neuroleptic is decreased or stopped. When these interventions are not effective or are not possible due to the severity of the patient's disorder, olanzapine is the treatment of choice. All the other medications listed are typical antipsychotics, which have just as high a risk for TD as haloperidol.

1-13. The answer is e. *(Cunningham, 21/e, pp 541–543. ACOG, Practice Bulletin 5.)* The desire for sterilization is not an indication for an elective repeat cesarean section. The morbidity of repeat cesarean section is greater than that of vaginal birth with postpartum tubal ligation. The risk of uterine rupture in a woman who undergoes a trial of labor and has had one prior cesarean section is approximately 0.6%. With a history of two prior cesarean sections, the risk of uterine rupture is about 1.8%. The risk of uterine rupture in someone who has had a classical or T-shaped uterine incision is 4 to 6%. The success rate for a trial of labor is generally about 60 to 80% Success rates are higher when the original cesarean section was performed for breech rather than dystocia. Induction of labor should not be performed without an obstetrical indication (e.g., preeclampsia); some studies suggest that high doses of oxytocin infusion increase a patient's risk of uterine rupture.

1-14.   The answer is c. (*Braunwald, 15/e, p 1525.*) When stupor and coma supervene in CO_2 retention, fatal arrhythmias, seizures, and death are likely to follow. Stopping oxygen is the worst course of action, as it will exacerbate life-threatening hypoxia. Intubation is the only good alternative. Bicarbonate plays no role in this acidosis, which is respiratory and caused by hypoventilation.

1-15.   The answer is e. (*Greenfield, 2/e, pp 827, 1092–1093.*) The film shows a markedly distended colon. The differential diagnosis includes tumor, foreign body, and colitis, but far more likely is either cecal or sigmoid volvulus. Sigmoid volvulus may be ruled out quickly by proctosigmoidoscopy, which is preferable to barium enema, since sigmoid volvulus may be treated successfully by rectal tube decompression via the sigmoidoscope. If sigmoidoscopy is negative, the working diagnosis, based on this classic film, must be cecal volvulus; barium enema would clinch the diagnosis, but the colon might rupture in the intervening 1 to 2 h. Emergency celiotomy should be done.

1-16.   The answer is c. (*Bradley, p 83.*) With the fragile X syndrome, the terminal elements of the long arm of the abnormal X chromosome appear stretched or broken away from the rest of the chromosome. Retardation usually becomes evident during childhood. Affected men have large ears, a high-arched palate, hypotelorism, and large testes. Autism also occurs among affected men.

1-17.   The answer is e. (*Tintinalli, 5/e, pp 539–541.*) The patient has a past medical history of appendectomy, which predisposes him to adhesions and

small bowel obstruction (SBO). Other etiologies for SBO include incarcerated hernia, stricture, and malignancy. The high-pitched bowel sounds, **peristaltic rushes,** and tympany with percussion are physical findings when air is under pressure in viscera and intestinal fluid is present (i.e., obstruction). The hallmarks of intestinal obstruction are abdominal pain, distension, vomiting, and obstipation. Abdominal radiographs may reveal dilated loops of bowel in a ladder-like pattern and **air-fluid levels. Large bowel obstruction (LBO)** is due to malignancy, diverticulitis, and volvulus. A mnemonic for abdominal distension is the **six F's:** Fat, Fluid, Food, Fetus, Feces, and Flatus.

1-18. The answer is a. *(Behrman, 16/e, pp 2152–2153, 2162. McMillan, 3/e, p 621. Rudolph, 21/e, pp 373–374.)* When the clinical signs of constricted pupils, bradycardia, and muscle fasciculations are associated with the sudden onset of neurologic symptoms, progressive respiratory distress, diaphoresis, diarrhea, and overabundant salivation, a diagnosis of organophosphate poisoning should be suspected. Intake of organophosphate agents can occur by ingestion, inhalation, or absorption through skin or mucosa. Organophosphates inhibit carboxylic esterase enzymes, including acetylcholinesterase and pseudocholinesterase; toxicity depends primarily on the inactivation or inhibition of acetylcholinesterase.

Treatment consists of gastric lavage, if the poison has been ingested, or decontamination of the skin, if exposure has been through contact. Maintenance of adequate ventilation and fluid and electrolyte balance also is indicated. All symptomatic children should receive atropine and, if severely affected, cholinesterase-reactivating oximes as well. Cholinesterase-reactivating oximes quickly restore consciousness by inhibiting muscarine- and nicotine-like synaptic actions of acetylcholine. Cholinesterase-reactivating oximes include pralidoxime chloride or obidoxime.

1-19. The answer is a. *(Braunwald, 15/e, pp 318, 323, 822, 1061, 1917–1918.)* Urticaria, or hives, is a common dermatologic problem characterized by pruritic, edematous papules and plaques that vary in size and come and go, often within hours. Mast cells may be stimulated by heat, cold, pressure, water, or exercise. Immunologic mechanisms can also cause mast cell degranulation. Folliculitis caused by *Pseudomonas aeruginosa* can cause a rash, often after exposure to hot tubs. The lesions would not be as diffuse, with a line of demarcation depending on the water level. These lesions are pustular and occur 8 to 48 h after soaking. Erythema multiforme produces target-like lesions and oral blisters often secondary to medications. Erythema chronicum migrans usually presents with a large, solitary annular lesion.

1-20. The answer is c. *(Hoskins, 2/e, p 728.)* Although rare, adenocarcinoma of the Bartholin's gland must be excluded in women over 40 years of age who present with a cystic or solid mass in this area. The appropriate treatment in these cases is surgical excision of the Bartholin's gland to allow for a careful pathologic examination. In cases of abscess formation, both marsupialization of the sac and incision with drainage as well as appropriate antibiotics are accepted modes of therapy. In the case of the asymptomatic Bartholin's cyst, no treatment is necessary.

1-21. The answer is c. *(Tierney, 42/e, pp 793–795.)* Since the patient has no neurologic compromise, the most likely diagnosis is **back strain.** Strain is common in people in their forties. It is exacerbated by activity and improves with rest. A **straight-leg maneuver** is positive for nerve root compression from disk herniation when pain is produced at less than 70° of elevation. **Crossover pain** (straight-leg maneuver of nonpainful leg worsens pain of involved leg) is also a strong indicator of nerve root compression, but only if pain is produced below the knee. **Paravertebral abscess** usually presents with fever and tenderness with percussion of the affected back area. Risk factors for osteoporosis include female gender, menopause, lack of activity, slim body habitus, older age, inadequate calcium intake, medications such as corticosteroids, and racial-ethnic background (Asian and northern European descent). **Paget's disease** (osteitis deformans) is a slowly progressing disease of bone that may be asymptomatic or may cause bone pain, deformities (such as a large skull or leg bowing), hearing loss, and fractures. It begins in middle-aged men and is thought to be due to an inborn error of metabolism causing the formation of poorly organized bone.

1-22. The answer is e. *(Behrman, 16/e, pp 1127–1128. Rudolph, 21/e, pp 1397–1398.)* Many types of objects produce esophageal obstruction in young children, including small toys, coins, and food. Most are usually lodged below the cricopharyngeal muscle at the level of the aortic arch. Initially, the foreign body may cause a cough, drooling, and choking. Later, pain, avoidance of food (liquids are tolerated better), and shortness of breath can develop. Diagnosis is by history (as outlined in the question) and by radiographs (especially if the object is radiopaque). The usual treatment is removal of the object via esophagoscopy.

1-23. The answer is b. *(Braunwald, 15/e, pp 1947–1949.)* The complaints described are characteristic of Sjögren syndrome, an autoimmune disease with presenting symptoms of dry eyes and dry mouth. The disease is caused by lymphocytic infiltration and destruction of lacrimal and salivary glands. Dry eyes can be measured objectively by the Schirmer test, which measures the amount of wetness of a piece of filter paper when exposed to the lower eyelid for 5 minutes. Most patients with Sjögren syndrome produce auto-antibodies, particularly anti-Ro (SSA). Lip biopsy is needed only to evaluate uncertain cases, such as when dry mouth occurs without dry eye symptoms. Mumps can cause bilateral parotitis, but would not explain the patient's dry eye syndrome. Corticosteroids are reserved for life-threatening vasculitis, particularly when renal or pulmonary disease is severe.

1-24. The answer is e. *(Victor, pp 1281–1282.)* Methacholine is a cholinergic agent and would be expected to worsen the symptoms exhibited by this man. Pyridostigmine, physostigmine, and edrophonium are all cholinesterase inhibitors used in the evaluation or treatment of myasthenia gravis, and they too would only hasten this man's deterioration. Atropine is usually given in combination with pralidoxime. This man is at most immediate risk of severe bronchospasm and diaphragmatic paralysis with subsequent respiratory arrest. Even if the patient does survive the acute poisoning, he is at risk for a delayed deterioration of the motor system, which may itself prove fatal and which does not respond to atropine treatment.

1-25. The answer is c. *(Schwartz, 7/e, p 1881.)* Epidural hematomas are typically caused by a tear of the middle meningeal artery or vein or a dural venous sinus. Ninety percent of epidural hematomas are associated with linear skull fractures, usually in the temporal region. Only 2% of patients admitted with craniocerebral trauma suffer epidural hematomas. The lesion appears as a hyperdense biconvex mass between the skull and brain on CT scan. Clinical presentation is highly variable and outcome largely depends on promptness of diagnosis and surgical evacuation. The typical history is one of head trauma followed by a momentary alteration in consciousness and then a lucid interval lasting for up to a few hours. This is followed by a loss of consciousness, dilation of the pupil on the side of the epidural hematoma, and then compromise of the brainstem and death. Treatment consists of temporal craniectomy, evaluation of the hemorrhage, and control of the bleeding vessel. The mortality associated with epidural hematoma is approximately 50%.

I-26. The answer is b. (*Victor, pp 1300–1301.*) High-dose intravenous methylprednisolone [30-mg/kg intravenous bolus followed by 5.4 mg/(kg·h) for 23 h] has been shown to have a statistically significant, if clinically modest, benefit on the outcome after spinal cord injury when given within 8 h of the injury. Naloxone hydrochloride and other agents, such as G_{M1} ganglioside, have not been shown to be of benefit. The role of surgical decompression, removal of hemorrhage, and correction of bone displacement is controversial. Most American neurosurgeons do not advocate surgery, and instead propose external spinal fixation.

I-27. The answer is b. (*Beckmann, 4/e, pp 166–169. Decherney, 9/e, pp 295–299. Cunningham, 21/e, pp. 1057–1059, 1066.*) During the first prenatal visit, all pregnant women are screened for the ABO blood group and the Rh group, which includes the D antigen. If the woman is Rh-negative, antibody screening is performed. If the antibody D titer is positive, the woman is considered sensitized because she has produced antibodies against the D antigen. Sensitization occurs as a result of exposure to blood from an Rh+ fetus in a prior pregnancy. A fetus that is Rh+ possesses red blood cells that express the D antigen. Therefore, the maternal anti-D antibodies can cross the placenta and cause fetal hemolysis. Once the antibody screen is positive for isoimmunization, the titer should be followed at regular intervals (about every 4 weeks). A titer of 1:16 or greater is usually indicative of the possibility of severe hemolytic disease of the fetus. Once the critical titer is reached, further evaluation is done by amniotic fluid assessment or analysis of fetal blood via PUBS. In the presence of fetal hemolysis, the amniotic fluid contains elevated levels of bilirubin that can be determined via spectrophotometric analysis. Cordocentesis, or percutaneous umbilical blood sampling, involves obtaining a blood sample from the umbilical cord under ultrasound guidance. The fetal blood sample can then be analyzed for Hct and determination of fetal blood type. Cordocentesis also allows the fetus with anemia to undergo a blood transfusion.

I-28. The answer is a. (*Tierney, 42/e, pp 331–332.*) The increased venous return of inspiration (the **Müller maneuver** is sucking in with the nares held closed) increases murmurs of the right side of the heart, and expiration increases murmurs of the left side of the heart. The murmur of **tricuspid regurgitation** is a holosystolic murmur heard best at the left lower sternal border that increases with inspiration. Other findings in tricuspid regurgitation include distended neck veins, prominent v waves, hepatomegaly, pulsatile liver, edema, and a positive hepatojugular reflex (pressure applied over the liver causes increased distension of the neck veins). Intravenous drug abusers are at risk for developing acute endocarditis of the tricuspid valve due to *Staphylococcus aureus* bacteria. Other signs of **bacterial endocarditis** include splinter hemorrhages (subungual streaks), **Roth spots** (oval retinal hemorrhages with a pale center), **Osler nodes** (tender nodules on finger or toe pads), **Janeway lesions** (small hemorrhages on the palms and soles), clubbing, and splenomegaly. Rheumatic heart disease predisposes patients to endocarditis; the organism is often *Streptococcus viridans*, and the mitral valve is most commonly involved. Mitral valve prolapse also predisposes patients to endocarditis.

I-29. The answer is c. (*Schwartz, 7/e, pp 1028–1030.*) This patient is at high risk for developing cellulitis of her right foot because her underlying problem is unilateral primary lymphedema. Hypoplasia of the lymphatic system of the lower extremity accounts for greater than 90% of cases of primary lymphedema. If edema is present at birth, it is referred to as congenital; if it starts early in life (as in this woman), it is called praecox; if it appears after age 35, it is tarda. The inadequacy of the lymphatic system accounts for the repeated episodes of cellulitis that these patients experience. Swelling is not seen with acute arterial insufficiency or with popliteal entrapment syndrome. Deep venous thrombophlebitis will result in tenderness and is generally not a predisposing factor for cellulitis of the foot.

I-30. The answer is c. (*Tierney, 42/e, pp 1258–1259.*) Pathogens that may cause an **inflammatory diarrhea** and produce **fecal leukocytes** include *Shigella, Salmonella, C. jejuni, Yersinia enterocolitica, Clostridium difficile, Vib-*

rio parahaemolyticus, enterohemorrhagic *Escherichia coli,* and enteroinvasive *E. coli.*

1-31. The answer is d. (*Rowland, pp 155–156.*) Adrenoleukodystrophy, MS, SSPE, PML, and metachromatic leukodystrophy are all demyelinating diseases, but PML is the only one confidently linked to a virus. The specific strains of papovavirus most often implicated in PML are BK, JC, and SV40. The patients at risk for this often lethal demyelinating process are those with lymphomas, leukemias, and AIDS. Patients on immunosuppressants face substantially less risk, but are at more risk than the general population.

1-32. The answer is c. (*Behrman, 16/e, pp 1892–1893. McMillan, 3/e, pp 1959–1965, 1972–1976. Rudolph, 21/e, pp 2281–2283.*) The paralysis of Guillain-Barré occurs about 10 days after a nonspecific viral illness. Weakness is gradual over days or weeks, beginning in the lower extremities and progressing toward the trunk. Later, the upper limbs and the bulbar muscles can become involved. Involvement of the respiratory muscles is life-threatening. The syndrome seems to be caused by a demyelination in the motor and, occasionally, the sensory nerves. Measurement of spinal fluid protein is helpful in the diagnosis; protein levels are increased to more than twice normal, while glucose and cell counts are normal. Hospitalization for observation is indicated. Treatment can consist of intravenous immunoglobulin, steroids, or plasmapheresis. Recovery is not always complete. Bell palsy usually follows a mild upper respiratory infection, resulting in the rapid development of weakness of the entire side of the face. Muscular dystrophy encompasses a number of entities that include weakness over months. Charcot-Marie-Tooth disease has a clinical onset including peroneal and intrinsic foot muscle atrophy, later extending to the intrinsic hand muscles and proximal legs. Werdnig-Hoffmann disease is an anterior horn disorder that presents either in utereo (in about one-third of cases) or by the first 6 months of life with hypotonia, weakness, and delayed developmental motor milestones.

1-33. The answer is c. (*Greenfield, 2/e, pp 825–826.*) Gallstone ileus is due to erosion of a stone from the gallbladder into the gastrointestinal tract (most commonly the duodenum). The stone becomes lodged in the small bowel (usually in the terminal ileum) and causes small-bowel obstruction. Plain films of the abdomen that demonstrate small-bowel obstruction and air in the biliary tract are diagnostic of the condition. Treatment consists of ileotomy, removal of the stone, and cholecystectomy if it is technically safe. If there is significant inflammation of the right upper quadrant, ileotomy for stone extraction followed by an interval cholecystectomy is often a safer alternative. Operating on the biliary fistula doubles the mortality rate compared with simple removal of the gallstone from the intestine.

1-34. The answer is e. (*Gleicher, 3/e, pp 27–31.*) Numerous changes occur in the cardiovascular system during pregnancy. Heart rate increases by about 10 to 15/min. Blood volume and cardiac output increase significantly. Many cardiac sounds that would be abnormal in a nonpregnant state are normal during pregnancy. All the findings listed in the question are normal. Ninety percent of pregnant women have systolic ejection murmurs. In approximately 20% of women, a soft diastolic murmur can be heard.

1-35. The answer is c. (*Behrman, 16/e, p 491. McMillan, 3/e, pp 164, 2122. Rudolph, 21/e, p 2447.*) In a difficult delivery in which traction is applied to the head and neck, several injuries, including all those listed in the question, may occur. Erb-Duchenne paralysis affects the fifth and sixth cervical nerves; the affected arm cannot be abducted or externally rotated at the shoulder, and the forearm cannot be supinated. Injury to the seventh and eighth cervical and first thoracic nerves (Klumpke paralysis) results in palsy of the hand and also can produce Horner's syndrome. Fractures in the upper limb are not associated with a characteristic posture, and passive movement usually elicits pain. Spinal injury causes complete paralysis below the level of injury.

When paralysis of an upper extremity from injury to the brachial plexus is found in a neonate, injury to the phrenic nerve should also be suspected because the nerve roots are close together and can be injured concurrently. The paralyzed diaphragm can be noted to remain elevated on a chest x-ray taken during deep inspiration when it will contrast with the opposite normal diaphragm in its lower normal position; on expiration, this asymmetry cannot be seen. On inspiration, not only is breathing impaired since the paralyzed diaphragm does not contract, but the negative pressure generated by the intact diaphragm pulls the mediastinum toward the normal side, impairing ventilation further. The diagnosis can easily be made by fluoroscopy, where these characteristic movements on inspiration and expiration can be seen. Rarely, both diaphragms can be paralyzed, producing much more severe ventilatory impairment. Fortunately, these injuries frequently improve spontaneously.

1-36. The answer is a. *(Kaplan, 8/e, p 269.)* Chronic subdural hematoma causes a reversible form of dementia. It frequently follows head trauma (60% of the cases) with tearing of the bridging veins in the subdural space. Ruptured aneurysms, rapid deceleration injuries, and arterovenous malformations (AVMs) of the pial surface account for the nontraumatic cases. The most common symptoms of chronic subdural hematomas are headache, confusion, inattention, apathy, memory loss, drowsiness, and coma. Lateralization signs, such as hemiparesis, hemianopsia, and cranial nerve abnormalities, are less prominent features. Epidural hematoma usually follows a temporal or parietal skull fracture that causes the laceration of the middle meningeal artery or vein. It is characterized by a brief period of lucidity followed by loss of consciousness, hemiparesis, cranial nerve palsies, and death unless the hematoma is surgically evacuated. Multi-infarct dementia and Alzheimer's disease are characterized by a slower onset and have a more chronic course, although diagnostic confusion is possible at times. Korsakoff's disorder is characterized by anterograde and retrograde memory deficits. Frontal lobe tumors mainly present with personality and behavioral changes, which differ depending on the localization.

1-37. The answer is b. *(Victor, p 1382.)* This patient's clinical course is consistent with a diagnosis of AIDP, also known as Guillain-Barré syndrome. Cerebrospinal fluid is typically under normal pressure in this syndrome, and contains no cells in up to 90% of patients. In 10% of patients, 10 to 50 WBCs, mostly lymphocytes, may appear. Protein levels are generally elevated, sometimes to extremely high levels, reflecting the degree of inflammatory activity taking place at the level of the spinal roots.

1-38. The answer is e. *(Behrman, 16/e, p 1893. McMillan, 3/e, p 1963. Rudolph, 21/e, p 2366.)* Bell palsy is an acute, unilateral facial nerve palsy that begins about 2 weeks after a viral infection. The exact pathophysiology is unknown, but it is thought to be immune or allergic. On the affected side, the upper and lower face are typically paretic, the mouth droops, and the patient cannot close the eye. Treatment consists of maintaining moisture to the affected eye (especially at night) to prevent keratitis. Complete, spontaneous resolution occurs in about 85% of cases, 10% of cases have mild residual disease, and about 5% of cases do not resolve.

1-39. The answer is a. *(Braunwald, 15/e, pp 2066–2069.)* This patient presents with classic features of hypothyroidism. Hypothyroidism is almost always caused by autoimmune disease, thyroid damage from surgery, or radiation therapy. Autoimmune thyroiditis usually occurs in women, has a genetic component, and is associated with other autoimmune conditions. Autoimmune thyroiditis may be present with a goiter (Hashimoto's thyroiditis) or with minimal residual thyroid tissue (atrophic thyroiditis). Primary hypothyroidism can result from surgery or radiation therapy, but there is no such history in this patient. Thyroid cancer does not cause hypothyroidism. It presents with neck mass, hoarse voice, or expanding nodule.

1-40. The answer is c. *(Braunwald, 15/e, pp. 2138–2142.)* This clinical picture and laboratory results suggest factitious hypoglycemia caused by self-administration of insulin. The diagnosis should be suspected in health care workers, patients or family members with diabetes, and others who have a history of malingering. Patients present with symptoms of hypoglycemia and low plasma glucose levels. Insulin levels will be high, but without a concomitant rise in C peptide. Endogenous hyperinsulinism, such as would be seen with an insulinoma, would result in elevated plasma insulin concentrations (>36 pmol/L) and elevated C peptide levels (>0.2 mmol/L). C peptide is derived from the breakdown of proinsulin, which is produced endogenously; thus C peptide will not rise in the patient who develops hypoglycemia from exogenous insulin. Reactive hypoglycemia occurs after meals and is self-limited. A rapid postprandial rise in glucose may induce a brisk insulin response that causes transient hypoglycemia hours later. It may be associated with gastric or intestinal surgery.

1-41. The answer is c. *(Kaplan, 8/e, pp 578–580.)* Cyclothymic disorder is characterized by recurrent periods of mild depression alternating with periods of hypomania. This pattern must be present for at least 2 years (1 year for children and adolescents) before the diagnosis can be made. During these 2 years, the symptom-free intervals should not be longer than 2 months. Cyclothymic disorder usually starts during adolescence or early adulthood and tends to have a chronic course. The marked shifts in mood of cyclothymic disorder can be confused with the affective instability of borderline personality disorder or may suggest a substance abuse problem.

1-42. The answer is d. *(Rowland, pp 679–682.)* The tremor is of a Parkinsonian type. The patient also has the classic findings of Parkinson's disease: asymmetric tremor, rigidity, and bradykinesia. Epilepsy is characterized by repeated unprovoked seizures. Hand shaking can be the result of a focal motor seizure, but the presentation overall makes epilepsy an unlikely diagnosis. Guillain-Barré syndrome is a peripheral demyelinating disease that usually presents as an ascending motor deficit. Multiple sclerosis is a central nervous system (CNS) demyelinating disease. It presents with individual episodes of CNS deficits, which usually recover to some extent. Stroke is characterized by the acute onset of a neurological deficit due to nerve infarction. Tremor would be an exceedingly rare presentation for stroke, and it would not evolve over 6 to 12 months.

1-43. The answer is d. *(Beckmann, 4/e, pp 157–158, 183–188. Cunningham, 21/e, pp 676–680.)* Metritis, or infection of the uterus, is the most common infection that occurs after a cesarean section. A long labor and prolonged rupture of membranes are predisposing factors for metritis. In the presence of a pelvic abscess, usually signs of peritoneal irritation such as rebound tenderness, ileus, and decreased bowel sounds are present. Wound infections occur with an incidence of about 6% following cesarean deliveries. Fever usually begins on the fourth or fifth postoperative day, and erythema around the incision along with pus drainage is often present. In the case of a wound infection, first-line treatment involves draining the incision. Atelectasis can be a cause of postoperative fever, but the fever occurs generally in the first 24 h. In addition, on physical exam, atelectasis is generally accompanied by decreased breath sounds at the lung bases on auscultation. It more commonly occurs in women who have had general anesthesia, not an epidural like the patient described here. Septic pelvic thrombophlebitis occurs uncommonly as a sequela of pelvic infection. Venous stasis occurs in dilated pelvic veins; in the presence of bacteria, it can lead to septic thromboses. Diagnosis is usually made when persistent fever spikes occur after treatment for metritis. The patient usually has no uterine tenderness, and bowel function tends to be normal. Treatment is with intravenous heparin.

1-44. The answer is b. (*Tierney, 42/e, pp 205–206.*) The patient has a **peritonsillar abscess,** which is an accumulation of pus between the tonsillar capsule and the superior constrictor muscle of the pharynx. Patients present with a hot potato voice, fever, cervical lymphadenopathy, trismus, and a displaced uvula due to a unilaterally enlarged tonsil. Patients complain of dysphagia, odynophagia, and otalgia. A **retropharyngeal abscess** is an infection of the deep spaces of the neck (from the base of the skull to the tracheal bifurcation); patients are often young children who present with fever, cervical lymphadenopathy, neck pain, neck swelling, torticollis (rotation to the affected side), difficulty breathing, and stridor. Patients with an **exudative pharyngitis** have fever, cervical lymphadenopathy, bilateral tonsillar enlargement, erythema, edema of the midline uvula, and discrete tonsillar exudate.

1-45. The answer is c. (*Greenfield, 2/e, pp 571–581.*) Hemodialysis, rather than management by dietary manipulation alone, should be instituted in patients with end-stage renal failure whose serum creatinine is over 15 mg/dL or whose creatinine clearance is less than 3 mL/min. It is important that hemodialysis be initiated prior to the onset of uremic complications. These complications include hyperkalemia, congestive heart failure, peripheral neuropathy, severe hypertension, pericarditis, bleeding, and severe anemia. The uremic hyperkalemic patient in congestive heart failure may require emergency dialysis in addition to the standard conservative measures, which include (1) limitation of protein intake to less than 60 g/day and restriction of fluid intake and (2) reduction of elevated serum potassium levels by insulin-glucose or sodium polystyrene sulfonate (Kayexalate) enema treatment. Arteriovenous fistulas require about 2 weeks to develop adequate size and flow. While awaiting maturation, temporary dialysis can be satisfactorily performed using either an external arteriovenous shunt or the peritoneal cavity. Renal biopsy would be performed in an attempt to obtain a diagnosis of the underlying renal disease. Patients who are acceptable candidates for kidney transplantation usually should undergo this form of treatment, after they are stabilized, rather than chronic hemodialysis, the mortality for which is now higher than for transplantation. Despite adequate dialysis, problems of neuropathy, bone disease, anemia, and hypertension remain difficult to manage. Compared with chronic dialysis, transplantation restores more patients to happier and more productive lives.

It had been conjectured that, all other issues being equal, sex matching was important in the graft survival and that a mother-daughter graft was preferred to a father-daughter graft. Review of the current data does not support such a conclusion. The best graft survival rates for living related transplants—over 90% at 5 years—are obtained when all six histocompatibility loci are identical. All family members of potential transplant recipients should be tissue typed and the donor should be selected on the basis of closest match, if psychological and medical evaluation makes this feasible. With the development of cyclosporine-based immunosuppression, cadaveric kidney graft survival has approached that of living-related transplantation. There are some transplanters who believe that the slight improvement with living-related kidneys does not justify the risk to the donor and that these transplantations should no longer be performed.

1-46. The answer is c. (*Gorbach, 2/e, pp 542–544.*) This patient, with the development of hoarseness, breathing difficulty, and stridor, is likely to have acute epiglottitis. Because of the possibility of impending airway obstruction, the patient should be admitted to an intensive care unit for close monitoring. The diagnosis can be confirmed by indirect laryngoscopy or soft tissue x-rays of the neck, which may show an enlarged epiglottis. Otolaryngology consult should be obtained. The most likely organism causing this infection is *Haemophilus influenzae*. Many of these organisms are β-lactamase-producing and would be resistant to ampicillin. The clinical findings are not consistent with the presentation of streptococcal pharyngitis. Lateral neck films would be more useful than a chest x-ray.

1-47. The answer is b. (*Behrman, 16/e, pp 1395–1398. McMillan, 3/e, pp 1322–1324. Rudolph, 21/e, pp 1823–1826.*) Transposition of the great vessels with an intact ventricular septum presents with early cyanosis, a normal-sized heart (classic "egg on a string" radiographic pattern in one-third of cases), normal or slightly increased pulmonary vascular markings, and an electrocardiogram showing right axis deviation and right ventricular hypertrophy. In tetralogy of Fallot, cyanosis is often not seen in the first few days of life. Tricuspid atresia, a cause of early cyanosis, causes diminished pulmonary arterial blood flow; the pulmonary fields on x-ray demonstrate a diminution of pulmonary vascularity. There is a left axis and left ventricular hypertrophy shown by electrocardiogram. Total anomalous pulmonary venous return below the diaphragm is associated with obstruction to pulmonary venous return and a classic radiographic finding of marked, fluffy-appearing venous congestion ("snowman"). In pulmonic atresia with intact ventricular septum, cyanosis appears early, the lung markings are normal to diminished, and the heart is large.

1-48. The answer is a. *(Beckmann, 4/e, pp 159–160. Cunningham, 21/e, pp 1421–1423.)* This patient is exhibiting classic symptoms of postpartum depression. Postpartum depression develops in about 8 to 15% of women and generally is characterized by an onset about 2 weeks to 12 months post delivery and an average duration of 3 to 14 months. Women with postpartum depression have the following symptoms: irritability, labile mood, difficulty sleeping, phobias, and anxiety. About 50% of women experience postpartum blues, or maternity blues, within 3 to 6 days after delivering. This mood disturbance is thought to be precipitated by progesterone withdrawal following delivery and usually resolves in 10 days. Maternity blues is characterized by mild insomnia, tearfulness, fatigue, irritability, poor concentration, and depressed affect. Postpartum psychosis usually has its onset within a few days of delivery and is characterized by confusion, disorientation, and loss of touch with reality. Postpartum psychosis is very rare and only occurs in 1 to 4 in 1000 births. Bipolar disorder or manic-depressive illness is a psychiatric disorder characterized by episodes of depression followed by mania.

1-49. The answer is b. *(Behrman, 16/e, pp 583–586, 829–832, 919–920. McMillan, 3/e, pp 561–562. Rudolph, 21/e, pp 260–270.)* Each year, a diagnosis of pelvic inflammatory disease (PID) is made in over 1 million women. Sexually active teenagers are at great risk of acquiring PID because of their high-risk behavior, exposure to multiple partners, and failure to use contraceptives. The strong likelihood of PID in the patient presented should not preclude consideration of serious conditions requiring surgical intervention, such as appendiceal abscess, ectopic pregnancy, and ovarian cyst. Renal cyst does not present in the manner described. An episode of PID raises the risk of ectopic pregnancy, and about 20% of women become infertile following one episode of PID. Other sequelae include dyspareunia, pyosalpinx, tuboovarian abscess, and pelvic adhesions. Endometriosis is not related to PID.

1-50. The answer is d. (*Ebert, pp 546–556.*) Patients diagnosed with Rett's disorder have normal prenatal and postnatal development but, between ages 5 to 30 months, they begin to lose previously acquired purposeful hand skills and develop stereotyped hand movements (hand wringing or hand washing) and poorly coordinated gait or trunk movements. These patients have severe to profound mental retardation and severe receptive and expressive language deficits. They also lose all interest in social interaction. Characteristically, head circumference is normal at birth, but between 5 months and 4 years of age the rate of the head growth decelerates rapidly. Rett's disorder has been described only in females and is very rare.

BLOCK 2

Answers

2-1. The answer is a. (*Behrman, 16/e, pp 704–709. McMillan, 3/e, pp 2156–2160. Rudolph, 21/e, pp 836–839.*) Pauciarticular rheumatoid arthritis asymmetrically involves large joints, especially the knee, and often has no other symptoms. The major morbidity of pauciarticular rheumatoid arthritis is blindness. About 20% of girls who have the monoarthritic or pauciarticular form of juvenile rheumatoid arthritis have iridocyclitis as their only significant systemic manifestation. Because this eye disorder can require treatment with local or systemic steroids and develop without signs or symptoms, it is recommended that all children with this form of arthritis have frequent slit-lamp eye examinations.

2-2. The answer is c. (*Braunwald, 15/e, p 1369.*) The history and physical are consistent with post–cardiac injury syndrome (in the past also known as Dressler syndrome or postmyocardial infarction syndrome). This generally benign self-limited syndrome comprises an autoimmune pleuritis, pneumonitis, or pericarditis characterized by fever and pleuritic chest pain, with onset days to 6 weeks post cardiac injury with blood in the pericardial cavity, as after a cardiac operation, cardiac trauma, or MI. Therefore the most effective therapy is a nonsteroidal anti-inflammatory drug or occasionally a glucocorticoid. Infection such as bacterial pneumonia, which would require antibiotics, would typically cause dyspnea, cough with sputum production, and rales on lung auscultation. Pulmonary embolus, which would require anticoagulation, would cause dyspnea and tachypnea, often in conjunction with physical findings of heat, swelling, and pain in the leg consistent with deep vein thrombosis. Angina or recurrent myocardial infarction is always a concern post MI (and what the patient usually fears in this situation), but the nature of the pain—here pleuritic rather than pressurelike—and the unchanged ECG are fairly reassuring and mitigate against an increase in antianginal therapy. Anxiety can be present but would not cause fever.

2-3. The answer is c. (*Cunningham, 21/e, pp 979–985, 989–991.*) The multiple marker screening test, also referred to as the expanded AFP test or triple screen, consists of maternal serum measurements of estriol, human chorionic gonadotropin, and α-fetoprotein. The multiple marker screening test is used to determine a pregnant patient's risk of having a baby with aneuploidy and a neural tube defect. The AFP test has the greatest sensitivity when done between 16 and 18 weeks. A maternal serum AFP level that is greater than or equal to 2.0 to 2.5 MOM indicates an elevated risk for a neural tube defect and indicates that further workup and evaluation are needed. The first step when an elevated serum AFP result is obtained is to have the patient undergo an ultrasound to verify that the gestational age of the pregnancy is correct. The sonogram can also identify a fetal death in utero, multiple gestation, or a neural tube or abdominal defect, which could all explain the elevated AFP level. A repeat serum AFP test can be done, because at a level of 2.0 MOM there is some overlap between normal and affected pregnancies. The repeat test should be done as soon as possible; waiting until 20 weeks decreases the sensitivity of the test and wastes valuable time in the workup. An amniocentesis is recommended if a neural tube defect is suspected, in order to measure amniotic fluid levels of AFP and therefore confirm the findings of the maternal serum AFP. The physician would not immediately refer the patient for a chorionic villus sampling because this procedure obtains placental tissue for fetal karyotyping and does not add to information regarding the presence of a neural tube defect. A cordocentesis or percutaneous umbilical cord blood sampling (PUBS) is a procedure whereby the umbilical vein is punctured under ultrasonic guidance and a fetal blood sample is obtained. Usually a PUBS is performed when rapid fetal karyotyping must be done, such as in a situation where severe growth restriction exists. PUBS is most commonly used in situations where fetal hydrops exists to obtain information regarding fetal platelet counts and fetal hematocrits.

2-4. The answer is d. (*Greenberg, 5/e, pp 241–243.*) This patient gives a typical history for early Parkinson's disease. The classic triad is asymmetric resting tremor, rigidity, and bradykinesia. The rigidity is generally severe later, not early in the disease. Parkinson's disease is not characterized by weakness.

2-5. The answer is b. (*Braunwald, 15/e, pp 1994–1995.*) The sudden onset and severity of this monoarticular arthritis suggests acute gouty arthritis, especially in a patient on diuretic therapy. However, an arthrocentesis is indicated in the first episode to document gout by demonstrating needle-shaped, negatively birefringent crystals and to rule out other diagnoses such as infection. For most patients with acute gout, NSAIDs are the treatment of choice. Colchicine is also effective, but causes nausea and diarrhea. Antibiotics should not be started for infectious arthritis before an arthrocentesis is performed. Hyperuricemia should never be treated in the setting of an acute attack of gouty arthritis. Long-term goals of management are to control hyperuricemia, prevent further attacks, and prevent joint damage. Long-term prophylaxis with a uricosuric agent or allopurinol is considered for repeated attacks of acute arthritis, urolithiasis, or formation of tophaceous deposits. Attempts to normalize serum uric acid prior to drug therapy should include control of body weight, avoidance of ethanol and diuretics, and perhaps low-purine diet. X-ray of the ankle would likely be inconclusive in this patient with no trauma history.

2-6. The answer is d. (*Cunningham, 21/e, pp 174, 569–574, 1021, 1235–1236.*) Increased fluid retention manifested by pitting edema of the ankles and legs is a normal finding in pregnancy. During pregnancy, there is a decrease in colloid osmotic pressure and a fall in plasma osmolality. Moreover, there is an increase in venous pressure created by partial occlusion of the vena cava by the gravid uterus, which also contributes to pedal edema. Diuretics are sometimes given to pregnant women who have chronic hypertension, but this is not the case in this patient. More commonly, Lasix is used in the acute setting to treat pulmonary edema. This patient is not hypertensive and does not have any other signs or symptoms of preeclampsia and therefore does not need to be admitted for a further workup. Trace protein in the urine is common in normal pregnancies and is not of concern. Doppler studies of the lower extremities are not indicated in this patient since the history and exam (specifically, the lack of calf tenderness) are consistent with physiologic edema. The normal swelling detected in pregnancy is not prevented by a low-sodium diet or improved with a lower intake of salt.

2-7. The answer is b. (*Sabiston, 15/e, pp 332–333.*) The **five P's** of arterial injury include **p**ain, **p**aresthesias, **p**allor, **p**ulselessness, and **p**aralysis. In the extremities, the tissues most sensitive to anoxia are the peripheral nerves and striated muscle. The early developments of paresthesias and paralysis are signals that there is significant ischemia present, and immediate exploration and repair are warranted. The presence of palpable pulses does not exclude an arterial injury because this presence may represent a transmitted pulsation through a blood clot. When severe ischemia is present, the repair must be completed within 6 to 8 h to prevent irreversible muscle ischemia and loss of limb function. Delay to obtain an angiogram or to observe for change needlessly prolongs the ischemic time. Fasciotomy may be required but should be done in conjunction with and after reestablishment of arterial flow. Local wound exploration is not recommended because brisk hemorrhage may be encountered without the securing of prior vascular control.

2-8. The answer is b. *(Behrman, 16/e, pp 1025–1028. McMillan, 3/e, p 870. Rudolph, 21/e, pp 1046–1048.)* This child is presenting with failure to thrive (FTT), and the differential diagnosis of this problem is extensive. While any of the answers provided may have a place in an FTT evaluation, the best single recommendation in this case would be to evaluate for HIV. With a mother in jail for unknown reasons (possibly for prostitution, drugs, or other high-risk activities), this child has increased risk for congenital HIV. In addition, the presenting symptoms are most consistent with HIV.

2-9. The answer is c. *(Shuaib, p 58.)* This is a good history for cardioembolic stroke—sudden onset, cortical symptoms, atrial fibrillation, and subtherapeutic INR. The immediate goal should be to rule out an intracranial hemorrhage and confirm the diagnosis. Tissue plasminogen activator is the treatment for acute stroke in specific circumstances. However, it is not yet certain that this is a stroke. It may be an intracranial hemorrhage, which would be a contraindication for tissue plasminogen activator. Additionally, an elevated INR in a patient on warfarin is a contraindication for tissue plasminogen activator. Carotid endarterectomy is indicated for some cases when a transient ischemic attack or stroke is believed to be caused by carotid artery narrowing. It is not yet known what caused this patient's event, and this procedure would rarely be done emergently. A cerebral angiogram would be indicated if you had strong suspicion of an aneurysm or vascular malformation. There is no reason to believe one of these is causing the patient's symptoms. Heparin may be indicated if there is not an intracranial hemorrhage. This must first be established by CT or MRI.

2-10. The answer is b. (*Kaplan, 8/e, p 775.*) The essential feature of obsessive-compulsive personality disorder is a preoccupation with perfection, orderliness, and control. Individuals with this disorder lose the main point of an activity and miss deadlines because they pay too much attention to rules and details and are not satisfied with anything less than "perfection." As in other personality disorders, symptoms are ego-syntonic and create interpersonal, social, and occupational difficulties. Obsessive-compulsive disorder is differentiated from obsessive-compulsive personality disorder by the presence of obsessions and compulsions. Patients with borderline personality disorder present with a history of pervasive instability of mood, relationships, and self-image beginning by early adulthood. Their behavior is often impulsive and self-damaging. Patients with bipolar disorder present with problems with mood stability; mood may be depressed for several weeks at a time, then euphoric. Patients with an anxiety disorder not otherwise specified present with anxiety as a main symptom, though they do not specifically fit any other more specific anxiety disorder as per DSM-IV-TR.

2-11. The answer is b. (*Seidel, 5/e, p 673.*) **Klinefelter syndrome,** the most common (1 in 500) disorder of sexual differentiation, is associated with XXY chromosomal inheritance and is characterized by tall stature, hypogonadism or small scrotum with pea-sized testes (normal testes are 5 cm long), a female distribution of pubic hair, and gynecomastia. Newborns require prompt chromosomal studies if born with ambiguous genitalia (small penis with hypospadias or enlarged clitoris). Patients with gonadal dysgenesis or **Turner syndrome** are 45,X0; the syndrome is characterized by primary amenorrhea, short stature, webbed neck, and multiple congenital abnormalities.

2-12. The answer is e. (*Cunningham, 21/e, pp 1095–1107.*) Maternal perception of decreased fetal movement has preceded fetal death in utero. Therefore, kick counts have been employed as a method of antepartum assessment. The optimal number of fetal movements that should be perceived per hour has not been determined. However, studies indicate that the perception of 10 distinct movements in a period of up to 2 h is reassuring. Since this patient is only experiencing one movement per hour and this movement is decreased from her previous baseline, further antepartum testing is indicated. A nonstress test is the preferred modality, because a contraction stress test involves giving a preterm pregnancy uterine contractions. Delivery is not indicated until nonreassuring fetal status can be documented.

2-13. The answer is d. (*Braunwald, 15/e, pp 554–557.*) The lesion has characteristics of melanoma (pigmentation, asymmetry, irregular border), and a full-thickness excisional biopsy is required. Shave biopsy of a suspected melanoma is always contraindicated. Diagnosis is urgent; the lesion cannot be observed over time. Once the diagnosis of melanoma is made, the tumor must then be staged to determine prognosis and treatment.

2-14. The answer is d. (*Victor, pp 961–962.*) This is a typical history for multiple sclerosis (MS). Multiple sclerosis is a progressive demyelinating disease of the central nervous system. Risk factors include a first time demyelinating episode such as optic neuritis. Patients are more commonly in the 20 to 30 age range, with a higher incidence in women. A transient ischemic attack is a brief period of brain ischemia causing neurological deficits that resolve within 24 h. Patients who have a transient ischemic attack are at increased risk for stroke. A seizure is abnormal rhythmic electrical brain activity with a clinical correlation. There is nothing in the history that suggests that this patient had a seizure or a seizure predisposing factor. Seizure predisposing factors include previous seizure, brain trauma, brain hemorrhage, and encephalitis. An anaplastic astrocytoma is a malignant high-grade brain tumor. These often present with a seizure or hemorrhage. Risk factors include previous brain tumor. Parkinson's disease is caused by a loss of dopaminergic neurons. It is characterized by asymmetric slowness, rigidity, and tremor. Risk factors include family history.

2-15. The answer is d. (*Cunningham, 21/e, pp 704–718.*) This patient with premature rupture of membranes (PROM) has a physical exam consistent with an intrauterine infection or chorioamnionitis. Chorioamnionitis can be diagnosed clinically by the presence of maternal fever, tachycardia, and uterine tenderness. Leukocyte counts are a nonspecific indicator of infection because they can be elevated with labor and the use of corticosteroids. When chorioamnionitis is diagnosed, fetal and maternal morbidity increases and delivery is indicated regardless of the fetus's gestational age. In the case described, antibiotics need to be administered to avoid neonatal sepsis. Ampicillin is the drug of choice to treat group B streptococcal infection. Since the fetal heart rate is reactive, there is no indication for cesarean section. Augmentation with Pitocin should be instituted as indicated. There is no role for tocolysis in the setting of chorioamnionitis, since delivery is the goal. There is also no role for the administration of steroids since delivery is imminent. In addition, steroids are only indicated at 32 weeks gestational age or less with PROM. A cerclage (cervical stitch) would be placed in a previable pregnancy where an incompetent cervix is diagnosed in the absence of ruptured membranes.

2-16. The answer is a. (*Behrman, 16/e, p 1279, McMillan, 3/e, p 1309, Rudolph, 21/e, p 1944.*) Bacterial tracheitis is an uncommon but severe and life-threatening sequella of a viral laryngotracheobronchitis. The typical story is that presented in the case, with several days of viral upper respiratory symptoms, followed by an acute elevation of temperature and an increase in respiratory distress. Children may also present acutely and without the initial viral symptoms. The differential must include epiglottitis; the lack of drooling and dysphagia help make this a case of tracheitis. Management includes establishing an airway with endotracheal intubation and IV antibiotics. Special attention is focused on preservation of the airway, as even intubated children with tracheitis can have secretions thick and copious enough to occlude the airway.

2-17. The answer is a. (*Behrman, 16/e, pp 946–953, 964–966, 984–986, 1989–1990. McMillan, 3/e, pp 721–722, 1098–1100, 1124–1125, 1134–1140. Rudolph, 21/e, pp 1039–1040, 1053–1056, 1058–1059, 1075–1079, 1195–1197.*) Symptoms of rubella, usually a mild disease, include a diffuse maculopapular rash that lasts for 3 days, marked enlargement of the posterior cervical and occipital lymph nodes, low-grade fever, mild sore throat, and, occasionally, conjunctivitis, arthralgia, or arthritis. Persons with rubeola develop a severe cough, coryza, photophobia, conjunctivitis, and a high fever that reaches its peak at the height of the generalized macular rash, which typically lasts for 5 days. Koplik spots on the buccal mucosa are diagnostic. Roseola is a viral exanthem of infants, in which the high fever abruptly abates as a rash appears. Erythema infectiosum (fifth disease) begins with bright erythema on the cheeks ("slapped cheek" sign), followed by a red maculopapular rash on the trunk and extremities, which fades centrally at first. Erythema multiforme is a poorly understood syndrome consisting of skin lesions and involvement of mucous membranes. A number of infectious agents and drugs have been associated with this syndrome.

2-18. The answer is c. (*Harrison's Online.*) Acute arsenic poisoning from ingestion results in increased permeability of small blood vessels and inflammation and necrosis of the intestinal mucosa; these changes manifest as hemorrhagic gastroenteritis, fluid loss, and hypotension. Symptoms include nausea, vomiting, diarrhea, abdominal pain, delirium, coma, and seizures. A garlicky odor may be detectable on the breath. Arsenic is found in herbal and homeopathic remedies, insecticides, rodenticides, and wood preservatives, and it has a variety of other industrial applications.

2-19. The answer is c. (*Sabiston, 15/e, pp 269–270.*) Necrotizing skin and soft tissue infections may produce insoluble gases (hydrogen, nitrogen, methane) through anaerobic bacterial metabolism. While the term "gas gangrene" has come to imply clostridial infection, gas in tissues is more likely not to be due to *Clostridium* species but rather to other facultative and obligate anaerobes, particularly streptococci. Though fungi have also been implicated, they are less often associated with rapidly progressive infections. Treatment for necrotizing soft tissue infections includes repeated wide debridement, with wound reconstruction delayed until a stable, viable wound surface has been established. The use of hyperbaric oxygen in the treatment of gas gangrene remains controversial, due to lack of proven benefit, difficulty in transporting critically ill patients to hyperbaric facilities, and the risk of complications. Antitoxin has neither a prophylactic nor a therapeutic role in the treatment of myonecrosis.

2-20. The answer is b. (*Braunwald, 15/e, pp 605–608.*) Renal carcinoma is twice as common in men as women and tends to occur in the 50- to 70-year age group. Many patients present with a hematuria or flank pain, but the classic triad of hematuria, flank pain, and a palpable flank mass occurs in only 10 to 20% of patients. Paraneoplastic syndromes such as erythrocytosis, hypercalcemia, hepatic dysfunction, and fever of unknown origin are common. Surgery is the only potentially curable therapy; the results of treatment with chemotherapy or radiation therapy for nonresectable disease have been disappointing. Interferon α and interleukin 2 produce responses (but no cures) in 10 to 20% of patients. The prognosis for metastatic renal cell carcinoma is dismal.

2-21. The answer is d. (*Schwartz, 7/e, pp 97–98.*) Most transfusion reactions are hemolytic and are due to clerical errors that result in administration of blood with major (ABO) and minor antigen incompatibility. Interestingly, Rh incompatibility is not associated with intravascular hemolysis. Administration of blood through hypotonic solutions such as 5% dextrose and water results in swelling of the erythrocytes and hemolysis. Calcium-containing solutions such as Ringer's lactate cause clotting within the intravenous line rather than hemolysis and may lead to pulmonary embolism. Delayed transfusion reactions, caused by a presumed anamnestic immune response that occurs 3 to 21 days after blood is infused, result in a hemolytic anemia.

2-22. The answer is e. (*Greenberg, 2/e, p 601.*) All of these disturbances will produce intracranial calcifications in some cases. The calcifications in Sturge-Weber syndrome follow the gyral pattern of the cerebral cortex and consequently produce the railroad track pattern that is evident on plain x-ray of the skull. Calcium is deposited in the brain of the patient with Sturge-Weber syndrome, presumably because the abnormal vessels overlying the brain allow calcium, as well as iron, across the defective blood-brain barrier. Craniopharyngioma and acoustic schwannoma produce calcifications, but these are obviously outside the cerebral cortex.

2-23. The answer is e. (*Cunningham, 21/e, pp 428–429.*) This patient is either experiencing prolonged latent labor or is in false labor. The latent phase of labor begins with the onset of regular uterine contractions and is accompanied by progressive but slow cervical dilation. The latent phase ends when the cervical dilation rate reaches about 1.2 cm/h in nulliparous patients and 1.5 cm/h in multiparous patients; this normally occurs when the cervix is about 3 to 4 cm dilated. In nulliparous patients, the latent phase of labor usually lasts less than 20 h (in multiparous patients, it lasts less than 14 h.) To correct prolonged latent labor, it is generally recommended that a strong sedative such as morphine be administered to the patient. This is preferred over augmentation with Pitocin or performing an amniotomy, because 10% of patients will actually have been in false labor and these patients will stop contracting after administration of morphine. If a patient truly is in labor, then, after the sedative wears off, she will have undergone cervical change and will have benefited from the rest in terms of having additional energy to proceed with labor. An epidural would not be recommended because the patient may be in false labor. There is no role for cervical ripening in this patient because of the fact that she might be in false labor and can go home and wait for natural cervical ripening if her uterine contractions resolve with a therapeutic rest with morphine.

2-24. The answers are 393-c, 394-a. *(Behrman, 16/e, pp 1520–1522. McMillan, 3/e, pp 367, 1477–1479. Rudolph, 21/e, pp 1556–1557.)* In children, idiopathic or immune thrombocytopenic purpura (ITP) is the most common form of thrombocytopenic purpura. In most cases a preceding viral infection can be noted. No diagnostic test exists for this disease; exclusion of the other diseases listed in the question is necessary. In this disease, the platelet count is frequently less than 20,000/μL, but other laboratory tests yield essentially normal results, including the bone marrow aspiration (if done). For ITP, platelets are sequestered and destroyed at the spleen by the reticuloendothelial system (RES) that binds self-immunoglobulins attached to the platelet. Exogenous IV gamma globulin can work to saturate the RES binding sites for platelet-bound self-immunoglobulin. Thus, there is less platelet uptake and destruction by the spleen.

Aplastic anemia is unlikely if the other cell lines are normal. Von Willebrand disease might be expected to present with bleeding and not just bruising. It is unlikely that acute leukemia would present with thrombocytopenia only. Thrombotic thrombocytopenic purpura is rare in children. Treatment for ITP consists of observation and/or gamma globulin and steroids. Splenectomy is reserved for the most severe and chronic forms.

2-25. The answer is a. *(Braunwald, 15/e, p 1428.)* The most common cause of refractory hypertension is nonadherence to the medication regimen. A history from the patient is useful, and pill count is the best compliance check. Cushing's disease, coarctation of the aorta, renal artery stenosis, and primary aldosteronism are secondary causes that could result in refractory hypertension, but no clues to these diagnoses are apparent on physical exam or lab.

2-26. The answer is b. *(Braunwald, 15/e, p 1513.)* Classifying a pleural effusion as either a transudate or an exudate is useful in identifying the underlying disorder. Pleural fluid is exudative if it has any one of the following three properties: a ratio of concentration of total protein in pleural fluid to serum greater than 0.5, an absolute value of LDH greater than 200 IU, or a ratio of LDH concentration in pleural fluid to serum greater than 0.6. Causes of exudative effusions include malignancy, pulmonary embolism, pneumonia, tuberculosis, abdominal disease, collagen vascular diseases, uremia, Dressler syndrome, and chylothorax. Exudative effusions may also be drug-induced. If none of the aforementioned properties are met, the effusion is a transudate. Differential diagnosis includes congestive heart failure, nephrotic syndrome, cirrhosis, Meigs syndrome (benign ovarian neoplasm with effusion), and hydronephrosis.

2-27. The answer is e. (*Victor, pp 658–660, 684–686.*) The headache is typical of that caused by intracranial hypertension. Additionally, the patient has focal neurological symptoms and signs. This creates particular concern about a brain tumor or hemorrhage, and the patient should be evaluated as soon as possible. An appointment next month is too late. Intravenous prochlorperazine is a good treatment for status migrainosus; however, this history is atypical for such a diagnosis and more serious problems should be ruled out first in the emergency room. Zolmitriptan is a treatment for migraines. This history is not typical for migraine, and zolmitriptan is also relatively contraindicated in patients with complex migraine. This history is very atypical for seizures, and an electroencephalogram is not likely to provide useful information in this case.

2-28. The answer is c. (*Schwartz, 7/e, pp 462–465.*) There are several recommended interventions in cardiac patients who are undergoing noncardiac surgery. The two factors that correlate best with postoperative life-threatening or fatal cardiac complications are myocardial infarction (transmural or subendocardial) and uncontrolled congestive heart failure. Therefore, delay of elective surgery for 6 months after myocardial infarction and preoperative control of congestive heart failure with diuretics and digitalis in severe cases will have the greatest effect in decreasing the risks of surgery. A patient's cardiac medications should be continued preoperatively, including during the morning of surgery, to maintain adequate therapeutic levels. This is especially true for beta blockers, which can manifest withdrawal rebound hypertension and tachycardia approximately 24 h after discontinuation. Patients with prosthetic valves or valvular heart disease should be given prophylactic antibiotics to prevent seeding of their valves during episodes of significant bacteremia. This most commonly occurs during gastrointestinal or genitourinary procedures. Ampicillin and gentamicin cover the flora frequently encountered, including enterococci and gram-negative organisms.

2-29. The answers are 201-a, 202-d. *(Behrman, 16/e, pp 1285–1287. McMillan, 3/e, pp 1214–1216. Rudolph, 21/e, pp 1984–1985.)* Of the choices given, bronchiolitis is the most likely, although asthma, pertussis, and bronchopneumonia can present similarly. The family history of upper respiratory infections, the previous upper respiratory illness in the patient, and signs of intrathoracic airway obstruction make the diagnosis of bronchiolitis more likely. Viral croup, epiglottitis, and diphtheria are not reasonable choices because there are no signs of extrathoracic airway obstruction.

The most likely cause of the illness is infection by respiratory syncytial virus, which causes outbreaks of bronchiolitis of varying severity, usually in the winter and spring. Other viruses, such as parainfluenza and the adenoviruses, have also been implicated in producing bronchiolitis. Treatment is usually supportive in this usually self-limited condition.

2-30. The answer is c. *(Braunwald, 15/e, p 896.)* In the treatment of hospital-acquired staphylococcal pneumonia, the incidence of methicillin-resistant staph in the local facility will be very important. In most hospitals, methicillin-resistant staph is common enough to require initial therapy with vancomycin. Oxacillin would be the drug of choice only if the incidence of methicillin-resistant staph is very low. Quinolones are often useful in the treatment of community-acquired pneumonia, but they would not be effective against methicillin-resistant staph.

2-31. The answer is c. *(Schwartz, 7/e, p 64.)* Hypocalcemia is associated with a prolonged QT interval and may be aggravated by both hypomagnesemia and alkalosis. Serum calcium levels below 7.0 mg/dL, encountered most frequently following parathyroid or thyroid surgery or in patients with acute pancreatitis, should be treated with intravenous calcium gluconate or lactate. The myocardium is very sensitive to calcium levels; therefore calcium is considered a positive inotropic agent. Calcium increases the contractile strength of cardiac muscle as well as the velocity of shortening. In its absence, the efficiency of the myocardium decreases. Hypocalcemia often occurs with hypoproteinemia even though the ionized serum calcium fraction remains normal.

2-32. The answer is c. *(Victor, p 231.)* Ipsilateral optic atrophy and contralateral papilledema in association with an intracranial tumor constitute the Foster-Kennedy syndrome. A meningioma of the olfactory groove may produce this syndrome if it extends posteriorly to involve the ipsilateral optic nerve. Compression on the optic nerve by the tumor produces atrophy and interferes with transmission of the increased intracranial pressure down the optic sheath. The increased intracranial pressure is reflected in the papilledema apparent in the contralateral eye.

2-33. The answer is c. *(Cunningham, 21/e, pp 404–406. Beckmann, 2/e, pp 409–410, 571.)* The uterus achieves its previous nonpregnant size by about 4 weeks postpartum. Subinvolution (cessation of the normal involution) of the uterus can occur in cases of retained placenta or uterine infection. In such cases, the uterus is larger and softer than it should be on bimanual exam. In addition, the patient usually experiences prolonged discharge and excessive uterine bleeding. With endometritis, the patient will also have a tender uterus on exam, and will complain of fever and chills. In adenomyosis, portions of the endometrial lining grow into the myometrium, causing menorrhagia and dysmenorrhea. On physical exam, the uterus is usually tender to palpation, boggy, and symmetrically enlarged. The patient described here has a physical exam most consistent with fibroids. Uterine leiomyomas would cause the uterus to be firm, irregular, and enlarged.

2-34. The answer is c. *(Braunwald, 15/e, pp 2095–2096.)* The patient has diastolic hypertension with associated hypokalemia. She is not taking diuretics. There is no edema on physical exam. Excessive inappropriate aldosterone production will produce a hypertension with hypokalemia syndrome. Hypersecretion of aldosterone increases distal tubular exchange of sodium for potassium with progressive depletion of body potassium. The hypertension is due to increased sodium absorption. Very low plasma renin that fails to increase with appropriate stimulus (such as volume depletion) and hypersecretion of aldosterone suggest the diagnosis of primary hyperaldosteronism. Suppressed renin activity occurs in about 25% of hypertensive patients with essential hypertension. Lack of suppression of aldosterone is also necessary to diagnose primary aldosteronism. High aldosterone levels that are not suppressed by saline loading prove that there is a primary inappropriate secretion of aldosterone. A 24-h urine for free cortisol would be used in the workup of a patient with Cushing syndrome. Urinary metanephrine is a screening test for pheochromocytoma.

2-35. The answer is a. *(Braunwald, 15/e, pp 2524–2528.)* Polymyositis is an acquired myopathy characterized by subacute symmetrical weakness of proximal limb and trunk muscles that progresses over several weeks or months. When a characteristic skin rash occurs, the disease is known as dermatomyositis. In addition to progressive proximal limb weakness, the patient often presents with dysphagia and neck muscle weakness. Up to half of cases with polymyositis-dermatomyositis may have, in addition, features of connective tissue diseases (rheumatoid arthritis, lupus erythematosus, scleroderma, Sjögren syndrome). Laboratory findings include an elevated serum CK level, an EMG showing myopathic potentials with fibrillations, and a muscle biopsy showing necrotic muscle fibers and inflammatory infiltrates. Polymyositis is clinically distinguished from the muscular dystrophies by its less prolonged course and lack of family history. It is distinguished from myasthenia gravis by its lack of ocular muscle involvement, absence of variability in strength over hours or days, and lack of response to cholinesterase inhibitor drugs.

2-36. The answer is e. *(Kaplan, 8/e, pp 573–578.)* Dysthymia is defined as a chronic depression that lasts at least 2 years. Usually, it begins in late adolescence or early adulthood, and sometimes patients describe being depressed for as long as they can remember. Symptoms fluctuate but are usually not severe. Patients tend to have low self-esteem and perceive themselves as inadequate and inferior to others. The somatic symptoms characteristic of major depression or melancholia are less prominent in dysthymia.

2-37. The answer is b. *(Greenfield, 2/e, pp 919–923.)* Tumors arising from the pancreatic β cells give rise to hyperinsulinism. Seventy-five percent of these tumors are benign adenomas, and in 15% of affected patients the adenomas are multiple. Symptoms relate to a rapidly falling blood glucose level and are due to epinephrine release triggered by hypoglycemia (sweating, weakness, tachycardia). Cerebral symptoms of headache, confusion, visual disturbances, convulsions, and coma are due to glucose deprivation of the brain. Whipple's triad summarizes the clinical findings in patients with insulinomas: (1) attacks precipitated by fasting or exertion; (2) fasting blood glucose concentrations below 50 mg/dL; (3) symptoms relieved by oral or intravenous glucose administration. These tumors are treated surgically and simple excision of an adenoma is curative in the majority of cases.

2-38. The answer is c. *(ACOG, Practice Bulletin 6.)* Immune thrombocytopenic purpura (ITP) typically occurs in the second or third decade of life and is more common in women than in men. The diagnosis of ITP is one of exclusion, because there are no pathognomonic signs, symptoms, or diagnostic tests. Traditionally, ITP is associated with a persistent platelet count of less than 100,000 in the absence of splenomegaly. Most women have a history of easy bruising and nose and gum bleeds that precede pregnancy. If the platelet count is maintained above 20,000, hemorrhagic episodes rarely occur. In cases of ITP, the patient produces IgG antiplatelet antibodies that increase platelet consumption in the spleen and in other sites. Gestational thrombocytopenia occurs in up to 8% of pregnancies. Affected women are usually asymptomatic, have no prior history of bleeding, and usually maintain platelet counts above 70,000. In gestational thrombocytopenia, platelet counts usually return to normal in about 3 months. The cause of gestational thrombocytopenia has not been clearly elucidated. Antiplatelet antibodies are often detected in women with gestational thrombocytopenia. HELLP syndrome of severe preeclampsia is associated with thrombocytopenia, but this condition occurs in the third trimester and is associated with hypertension. In neonatal alloimmune thrombocytopenia, there is a maternal alloimmunization to fetal platelet antigens. The mother is healthy and has a normal platelet count, but produces antibodies that cross the placenta and destroy fetal/neonatal platelets.

2-39. The answer is d. (*Tierney, 42/e, p 1012.*) The patient has no risk factors for coronary artery disease, such as family history or tobacco or cocaine use, and her ECG is normal. Hyperthyroidism is unlikely without tachycardia and other physical examination findings. A click and murmur are often found on heart auscultation in patients with MVP. The patient has no previous traumatic event in her life to have caused PTSD. The patient has symptomatology consistent with panic disorder. Four of five criteria are needed for the diagnosis of panic disorder: **PANIC** = **P**alpitations; **A**bdominal pain; **N**ausea; **I**ncreased perspiration; and **C**hest pain, **C**hills, or **C**hoking.

2-40. The answer is d. (*Behrman, 16/e, pp 1911–1914. McMillan, 3/e, pp 668–669. Rudolph, 21/e, p 2370.*) The time of onset of symptoms is somewhat helpful in the diagnosis of ophthalmia neonatorum. Chemical conjunctivitis is a self-limited condition that presents within 6 to 12 h of birth as a consequence of silver nitrate or erythromycin prophylaxis. Silver nitrate is no longer made for ocular prophylaxis in the United States. Gonococcal conjunctivitis has its onset within 2 to 5 days after birth and is the most serious of the bacterial infections. Prompt and aggressive topical treatment and systemic antibiotics are indicated to prevent serious complications such as corneal ulceration, perforation, and resulting blindness. Parents should be treated to avoid the risk to the child of reinfection. Silver nitrate is believed by some to be ineffective prophylaxis against chlamydial conjunctivitis, which occurs 5 to 14 days after birth. To avoid the risk of chlamydial pneumonia, treatment with systemic antibiotics is indicated for the infant as well as both parents in cases of chlamydial conjunctivitis.

2-41. The answer is c. (*Ebert, pp 472–474.*) Schizotypal personality disorder, a cluster A disorder, is characterized by acute discomfort in close relationships, cognitive and perceptual distortions, and eccentric behavior beginning in early adulthood and present in a variety of contexts. Individuals with schizoid personality disorder do not present with the magical thinking, oddity, unusual perceptions, and odd appearance typical of schizotypal individuals. In schizophrenia, psychotic symptoms are much more prolonged and severe. Avoidant individuals avoid social interaction out of shyness and fear of rejection and not out of disinterest or suspiciousness. In autism, social interactions are more severely impaired and stereotyped behaviors are usually present.

2-42. The answer is e. (*Victor, pp 265–266.*) Tunnel vision must be distinguished from concentric constriction. In the latter, the area perceived enlarges as the test screen is moved farther away from the patient, but the overall visual field is always smaller than the normal visual field. Concentric constriction associated with optic atrophy may develop with neurosyphilis. Tunnel vision, on the other hand, is characterized by the patient reporting the same size field even as the test screen is removed further away. Tunnel vision is not a physiologic pattern of visual loss, and should suggest either conversion disorder or malingering. Significant spiraling of the visual field, in which repeat testing of the same part of the visual field during the same examination leads to a successively smaller field each time, similarly may reflect conversion or malingering, although stress or panic may lead to mild effects of this sort.

2-43. The answers are 183-c, 184-b. (*Behrman, 16/e, pp 725–727. McMillan, 3/e, pp 924–932. Rudolph, 21/e, pp 844–845.*) Many conditions can be associated with prolonged fever, a limp caused by arthralgia, exanthem, adenopathy, and pharyngitis. Conjunctivitis, however, is suggestive of Kawasaki disease. The fissured lips, although common in Kawasaki disease, could occur after a long period of fever from any cause if the child became dehydrated. The predominance of neutrophils and high sedimentation rate are common to all. An increase in platelets within this constellation of symptoms, however, is found only in Kawasaki disease. Kawasaki disease presents a picture of prolonged fever, rash, epidermal peeling on the hands and feet (especially around the fingertips), conjunctivitis, lymphadenopathy, fissured lips, oropharyngeal mucosal erythema, and arthralgia or arthritis. The diagnosis is still possible in the absence of one or two of these physical findings. Coronary artery aneurysms can develop, as can aneurysms in other areas.

Initial treatment is typically IVIG and high-dose aspirin. The child will usually defervesce shortly after the infusion. Aspirin is typically kept at a higher dose until the platelet count begins to decrease, and then is continued at a lower dose for several weeks. While bacterial infection is in the differential diagnosis for this patient's presentation and blood cultures are usually part of the evaluation, intravenous vancomycin should be reserved for a culture-proven susceptible organism resistant to other antibiotics, or as emperic therapy in a critically ill patient.

2-44. The answer is c. (*Gaster, pp 152–156.*) The patient is attempting to self-treat her depressive symptoms with St. John's wort, which has been reported to interact with certain prescription medications, including digoxin. St. John's wort may lower levels of digoxin by 25%. Another interaction that could be important in this case is bleeding, which has been reported in patients taking warfarin and Ginkgo biloba.

2-45. The answer is b. (*Schwartz, 7/e, pp 1744–1745, 1810–1811.*) By the second year, a testicle not in the cooler environment of the scrotal sac will begin to undergo histologic changes characterized by reduced spermatogonia. Testicles left longer in the undescended state not only have a higher incidence of malignant degeneration, but are inaccessible for examination. If a malignancy should occur, diagnosis will be delayed. There is also a substantial psychological burden when children reach school age or are otherwise subjected to exposure of their deformed genitalia. Gel-filled prostheses are generally inserted when a testicle cannot be placed in the scrotum. Close follow-up by a physician until the late teens is indicated in all patients who have had an undescended testicle. Since these patients may be at increased risk for malignancy throughout life, careful training should be given in self-examination.

2-46. The answer is a. (*Kaplan, 8/e, p 821.*) Multi-infarct dementia results from the cumulative effects of multiple small- and large-vessel occlusions in cortical and subcortical regions. Most cases are caused by hypertensive cerebrovascular disease and thrombo-occlusive disease. It is the second most common cause of dementia in the elderly, accounting for 8 to 35% of the cases. Clinically, it is characterized by memory and cognitive deficits accompanied by focal neurologic signs (muscle weakness, spasticity, dysarthria, extensor plantar reflex, etc.). Unlike Alzheimer's disease, multi-infarct dementia is characterized by sudden onset and a stepwise progression.

2-47. The answer is b. (*Braunwald, 15/e, p 300.*) The symptoms of masculinization (e.g., alopecia, deepening of voice, clitoral hypertrophy) in the patient presented in the question are characteristic of active androgen-producing tumors. Such extreme virilization is very rarely observed in polycystic ovary syndrome or in Cushing syndrome; moreover, the presence of normal cortisol and markedly elevated plasma testosterone levels indicates an ovarian rather than adrenal cause of the findings. Arrhenoblastomas are the most common androgen-producing ovarian tumors. Their incidence is highest during the reproductive years. Composed of varying proportions of Leydig's and Sertoli cells, they are generally benign. In contrast to arrhenoblastomas, granulosa-theca cell tumors produce feminization, not virilization.

2-48. The answer is b. (*Rowland, p 646.*) More than 10% of patients with Friedreich's disease develop diabetes mellitus. A more life-threatening complication of this degenerative disease is the disturbance of the cardiac conduction system that often develops. Visual problems occur with the hyperglycemia of uncontrolled diabetes mellitus, but even Friedreich's patients without diabetes develop optic atrophy late in the course of the degenerative disease.

2-49. The answer is b. (*Behrman, 16/e, pp 1636–1637. McMillan, 3/e, pp 1549–1551. Rudolph, 21/e, p 1737.*) The constellation of findings described points to posterior urethral valves. The clinical picture may range from that described in the question to severe renal obstruction with renal failure and pulmonary hypoplasia. Urinary tract infections are common complications in older children, and sepsis can occasionally be the presenting sign in afflicted newborns. Despite early recognition and correction of the obstruction, the prognosis for normal renal function is guarded. Prenatal diagnosis is often accomplished secondary to ultrasound diagnosis.

2-50. The answer is d. (*Cunningham, 20/e, pp 746–754.*) The patient described in the question presents with a classic history for abruption—that is, the sudden onset of abdominal pain accompanied by bleeding. Physical examination reveals a firm, tender uterus with frequent contractions, which confirms the diagnosis. The fact that a clot forms within 4 min suggests that coagulopathy is not present. Because abruption is often accompanied by hemorrhaging, it is important that appropriate fluids (i.e., lactated Ringer solution and whole blood) be administered immediately to stabilize the mother's circulation. Cesarean section may be necessary in the case of a severe abruption, but only when fetal distress is evident or delivery is unlikely to be accomplished vaginally. Internal monitoring equipment should provide an early warning that the fetus is compromised. The internal uterine catheter provides pressure recordings, which are important if oxytocin stimulation is necessary. Generally, however, patients with abruptio placentae are contracting vigorously and do not need oxytocin.

BLOCK 3

Answers

3-1. The answer is d. (*Ebert, p 475.*) Individuals with borderline personality disorder characteristically form intense but very unstable relationships. Since they tend to perceive themselves and others as either totally bad or perfectly good, borderline individuals either idealize or devalue any person who occupies a significant place in their lives. Usually these perceptions do not last, and the person idealized one day can be seen as completely negative the next day.

3-2. The answer is e. (*Kaplan, 8/e, p 956.*) The boy in the question experienced an acute dystonic reaction, an adverse effect of neuroleptic medications secondary to blockage of dopamine receptors in the nigrostriatal system. Dystonic reactions are sustained spasmodic contractions of the muscles of the neck, trunk, tongue, face, and extraocular muscles. They can be quite painful and frightening. They usually occur within hours to 3 days after the beginning of the treatment and are more frequent in males and young people. They are also usually associated with high-potency neuroleptics. Occasionally, dystonic reactions are seen in young people who have ingested a neuroleptic medication, mistaking it for a drug of abuse. Administration of anticholinergic drugs provides rapid treatment of acute dystonia.

3-3. The answer is b. (*Fitzpatrick, 4/e, p 675.*) The rash described is **erythema migrans (EM)**, the early pathognomonic eruption of Lyme disease, a spirochetal infection transmitted to humans by the bite of an infected ixodid deer tick. Most cases in the United States involve the northeast or north central areas of the country. The rash typically occurs 1 to 2 weeks after the bite, but less than 20% of patients recall a bite. *R. rickettsii*, transmitted by dog or wood ticks, is the etiologic agent of **Rocky Mountain spotted fever.** The characteristic maculopapular rash begins peripherally and often involves the palms and soles. *B. henselae* (formerly *Rochalimaea henselae*) is the etiologic agent responsible for **cat-scratch disease (CSD)**. *M. marinum* infections follow a traumatic inoculation in aquariums and swimming pools. The bite of the **brown recluse spider** (*Loxosceles*) begins as an area of erythema. In some cases, the bite progresses to become a painful bulla and deep necrotic ulcer.

3-4. The answer is b. *(Cunningham, 21/e, pp 242–243.)* Lower back pain is a common symptom of pregnancy and is reported by about 50% of pregnant women. It is caused by stress placed on the lower spine and associated muscles and ligaments by the gravid uterus, especially in late pregnancy. The pain can be exacerbated with excessive bending and lifting. In addition, obesity predisposes the patient to lower back pain in pregnancy. Treatment options include heat, massage, and analgesia. This patient has no evidence of labor since she is lacking regular uterine contractions and cervical change. Without any urinary symptoms or a urinalysis suggestive of infection, cystitis is unlikely. The diagnosis of chorioamnionitis does not fit since the patient has intact membranes, no fever, and a nontender uterus. Round ligament pain is characterized by sharp groin pain.

3-5. The answer is e. *(Victor, p 296.)* Sympathetic innervation of the iris is required for the change in the color of the iris to occur after birth and infancy. Congenital Horner syndrome, which may be inherited as an autosomal dominant trait, is characterized by failure of one eye to develop normal iris color (heterochromia iridis). Any injury to the eye after this early developmental period would not be expected to leave a difference in eye color from one side to the other.

3-6. The answer is a. *(Schwartz, 7/e, p 63.)* The electrocardiogram demonstrates changes that are essentially diagnostic of severe hyperkalemia. Correct treatment for the affected patient includes administration of a source of calcium ions (which will immediately oppose the neuromuscular effect of potassium) and administration of sodium ions (which, by producing a mild alkalosis, will shift potassium into cells); each will temporarily reduce serum potassium concentration. Infusion of glucose and insulin would also effect a temporary transcellular shift of potassium. However, these maneuvers are only temporarily effective; definitive treatment calls for removal of potassium from the body. The sodium-potassium exchange resin sodium polystyrene sulfonate (Kayexalate) would accomplish this removal, but over a period of hours and at the price of adding a sodium ion for each potassium ion that is removed. Hemodialysis or peritoneal dialysis is probably required for this patient, since these procedures also rectify the other consequences of acute renal failure, but they would not be the first line of therapy given the acute need to reduce the potassium level. Both lidocaine and digoxin would not only be ineffective but contraindicated, since they would further depress the myocardial conduction system.

3-7. The answer is a. *(Behrman, 16/e, pp 559–560. McMillan, 3/e, pp 810–812. Rudolph, 21/e, pp 501–503.)* The adolescent who has attempted suicide should be hospitalized so that a complete medical, psychological, and social evaluation can be performed and an appropriate treatment plan developed. Hospitalization also emphasizes the seriousness of the adolescent's action to her and to her family and the importance of cooperation in carrying out the recommendations for ongoing future therapy. The treatment plan may include continued counseling or supportive therapy with a pediatrician, outpatient psychotherapy with a psychiatrist or other mental health worker, or family therapy.

3-8. The answer is d. *(Seidel, 5/e, pp 295–297.)* Normal **intraocular pressure (IOP)** is in the range of 10 to 21.5 mmHg. IOP is determined by the outflow of aqueous humor from the eye; the greater the resistance to outflow, the higher the IOP. IOP is important in the diagnosis of glaucoma. A **Schiotz tonometer** is used to measure IOP. The **red reflex** represents the light reflected from the retina; it means that all of the light-transmitting media of the eye will be transparent and visible. Cataracts and retinal detachment obscure the presence of a red reflex. The **light reflex** is emitted from the retinal arterioles; their walls are transparent and the bright light occupies approximately 25% of the diameter of the arterial column of blood. Changes in the light reflex occur with hypertension or with aging (walls thicken and more light is reflected, resembling copper wires). **Cotton-wool spots** (these are misnamed soft exudates) are white, indistinct, opaque areas of the inner or superficial retina. They represent microinfarctions and are due to hypertension, diabetes mellitus, infections, collagen vascular diseases, AIDS, and severe anemia. **Hard exudates** are yellowish, well-demarcated, deep retinal lesions. They are the result of leaky and damaged vessels, not of microinfarcts; they are most commonly due to hypertension and diabetes. **Drusen bodies** are yellow, deep epithelial pigment deposits located in the macula; they are the earliest sign of macular degeneration. The optic cup is enlarged to >30% of the disc in glaucoma. **Retinal hemorrhages** are due to leaky and damaged retinal capillaries. Depending on their retinal layer location, they may be blot-and-dot (due to diabetes and hypertension), flame-and-splinter (due to intracranial hemorrhage, papilledema, and glaucoma), or white-centered (**Roth spots** seen in endocarditis, leukemia, and diabetes). **Microaneurysms** are outpouchings of the retinal capillaries and are almost always associated with diabetes mellitus. In **retinitis pigmentosa,** the fundi are covered with a bony spicule formation.

3-9. The answer is c. (*Schwartz, 7/e, pp 1452–1454.*) The development of acute postoperative cholecystitis is an increasingly recognized complication of the severe illnesses that precipitate admissions to the intensive care unit. The causes are obscure but probably lead to a common final pathway of gallbladder ischemia. The diagnosis is often extremely difficult because the signs and symptoms may be those of occult sepsis. Moreover, the patients are often intubated, sedated, or confused as a consequence of the other therapeutic or medical factors. Biochemical tests, though frequently revealing abnormal liver function, are nonspecific and nondiagnostic. Bedside ultrasonography is usually strongly suggestive of the diagnosis when a thickened gallbladder wall or pericholecystic fluid is present, but radiologic findings may also be nondiagnostic. If diagnosis is delayed, mortality and morbidity are very high. Percutaneous drainage of the gallbladder is usually curative of acalculous cholecystitis and affords stabilizing palliation if calculous cholecystitis is present. Some authors have recommended prophylactic percutaneous drainage of the gallbladder under CT guidance in any ICU patient who is failing to thrive or has other signs of low-grade sepsis after appropriate therapy for the primary illness has been provided. The other choices are all either too aggressive to be safely done in critically ill patients or too cautious for a patient with a potentially fatal complication.

3-10. The answer is d. (*Stoudemire, 3/e, p 579.*) Vocal tics such as grunting, barking, throat clearing, coprolalia (the repetitive speaking of vulgarities), and shouting and simple and complex motor tics are characteristic findings of Tourette's syndrome. Pharmacological treatment of this disorder includes neuroleptics and α_2 agonists (clonidine, guanfacine).

3-11. The answer is a. (*Victor, p 170.*) Hemisection of the spinal cord results in a contralateral loss of pain and thermal sensation due to spinothalamic damage, and ipsilateral loss of proprioception due to posterior column damage. There is also an ipsilateral motor paralysis due to destruction of the corticospinal and rubrospinal tracts as well as motor neurons. Complete transection of the spinal cord would cause a bilateral spastic paralysis, and there would be no conscious appreciation of any cutaneous or deep sensation in the area below the transection. Posterior column syndrome would result in a bilateral loss of proprioception below the lesion, with relative preservation of pain and temperature sensation. Syringomyelic syndrome results from a lesion of the central gray matter. Pain and temperature fibers that cross at the anterior commissure are affected, which may result in bilateral loss of these sensations over several dermatomes. However, tactile sensation is spared. The most common cause of this type of syndrome is syringomyelia. Trauma, hemorrhage, or tumors are other possible etiologies. If the lesion becomes large enough, then other spinal cord systems become affected as well. Tabetic syndrome results from damage to proprioceptive and other dorsal root fibers. It is classically caused by syphilis. Symptoms include paresthesias, pain, and abnormalities of gait. Vibration sense is most affected.

3-12. The answer is a. (*Braunwald, 15/e, pp 1692–1694.*) This patient meets the Rome criteria for irritable bowel syndrome. The major criterion is abdominal pain relieved with defecation and associated with change in stool frequency or consistency. In addition, these patients often complain of difficult stool passage, a feeling of incomplete evacuation, and mucus in the stool. In this young patient with long-standing symptoms and no evidence of organic disease on physical and laboratory studies, no further evaluation is necessary. Irritable bowel syndrome is a motility disorder associated with altered sensitivity to abdominal pain and distention. It is the commonest cause of chronic GI symptoms and is three times more common in women than in men. Associated lactose intolerance may cause similar symptoms and should be considered in all cases. Patients older than 40 years with new symptoms, weight loss, or positive family history of colon cancer should have further workup, usually with colonoscopy.

3-13. The answer is b. (*Kaplan, 8/e, pp 1294–1295.*) Pick's disease accounts for 2.5% of cases of dementia. Clinically it is distinguishable from Alzheimer's disease due to the prominence and early onset of personality changes, disinhibition or apathy, socially inappropriate behavior, mood changes (elation or depression), and psychotic symptoms. Language is affected early in the disease, but the memory loss, apraxia, and agnosia characteristic of Alzheimer's disease are not prominent until the late stages of the disorder. Temporofrontal atrophy, demyelination and gliosis of the frontal lobes, Pick bodies (intracellular inclusions), and Pick cells (swollen neurons) are the characteristic pathological findings.

3-14. The answer is c. (*Greenfield, 2/e, pp 284, 337.*) The finding of an air-fluid level in the left lower chest with a nasogastric tube entering it after blunt trauma to the abdomen is diagnostic of diaphragmatic rupture with gastric herniation into the chest. This lesion needs to be fixed immediately. With continuing negative pressure in the chest, each breath sucks more of the abdominal contents into the chest and increases the likelihood of vascular compromise of the herniated viscera. While the diaphragm is easily fixed from the left chest, this injury should be approached from the abdomen. The possibility of injury below the diaphragm after sufficient blunt injury to rupture the diaphragm mandates examination of the intraabdominal solid and hollow viscera; adequate exposure of the diaphragm to allow secure repair is possible from this approach.

3-15. The answer is d. (*Tierney, 42/e, p 217.*) The most common cause of **chronic cough** in adults is postnasal drip due to sinusitis or rhinitis (allergic, vasomotor, irritant, perennial nonallergic). Patients typically complain of having to clear the throat or a feeling of something dripping in the back of the throat. Physical examination reveals mucopurulent secretions and a cobblestone appearance of the mucosa. Asthma is more of an episodic disease with wheezing, but occasionally patients complain of only cough. Gastroesophageal reflux disease (GERD) must be considered in patients who complain of heartburn or regurgitation. Other causes of chronic cough include bronchitis, congestive heart failure, and use of angiotensin converting enzyme (ACE) inhibitors.

3-16. The answer is e. (*Behrman, 16/e, p 1679. McMillan, 3/e, pp 1775–1780. Rudolph, 21/e, p 2103.*) A record of the sequential pattern of growth in height is very helpful in the differential diagnosis of a child with short stature. A child with constitutionally short stature and delayed puberty will have a consistent rate of growth below but parallel to the average for his or her age, whereas patients with organic disease do not follow a given percentile but progressively deviate from their prior growth percentile. A knowledge of the patterns of growth and sexual maturation of family members is helpful because such patterns are often familial. Puberty is said to be delayed in males if physical changes are not apparent by 14 years of age. Identification of the earliest signs of sexual maturation by means of careful physical examination avoids unnecessary workup. In this case, measurement of pituitary gonadotropins is unnecessary because the child already shows evidence of pubertal development (a testicular length of more than 2.5 cm, volume 3.0 cm³). The single most useful laboratory test is the determination of bone age. In those of constitutionally short stature with delayed pubertal maturation, the bone age is equal to the height age, both of which are behind chronologic age. In familial short stature, bone age is greater than height age and equal to chronologic age. In a child at any age, the administration of human chorionic gonadotropin (hCG) will stimulate interstitial cells of testes to produce testosterone, thereby serving as a method of assessing testicular function. The finding of testicular enlargement is evidence of pituitary secretion of gonadotropins and of testicular responsiveness and obviates the need for administration of hCG. Elevated serum gonadotropins are found in children 12 years of age or older who have primary hypogonadism (Klinefelter syndrome, bilateral gonadal failure from trauma or infection). Because the secretion of gonadotropins is not constant but occurs in spurts, children with constitutional delay of puberty may have normal or low levels of gonadotropins.

3-17. The answer is c. *(Tierney, 42/e, pp 348–349.)* **Myocardial infarction** occurs when an atherosclerotic plaque ruptures or ulcerates. Patients having a myocardial infarction are typically anxious, restless, and uncomfortable secondary to the extreme pain. They may be demonstrating the **Levine sign** (clenching of the fist over sternum to demonstrate the severity of the pain). Risk factors for this patient include male gender, positive family history, hypertension, diabetes mellitus, tobacco use, and hyperlipidemia. ECG will show ST elevations, and cardiac isoenzymes (troponin, CPK-MB fraction, and LDH) will be elevated. Patients with **Prinzmetal's angina** have recurrent attacks of chest pain at rest or while asleep (unstable angina) due to a focal spasm of an epicardial coronary artery. The diagnosis is confirmed by detecting the spasm after provocation during coronary arteriography. **Cardiogenic shock** is a form of severe left ventricular heart failure; patients are typically hypotensive. Right ventricular infarction is a complication of inferoposterior myocardial infarction;

patients present with JVD, the **Kussmaul sign,** and hypotension. Diagnosis is made by a right-sided electrocardiogram in which the leads are placed to the right of the sternum instead of the left.

3-18. The answer is e. *(Bradley, p 1439.)* The test performed is usually called the swinging flashlight test, and the pupillary finding is a Marcus Gunn, or afferent pupillary, defect. It commonly develops in persons with MS as a sequela of optic neuritis. Damage to the optic nerve reduces the light perceived with the affected eye. If the other eye has less or no optic atrophy, the consensual response of the pupil to light perceived by the better eye will constrict the pupil in the atrophic eye, even though direct light to the injured eye does not elicit a strong pupillary constriction.

3-19. The answer is c. *(Braunwald, 15/e, pp 1995–1996.)* The acute monoarticular arthritis in association with linear calcification of the cartilage of the knee suggests the diagnosis of pseudogout, also called calcium pyrophosphate dihydrate deposition disease. The disease resembles gout. Positive birefringent crystals (looking blue when parallel to the axis of the red compensator on a polarizing microscope) can be demonstrated in joint fluid. Serum uric acid and calcium levels are normal, as is the rheumatoid factor. Pseudogout is about half as common as gout but becomes more common after age 65. Calcium pyrophosphate dihydrate deposition disease is diagnosed in symptomatic patients by characteristic x-ray findings or crystals in synovial fluid. The disease is treated with NSAIDs or colchicine. Linear calcifications or chondrocalcinosis are often found in the joints of elderly patients who do not have symptomatic joint problems; such patients do not require treatment.

3-20. The answer is b. *(Droegemueller, 3/e, pp 357–360. Beckmann, 4/e, pp 420–421.)* This patient's breast mass is characteristic of a fibroadenoma. Fibroadenomas are the second most common benign breast disorder, after fibrocystic changes. They are characterized by being firm, solid, nontender, and freely mobile. Fibroadenomas have an average size diameter of 2.5 cm and are well circumscribed. These lesions most commonly occur in adolescents and women in their twenties. Fibrocystic changes occur in about one-third to one-half of reproductive-age women and represent an exaggerated response of the breast tissue to hormones. Patients with fibrocystic changes complain of bilateral mastalgia and breast engorgement preceding menses.

On physical exam, diffuse bilateral nodularity is typically encountered. Cystosarcoma phyllodes are rare fibroepithelial tumors that constitute 1% of breast malignancies. These rapidly growing tumors are the most frequent breast sarcoma and occur most frequently in women in the fifth decade of life. Trauma to the breast can result in fat necrosis. Women with fat necrosis commonly present to the physician with a firm, tender mass that is surrounded by ecchymosis. Occasional skin retraction can occur, making this lesion difficult to differentiate from cancer. It is unlikely that this patient who presents in her twenties has breast cancer. Fine-needle aspiration or excisional biopsy must be performed to rule out the rare chance of malignancy, but breast cancer is not the most likely diagnosis based on the patient's age and lack of any other breast changes consistent with carcinoma (such as a fixed mass, skin retraction, or lymphadenopathy).

3-21. The answer is c. *(Kaplan, 8/e, p 821.)* Impaired naming, memory deterioration, poor calculation, poor judgment, and disinhibition are characteristic symptoms of Alzheimer's disease. This progressive dementia develops in all individuals with trisomy 21 (Down syndrome) who survive beyond 30 years. Neurofibrillary tangles, neuritic plaques, and loss of acetylcholine neurons in the nucleus basalis of Meynert—characteristic pathological changes of Alzheimer's disease—develop in patients with Down syndrome at a relatively young adult age.

3-22. The answer is a. *(Schwartz, 7/e, pp 688–689.)* Flail chest is diagnosed in the presence of paradoxical respiratory movement in a portion of the chest wall. At least two fractures in each of three adjacent rib or costal cartilages are required to produce this condition. Complications of flail chest include segmental pulmonary hypoventilation with subsequent infection and ultimately respiratory failure. Management of flail chest should be individualized. If adequate pain control and pulmonary toilet can be provided, patients may be managed without stabilization of the flail. Often, intercostal nerve blocks and tracheostomy aid in this form of management. If stabilization is required, external methods such as sandbags or towel clips are no longer used. Surgical stabilization with wires is used if thoracotomy is to be performed for another indication. If this is not the case, internal stabilization is performed by placing the patient on mechanical ventilation with positive end-expiratory pressure. Tracheostomy is recommended because these patients usually require 10 to 14 days to stabilize their flail segment and postventilation pulmonary toilet is simplified by tracheostomy. Indications for mechanical ventilation include significant impedance to ventilation by the flail segment, large pulmonary contusion, an uncooperative patient (e.g., owing to head injury), general anesthesia for another indication, more than five ribs fractured, and the development of respiratory failure.

3-23. The answer is e. *(Behrman, 16/e, pp 1829–1830. Rudolph, 21/e, p 2274.)* The child in this question most likely has breath-holding spells. Two forms exist. Cyanotic spells consist of the symptoms outlined and are predictable upon upsetting or scolding the child. They are rare before 6 months of age, peak at about 2 years of age, and resolve by about 5 years of age. Avoidance of reinforcing this behavior is the treatment of choice. Pallid breath-holding spells are less common and are usually caused by a painful experience (such as a fall). With these events, the child will stop breathing, lose consciousness, become pale and hypotonic, and may have a brief tonic episode. These, too, resolve spontaneously. Again, avoidance of reinforcing behavior is indicated.

3-24. The answer is d. *(Greenfield, 2/e, pp 578–581.)* The patient is experiencing an acute rejection episode. Seventy-four percent of all acute rejection episodes occur between 1 and 6 months after transplantation. For cadaveric renal transplant recipients, 63% of patients will never have an acute rejection episode, 17% will have only one rejection episode, and 19% will have two or more rejections. In order to grade the rejection as well as to follow the response to treatment, a percutaneous renal biopsy should be performed. The three treatment modalities used for acute rejection are high-dose steroids alone, high-dose steroids plus antilymphocyte globulin (equine serum hyperimmunized to human lymphocytes), or high-dose steroids plus OKT3 (murine monoclonal antibody to the human CD3 complex).

3-25. The answer is a. *(Kaplan, 8/e, p 819.)* Patients with hyperthyroidism complain of heat intolerance and excessive sweating, as well as diarrhea, weight loss, tachycardia, palpitations, and vomiting. Psychiatric complaints can include nervousness, excitability, irritability, pressured speech, insomnia, psychosis, and a fear of impending death or doom. Decreased concentration, hyperactivity, and a fine tremor may also be found.

3-26. The answer is c. *(Tintinalli, 5/e, pp 588–592.)* The patient most likely has **necrotizing pancreatitis,** which is a complication of acute pancreatitis. Other complications of pancreatitis include **pseudocyst, abscess,** and **phlegmon.** The periumbilical discoloration (**Cullen sign**) suggests a hemoperitoneum. Discoloration of the flanks would be a positive **Turner sign.** When the patient experiences pain as the hands of the examiner are abruptly withdrawn from the abdomen, he or she is said to have rebound tenderness (a sign of peritonitis). Decreased bowel sounds are another sign of peritonitis. Risk factors for acute pancreatitis include alcohol use, trauma, hyperlipidemia, gallstones, and medications. An abdominal radiograph in acute pancreatitis might show a **sentinel loop** (air-filled small intestine in the LUQ) and **colon cutoff sign** (air in the transverse colon). Patients with **chronic pancreatitis** present with bouts of abdominal pain and signs of pancreatic insufficiency (weight loss, steatorrhea, and diabetes). The abdominal radiograph in patients with chronic pancreatitis demonstrates calcifications in the pancreas (pathognomonic).

3-27. The answer is d. (*Ebert, p 138.*) Neuroleptic malignant syndrome (NMS) is a relatively rare but potentially fatal complication of neuroleptic treatment. Its main features are hyperthermia, severe muscular rigidity, autonomic instability, and changes in mental status. Associated findings are increased CPK, increased liver transaminase activity, leukocytes, and myoglobinuria. The mortality rate can be as high as 30% and can be higher when the syndrome is precipitated by depot forms. Neuroleptic malignant syndrome is more common in young males when high-potency neuroleptics are used in high doses and when dosage is escalated rapidly.

3-28. The answer is b. (*Cunningham, 21/e, pp 22–29.*) Nausea, fatigue, breast tenderness, and urinary frequency are all common symptoms of pregnancy, but their presence cannot definitively make the diagnosis of pregnancy because they are nonspecific symptoms that are not consistently found in early pregnancy. On physical exam, the pregnant uterus enlarges and becomes more boggy and soft, but these changes are not usually apparent until after 6 weeks gestational age. In addition, other conditions such as adenomyosis, fibroids, or previous pregnancies can result in an enlarged uterus being palpated on physical exam. Abdominal ultrasound will not demonstrate a gestational sac until a gestational age of 5 to 6 weeks is reached. A Doppler instrument will detect fetal cardiac action usually no sooner than 10 weeks. A sensitive serum pregnancy test can detect placental HCG levels by 8 to 9 days post-ovulation, and it is therefore the most sensitive modality for detecting and diagnosing pregnancy.

3-29. The answer is d. *(Tierney, 42/e, pp 1095–1096.)* Symptoms of **hypothyroidism** include constipation, depression, edema, tongue thickening, cold intolerance, Queen Anne sign (missing lateral one-third of eyebrows), muscle cramps, weight gain, goiter, amenorrhea, galactorrhea, pleural effusion, pericardial effusion, cardiomegaly, bradycardia, hypothermia, hyponatremia, anemia, and hypertension. Patients are said to have **hung-up** reflexes (a prolonged relaxation phase). Amiodarone has high iodine content and causes hypothyroidism in 8% of patients. **Myxedema** is a rare complication of hypothyroidism; patients present with coma, severe hypotension, hypothermia, hypoventilation, and hypoxemia. **Cretinism** is congenital (infantile) hypothyroidism.

3-30. The answer is c. *(Kaplan, 8/e, p 572.)* Sleep deprivation has an antidepressant effect in depressed patients and may trigger a manic episode in bipolar patients. The patient is not ill enough to require hospitalization. The use of a long-acting benzodiazepine will allow the patient to return to a normal sleep pattern and generally will abort the manic episode.

3-31. The answer is c. *(Sabiston, 15/e, pp 131–133.)* Whenever significant bleeding is noted in the early postoperative period, the presumption should always be that it is due to an error in surgical control of blood vessels in the operative field. Hematologic disorders that are not apparent during the long operation are most unlikely to surface as problems postoperatively. Blood transfusion reactions can cause diffuse loss of clot integrity; the sudden appearance of diffuse bleeding during an operation may be the only evidence of an intraoperative transfusion reaction. In the postoperative period, transfusion reactions usually present as unexplained fever, apprehension, and headache—all symptoms difficult to interpret in the early postoperative period. Factor VIII deficiency (hemophilia) would almost certainly be known by history in a 65-year-old man, but if not, intraoperative bleeding would have been a problem earlier in this long operation. Severely hypothermic patients will not be able to form clots effectively, but clot dissolution does not occur. Care should be taken to prevent the development of hypothermia during long operations through the use of warmed intravenous fluid, gas humidifiers, and insulated skin barriers.

3-32. The answer is b. *(Greenberg, 5/e, p 267.)* This history is typical of a simple partial seizure. A focal brain lesion must be ruled out. It would be wrong to discharge the patient to follow up in clinic in 2 weeks without at least a CT scan and preferably an MRI. Although he probably had a seizure, obtaining an electroencephalogram at this point will not be as helpful as an MRI. This is unlikely to be a peripheral nerve problem, and therefore an orthopedic consult or electromyography and nerve conduction studies are not indicated.

3-33. The answer is d. (*Scott, 8/e, pp 155–168.*) The photomicrograph shows villi within a tubular structure; the villi are easily identified by the presence of cytotrophoblasts. The diagnosis is tubal ectopic pregnancy. Molar pregnancy, incomplete abortion, and missed abortion can also be associated with the presence of villi, but specimens from these disorders would not be obtained at laparotomy.

3-34. The answer is b. (*Cunningham, 21/e, pp 1275–1276, 1283–1293.*) Acute fatty liver of pregnancy is a rare complication of pregnancy. Estimates of its incidence range from 1 in 7,000 to 1 in 15,000 pregnancies. This disorder is usually fatal for both mother and baby. Recently it has been suggested that recessively inherited mitochondrial abnormalities of fatty acid oxidation predispose a woman to fatty liver in pregnancy. This disorder usually manifests itself late in pregnancy and is more common in nulliparous women. Typically, a patient will present with a several-day or -week history of general malaise, anorexia, nausea, emesis, and jaundice. Liver enzymes are usually not elevated above 500. Indications of liver failure are present, manifested by elevated PT/PTT, bilirubin, and ammonia levels. In addition, there is marked hypoglycemia. Low fibrinogen and platelet levels occur secondary to a consumptive coagulopathy. In cases of viral hepatitis, serum transaminase levels are usually much higher and marked hypoglycemia or elevated serum ammonia levels would not be seen. Sometimes the HELLP syndrome can initially be difficult to differentiate from acute fatty liver, but in this case the patient has a normal blood pressure. In addition, hepatic failure is not characteristic of severe preeclampsia. Hyperemesis gravidarum is characterized by nausea and vomiting unresponsive to simple therapy. It usually occurs early in the first trimester and resolves by about 16 weeks. In some cases, there can be a transient hepatic dysfunction. Intrahepatic cholestasis of pregnancy is characterized by pruritus and/or icterus. Some women develop cholestasis in the third trimester secondary to estrogen-induced changes. There is an accumulation of serum bile salts, which causes the pruritus. Liver enzymes are seldom elevated above 250 U/L.

3-35. The answer is c. *(Ebert, pp 330–334.)* The patient in the question displays typical symptoms of recurrent panic attacks. Panic attacks can occur under a wide variety of psychiatric and medical conditions. The patient is diagnosed with panic disorder when there are recurrent episodes of panic and there is at least 1 month of persistent concern, worry, or behavioral change associated with the attacks. The attacks are not due to the direct effect of medical illness, medications, or substance abuse and are not better accounted for by another psychiatric disorder. While anxiety can be intense in generalized anxiety disorder, major depression, acute psychosis, and hypochondriasis, it does not have the typical presentation (i.e., a discrete episode or panic attack) described in the question.

3-36. The answer is b. *(Schwartz, 7/e, pp 1158–1161.)* Corrosive injuries of the esophagus most frequently occur in young children due to accidental ingestion of strong alkaline cleaning agents. Significant esophageal injury occurs in 15% of patients with no oropharyngeal injury, while 70% of patients with oropharyngeal injury have no esophageal damage. Signs of airway injury or imminent obstruction warrant close observation and possibly tracheostomy. The risk of adding injury, particularly in a child, makes esophagoscopy contraindicated in the opinion of most surgeons. Administration of oral antidotes is ineffective unless given within moments of ingestion; even then, the additional damage potentially caused by the chemical reactions of neutralization often makes use of them unwise. A barium esophagogram is usually done within 24 h unless evidence of perforation is present. In most reports, steroids in conjunction with antibiotics reduce the incidence of formation of strictures from about 70% to about 15%. Vomiting should be avoided, if possible, to prevent further corrosive injury and possible aspiration. It is probably wise to avoid all oral intake until the full extent of injury is ascertained.

3-37. The answer is d. *(Tierney, 42/e, pp 783–785.)* **Osteoarthritis** most often affects the weight-bearing joints and is associated with obesity or other forms of mechanical stress. It has no systemic manifestations. It is more common in women, and onset is usually after the age of 50. Pain often occurs on exertion and is relieved with rest, after which the joint may become stiff. Distal interphalangeal joints may be involved, with the production of **Heberden nodes**. **Bouchard nodes** are often found at the proximal interphalangeal joint. Crepitus (the sensation of bone rubbing against bone) is often felt on examination of the involved joint. **Rheumatoid arthritis** is a systemic disease of women under the age of 40. Joint involvement is usually symmetric, involving the proximal interphalangeal and metacarpophalangeal joints. Ninety-five percent of **gouty arthritis** occurs in men and often involves the great toe. Chondromalacia patellae or **chondromalacia** means softening of the cartilage. Patients present with anterior knee pain and tenderness over the undersurface of the patella. Pain is worse when sitting for long periods of time or when climbing stairs. **Psoriatic arthritis** is an asymmetric oligoarthritis that involves the knees, ankles, shoulders, or digits of the hands and feet and occurs in 50% of patients with psoriasis.

3-38. The answer is b. *(Behrman, 16/e, pp 272–273. McMillan, 3/e, pp 614–615. Rudolph, 21/e, pp 2246–2248.)* Compression of cranial nerve III and distortion of the brainstem, resulting in unilateral pupillary dilatation, hemiplegia, focal seizures, and depressed consciousness, suggest a progressively enlarging mass, most likely a subdural hematoma. Such a hematoma displaces the temporal lobe into the tentorial notch and presses on the ipsilateral cranial nerve III. Brainstem compression by this additional tissue mass leads to progressive deterioration in consciousness. Rising blood pressure and falling pulse rate are characteristic of increasing intracranial pressure. The most urgent test to diagnose this condition is a CT scan.

3-39. The answer is a. *(Behrman, 16/e, pp 1191–1193. McMillan, 3/e, pp 1711–1712. Rudolph, 21/e, pp 1466–1467.)* The causes of pancreatitis in children are varied, with about one-fourth of cases without predisposing etiology and about one-third of cases as a feature of another systemic disease. Traumatic cases are usually due to blunt trauma to the abdomen. Acute pancreatitis is difficult to diagnose; a high index of suspicion is necessary. Common clinical features include severe pain with nausea and vomiting. Tenderness, guarding or rebound pain, abdominal distention, and a paralytic ileus are signs and symptoms often seen. No diagnostic test is completely accurate. An elevated total serum amylase with the correct clinical history and signs and symptoms is the best diagnostic tool. Plain films of the abdomen exclude other diagnoses; ultrasonography of the pancreas can reveal enlargement of the pancreas, gallstones, cysts, and pseudocysts. Supportive care is indicated until the condition resolves.

3-40. The answer is b. (*Schwartz, 7/e, pp 1231–1232, 1387.*) Patients with regional enteritis usually have a chronic and slowly progressive course with intermittent symptom-free periods. The usual symptoms are anorexia, abdominal pain, diarrhea, fever, and weight loss. Extraintestinal syndromes that may be seen include ankylosing spondylitis; polyarthritis; erythema nodosum; pyoderma gangrenosum; gallstones; hepatic fatty infiltration; and fibrosis of the biliary tract, pancreas, and retroperitoneum. However, in about 10% of patients, especially those who are young, the onset of the disease is abrupt and may be mistaken for acute appendicitis. Appendectomy is indicated in such patients as long as the cecum at the base of the appendix is not involved; otherwise the risk of fecal fistula must be considered. Interestingly, about 90% of patients who present with the acute appendicitis-like form of regional enteritis will not progress to development of the full-blown chronic disease. Thus, resection or bypass of the involved areas is not indicated at this time.

3-41. The answer is a. (*Hankins, pp 273–279.*) If attached, the placenta is not removed until the infusion systems are operational, fluids are being given, and anesthesia (preferably halothane) has been administered. To remove the placenta before this time increases hemorrhage. As soon as the uterus is restored to its normal configuration, the anesthetic agent used to provide relaxation is stopped and simultaneously oxytocin is started to contract the uterus.

3-42. The answer is c. (*Braunwald, 15/e, pp 2058–2059.*) The patient described has hyponatremia, normovolemia, and concentrated urine. These features are sufficient to make a diagnosis of inappropriate antidiuretic hormone secretion. Inappropriate ADH secretion occurs, in some cases, due to ectopic production by neoplastic tissue. Treatment necessitates restriction of fluid intake. A negative water balance results in a rise in serum Na^+ and serum osmolality and symptom improvement. This syndrome can occur as a side effect of many drugs or from carcinoma, head trauma, infections, neurologic diseases, or stroke.

3-43. The answer is a. *(Behrman, 16/e, pp 497–498. McMillan, 3/e, pp 265–266. Rudolph, 21/e, p 1934.)* Apneic episodes are characterized by an absence of respirations for more than 20 s and may be accompanied by bradycardia and cyanosis. A large number of conditions can cause apnea. Periods of apnea are generally thought to be secondary to an incompletely developed respiratory center, particularly when they are seen, as is common, associated with prematurity. Although seizures, hypoglycemia, and pulmonary disease accompanied by hypoxia can lead to apnea, these causes are less likely in the infant described, given that no unusual movements occur during the apneic spells, that the blood sugar level is more than 40 mg/dL, and that the child appears well between episodes. Periodic breathing, a common pattern of respiration in low-birth-weight babies, is characterized by recurrent breathing pauses of 3 to 10 s.

3-44. The answer is h. *((Cunningham, 21/e, pp 287–288.)* The Apgar scoring system, applied at 1 min and again at 5 min, was developed as an aid to evaluate infants that require resuscitation. Heart rate, respiratory effort, muscle tone, reflex, irritability, and color are the five components of the Apgar score. A score of 0, 1, or 2 is given for each of the five components and the total is added up to give one score. The table below demonstrates the scoring system.

Sign	0 Points	1 Point	2 Points
Heart rate	Absent	Below 100	Over 100
Respiratory effort	Absent	Slow, irregular	Good, crying
Muscle tone	Flaccid	Some extremity flexion	Active motion
Reflex irritability	No response	Grimace	Vigorous cry
Color	Blue, pale	Body pink, extremities blue	Completely pink

The baby described here receives an Apgar score of 9. One point is deducted for the baby not being completely pink and having blue extremities.

3-45. The answer is d. *(Kaplan, 8/e, p 27.)* Postpartum blues are very frequent, with a prevalence estimated between 20 and 40%. Symptoms include tearfulness, irritability, anxiety, and mood lability. Symptoms usually emerge during the first 2 to 4 days after birth, peak between days 5 and 7, and resolve by the end of the second week postpartum. This condition resolves spontaneously, and usually the only interventions necessary are support and reassurance.

3-46. The answer is d. (*Schwartz, 7/e, pp 552–553.*) Fibroadenomas occur infrequently before puberty but are the most common breast tumors between puberty and the early thirties. They usually are well demarcated and firm. Although most fibroadenomas are no larger than 3 cm in diameter, giant or juvenile fibroadenomas frequently are very large. The bigger fibroadenomas (greater than 5 cm) occur predominantly in adolescent black girls. The average age at onset of juvenile mammary hypertrophy is 16 years. This disorder involves a diffuse change in the entire breast and does not usually manifest clinically as a discrete mass; it may be unilateral or bilateral and can cause an enormous and incapacitating increase in breast size. Regression may be spontaneous and sometimes coincides with puberty or pregnancy. Cystosarcoma phyllodes may also cause a large lesion. Together with intraductal carcinoma, it characteristically occurs in older women. Lymphomas are less firm than fibroadenomas and do not have a whorl-like pattern. They display a characteristic fish flesh texture.

3-47. The answer is a. (*Hoskins, 2/e, pp 827–828.*) Cervical cancer is still staged clinically. Physical examination, routine x-rays, barium enema, colposcopy, cystoscopy, proctosigmoidoscopy, and IVP are used to stage the disease. CT scan results, while clinically useful, are not used to stage the disease. Stage I disease is limited to the cervix. Stage Ia disease is preclinical (i.e., microscopic), while stage Ib denotes macroscopic disease. Stage II involves the vagina, but not the lower one-third, or infiltrates the parametrium but not out to the pelvic side wall. IIa denotes vaginal but not parametrial extension, while IIb denotes parametrial extension. Stage III involves the lower one-third of the vagina or extends to the pelvic side wall; there is no cancer-free area between the tumor and the pelvic wall. Stage IIIa lesions have not extended to the pelvic wall, but involve the lower one-third of the vagina. Stage IIIb tumors have extension to the pelvic wall, and/or are associated with hydronephrosis or a nonfunctioning kidney caused by tumor. Stage IV is outside the reproductive tract.

3-48. The answer is d. (*Victor, pp 258–260, 684–686.*) The presentation with subacute onset of morning headaches culminating in confusion, right hemiparesis, and seizure in a young person suggests an expanding mass lesion, most likely a tumor. The weakness of eye abduction bilaterally is what may be referred to as a false localizing sign. Although this suggests injury to the sixth cranial nerves bilaterally, the injury is not restricted to the sixth cranial nerve. The increase in intracranial pressure (ICP) from the mass causes stretching of the sixth-nerve fibers, which consequently leads to their dysfunction. Diplopia may be appreciated only on lateral gaze, which requires full function of the sixth nerve. Funduscopic exam in such a case would most likely reflect changes of increased ICP. The first sign of this is usually blurring of the margins of the optic disc and elevation of the disc due to swelling. Changes in the optic disc—the area in which all the nerve fibers from the retina come together and exit as the optic nerve—occur with problems other than increased ICP (such as optic neuritis), but blurring of the margins should be routinely considered a sign of increased ICP. This is especially true if the appearance of the disc has changed in association with the development of headache, obtundation, and vomiting. Pigmentary degeneration of the retina may occur with some infections, such as congenital toxoplasmosis or cytomegalovirus, or as part of a hereditary metabolic disorder, as in retinitis pigmentosa. Hollenhorst plaques are cholesterol and calcific deposits seen in the retinal arterioles in the setting of atheroembolism to the eye, along with visual loss. Retinal venous pulsations are typically not present when there is increased ICP, although they may also be absent in up to 15% of normal individuals.

3-49. The answer is a. (*Kaplan, 8/e, pp 512–520.*) The main feature of delusional disorder is the presence of one or more nonbizarre delusions without deterioration of psychosocial functioning and in the absence of bizarre or odd behavior. Auditory and visual hallucinations, if present, are not prominent and are related to the delusional theme. Tactile and olfactory hallucinations may also be present if they are incorporated in the delusional system (such as feeling insects crawling over the skin in delusions of infestation). Subtypes of delusional disorder include erotomanic, grandiose, jealous, persecutory, and somatic (delusions of being infested with parasites, of emitting a bad odor, of having AIDS). Delusional disorder usually manifests in middle or late adult life and has a fluctuating course with periods of remissions and relapses.

3-50. The answer is b. (*Tierney, 42/e, pp 1193–1198.*) The surreptitious injection of insulin is just as common as insulinoma. Patients have low C-peptide levels with high insulin levels. **Factitious disease** should be suspected when hypoglycemic symptoms appear in health professionals or in relatives of patients with diabetes mellitus. Patients with **insulinoma** have high levels of both C peptide and insulin. Finding high levels of circulating insulin antibodies may help to make the diagnosis of factitious hypoglycemia.

BLOCK 4

Answers

4-1. The answer is e. *(Fuster, 10/e, pp 1616–1619.)* Cor pulmonale is characterized by the presence of pulmonary hypertension and consequent right ventricular dysfunction. Its causes include diseases leading to hypoxic vasoconstriction, as in cystic fibrosis; occlusion of the pulmonary vasculature, as in pulmonary thromboembolism; and parenchymal destruction, as in sarcoidosis. In the presence of a chronic increase in afterload, the right ventricle becomes hypertrophic, dilates, and fails. The electrocardiographic findings, as illustrated in the question, include tall, peaked P waves in leads II, III, and a VF, which indicate right atrial enlargement; tall R waves in leads V_1 to V_3 and a deep S wave in V_6 with associated ST-T wave changes, which indicate right ventricular hypertrophy; and right axis deviation. Right bundle branch block occurs in 15% of patients.

4-2. The answer is b. *(Behrman, 16/e, p 2031. McMillan, 3/e, pp 378–379, 418–420. Rudolph, 21/e, pp 1225–1226.)* Also known as Ritter disease, staphylococcal scalded skin disease is seen most commonly in children less than 5 years of age. The rash is preceded by fever, irritability, erythema, and extraordinary tenderness of the skin. Circumoral erythema; crusting of the eyes, mouth, and nose; and blisters on the skin can develop. Intraoral mucosal surfaces are not affected. Peeling of the epidermis in response to mild shearing forces (Nikolsky sign) leaves the patient susceptible to problems similar to those of a burn injury, including infection and fluid and electrolyte imbalance. Cultures of the bullae are negative, but the source site is often positive. Treatment includes antibiotics (to cover resistant *Staphylococcus aureus*) and localized skin care. Recovery without scarring can be expected.

4-3. The answer is b. *(Bradley, p 1758.)* Lennox-Gastaut syndrome is a disturbance seen in children. It is often difficult to control the seizures that develop in children with this combination of retardation and slow spike-and-wave discharges on EEG. Many affected children have a history of infantile spasms (West syndrome). Infants and children with infantile spasms exhibit paroxysmal flexions of the body, waist, or neck and usually have a profoundly disorganized EEG pattern called hypsarrhythmia.

4-4. The answer is b. *(Ransom 1997, p 53.)* Lymphogranuloma venereum (LGV) is a chronic infection produced by *C. trachomatis.* The primary infection begins as a painless ulcer on the labia or vaginal vestibule; the patient usually consults the physician several weeks after the development of painful adenopathy in the inguinal and perirectal areas. Diagnosis can be established by culture or by demonstrating the presence of antibodies to *C. trachomatis.* The Frei skin test is no longer used because of its low sensitivity. The differential diagnosis includes syphilis, chancroid, granuloma inguinale, carcinoma, and herpes. Chancroid is a sexually transmitted disease caused by *H. ducreyi* that produces a painful, tender ulceration of the vulva. Donovan bodies are present in patients with granuloma inguinale, which is caused by *C. granulomatis.* Therapy for both granuloma inguinale and LGV is administration of tetracycline. Chancroid is successfully treated with either azithromycin or ceftriaxone.

4-5. The answer is e. *(Beckmann, 4/e, pp 356–358.)* Approximately 0.5% of Pap smears come back with glandular cell abnormalities. These abnormalities can be associated with squamous lesions, adenocarcinoma in situ, or invasive adenocarcinoma. Therefore any patient with AGUS should undergo immediate colposcopy and ECC. In addition, postmenopausal women should have endometrial sampling. Hysterectomy or conization might be indicated based on results of the colposcopy; however, colposcopy must be performed initially.

4-6. The answer is b. *(Kaplan, 8/e, p 93.)* Temporal lobe epilepsy may often manifest as bizarre behavior without the classic grand mal shaking movements caused by seizures in the motor cortex. A TLE personality is characterized by hyposexuality, emotional intensity, and a perseverative approach to interactions, termed viscosity. Wernicke-Korsakoff syndrome is a neurologic condition manifested by confusion, ataxia, and nystagmus; thiamine deficiency is its direct cause. If thiamine is given during the acute stage of Wernicke's encephalopathy, Korsakoff's syndrome can be prevented. This syndrome is characterized by a severe anterograde learning defect associated with confabulations. Although Wernicke-Korsakoff's can be caused by malnutrition alone, it is usually associated with alcohol abuse and dependence. Pick's disease is a form of frontal lobe dementia in which Pick's cells and bodies (irregularly shaped, silver-staining, intracytoplasmic inclusion bodies that displace the nucelus toward the periophery) are present in the brain. There is an insidious onset and gradual progression, with early decline in social interpersonal conduct. Emotional blunting and apathy also occur early without insight into them. There is a marked decline in personal hygiene and significant distractibility and motor impersistence.

4-7. The answer is b. (*Behrman, 16/e, pp 2044–2046. McMillan, 3/e, pp 716–717. Rudolph, 21/e, pp 1153–1154, 1233–1234.*) Scabies is caused by the mite *Sarcoptes scabiei* var. *hominis*. Most older children and adults present with intensely pruritic and threadlike burrows in the interdigital areas, groin, elbows, and ankles; the palms, soles, face, and head are spared. Infants, however, usually present with bullae and pustules, and the areas spared in adults are often involved in infants. The clinical manifestations closely resemble those of atopic dermatitis. Because of the potential neurotoxic effect to infants of gamma benzene hexachloride through percutaneous absorption, an excellent alternative—5% permethrin cream (Elimite)—is available and is more often recommended.

4-8. The answer is c. (*Kaplan, 8/e, p 1033.*) Tardive dyskinesia (TD) is characterized by involuntary choreoathetoid movements of the face, trunk, and extremities. Tardive dyskinesia is associated with prolonged use of medications that block dopamine receptors, most commonly antipsychotic medications. Typical antipsychotic medications (such as perphenazine) and, in particular, high potency drugs carry the highest risk of TD. Atypical antipsychotics are thought to be less likely to cause this disorder.

4-9. The answer is e. (*Greenfield, 2/e, p 916.*) This woman has a cystadenocarcinoma arising from the pancreatic body and tail, which was successfully resected. About 90% of primary malignant neoplasms of the exocrine pancreas are adenocarcinomas of duct cell origin. The remaining neoplasms include adenosquamous carcinoma, mucinous carcinomas, microadenocarcinoma, giant cell carcinoma, and cystadenocarcinoma of uncertain histogenesis. The clinical presentation is usually quite subtle, with symptoms related primarily to the enlarging mass. There are no diagnostic laboratory findings, and definitive preoperative diagnosis is rare. An elderly patient with no history of pancreatitis is unlikely to have a pseudocyst, and a benign neoplasm is also less likely in this age group. These less common carcinomas are often several times the size of typical ductal cancers and often arise in the body or tail of the pancreas. They may become very large without invading adjacent viscera and do not generally cause significant pain or weight loss. Therefore, even large tumors may be cured by resection, and aggressive surgical management is indicated.

4-10. The answer is b. (*Braunwald, 15/e, pp 1340–1342.*) This 18-year-old presents with classic features of rheumatic fever. His clinical manifestations include arthritis, fever, and murmur. A subcutaneous nodule is noted, and a rash of erythema marginatum is described. These subcutaneous nodules are pea-sized and usually seen over extensor tendons. The rash is usually pink with clear centers and serpiginous margins. Laboratory data shows an elevated erythrocyte sedimentation rate as usually occurs in rheumatic fever. The ECG shows evidence of first-degree AV block. An antistreptolysin O antibody is necessary to diagnose the disease by documenting prior streptococcal infection. Most experts recommend the use of glucocorticoids when carditis is part of the picture of rheumatic fever. Therefore, in this patient with first-degree AV block, corticosteroids would be indicated. Penicillin should also be given to eradicate group A β-hemolytic streptococci.

4-11. The answer is d. (*Victor, pp 1482–1488.*) This woman presents with proximal muscle weakness and pain and a heliotrope rash about her eyes. The term heliotrope refers to the lilac color of the periorbital rash characteristic of dermatomyositis. This rash surrounds both eyes and may extend onto the malar eminences, the eyelids, the bridge of the nose, and the forehead. It is usually associated with an erythematous rash across the knuckles and at the base of the nails and may be associated with flat-topped purplish nodules over the elbows and knees. Men with dermatomyositis are at higher than normal risk of having underlying malignancies. Psoriatic arthritis may be associated with reddish discoloration of the knuckles and muscle weakness, but the heliotrope rash would not be expected with this disorder. The age of onset for a psoriatic myopathy is also atypical. Similarly, the patient's rashes are not suggestive of lupus erythematosus, although a myopathy may occur with this connective tissue disease as well.

4-12. The answer is c. (*ACOG, Practice Bulletin 17.*) Indications for an operative vaginal delivery with a vacuum extractor or forceps occur in situations where the fetal head is engaged, the cervix is completely dilated, and there is a prolonged second stage, suspicion of potential fetal compromise, or need to shorten the second stage for maternal benefit. In this situation, all the indications for operative delivery apply. This patient has been pushing for 3 h, which is the definition for prolonged second stage of labor in a nulliparous patient with an epidural. In addition, potential maternal and fetal compromise exists since the patient has the clinical picture of chorioamnionitis and the fetal heart rate is nonreassuring. It is best to avoid cesarean section since it would take more time to achieve and since the patient is infected.

4-13. The answer is c. (*Fitzpatrick, 4/e, pp 18–25.*) **Contact dermatitis** can be due to an allergen causing a type IV cell-mediated delayed hypersensitivity reaction. It may also be due to a nonallergen such as a chemical irritant. This patient presents with typical symptoms of acute contact dermatitis due to poison ivy resin. This results in sensitization within a week of exposure. Contact dermatitis due to poison ivy is usually pruritic, localized to one region, and often linear. **Impetigo** is an epidermal bacterial infection seen on the face characterized by vesicles that rupture and crust. **Erythema infectiosum** or **fifth disease** is a childhood disease due to parvovirus B19 and is characterized by edematous, erythematous plaques on the cheeks ("slapped cheek" disease). **Atopic dermatitis** or **eczema** is an autosomal dominant pruritic inflammation with a predilection for the neck, face, flexor areas, feet, wrists, and hands. Usually there is a personal or family history of asthma, allergic rhinitis, or hay fever. **Rubeola** (measles) is a viral infection characterized by **c**onjunctivitis, **c**oryza, and **c**ough (**the three C's**) and a confluent erythematous maculopapular rash that spreads centrifugally. **Koplik spots** (bright red spots with blue-white specks in the center), which appear on the buccal mucosa opposite the premolar teeth, are pathognomonic for rubeola.

4-14. The answer is d. (*Tierney, 42/e, pp 910–911.*) The patient presents with **pyelonephritis,** which is an infection of the kidney and renal pelvis. It is characterized by flank pain, fever, dysuria, and frequency. Patients often experience suprapubic and CVA tenderness. Patients with acute cystitis may present with dysuria, frequency, urgency, and suprapubic tenderness, but typically the patient is afebrile and the physical examination is normal. The organisms responsible for urinary tract infections are **SEEK PP** = **S**erratia marcescens, **E**scherichia coli, **E**nterobacter cloacae, **K**lebsiella pneumoniae, **P**roteus mirabilis, and **P**seudomonas aeruginosa.

4-15. The answer is b. (Behrman, 16/e, pp 526–527, 1101. McMillan, 3/e, p 360. Rudolph, 21/e, p 1372.) Hematemesis and melena are not uncommon in the neonatal period, especially if gross placental bleeding has occurred at the time of delivery. The diagnostic procedure that should be done first is the Apt test, which differentiates fetal from adult hemoglobin in a bloody specimen. If the blood in an affected infant's gastric contents or stool is maternal in origin, further workup of the infant is obviated.

4-16. The answer is d. (Braunwald, 15/e, pp 1495–1498.) This patient's chronic cough, hyperinflated lung fields, abnormal pulmonary function tests, and smoking history are all consistent with chronic bronchitis. A smoking cessation program can decrease the rate of lung deterioration and is successful in as many as 40% of patients, particularly when the physician gives a strong antismoking message and uses both counseling and nicotine replacement. Continuous low-flow oxygen becomes beneficial when arterial oxygen concentration falls below 55 mmHg. Antibiotics are indicated only for acute exacerbations of chronic lung disease, which might present with fever, change in color of sputum, and increasing shortness of breath. Oral corticosteroids are helpful in some patients, but are reserved for those who have failed inhaled bronchodilator treatments.

4-17. The answer is b. (Behrman, 16/e, pp 455, 1970. McMillan, 3/e, pp 372, 682. Rudolph, 21/e, p 1192.) Mongolian spots are bluish-gray lesions located over the buttocks, lower back, and occasionally, the extensor surfaces of the extremities. They are common in blacks, Asians, and Latin Americans. They tend to disappear by 1 to 2 years of age, although those on the extremities may not fully resolve. Child abuse is unlikely to present with bruises alone; children frequently present with more extensive injuries. Subcutaneous fat necrosis is usually found as a sharply demarcated, hard lesion on the cheeks, buttocks, and limbs. The lesion usually is red. Hemophilia and vitamin K deficiency rarely present with subcutaneous lesions as described and are more likely to present as a bleeding episode.

4-18. The answer is b. *(Kaplan, 8/e, p 754.)* The child in the question is experiencing episodes of sleep terror disorder, a dyssomnia characterized by sudden partial arousal accompanied by piercing screams, motor agitation, disorientation, and autonomic arousal. The episodes take place during the transition from deep sleep to REM sleep. Children do not report nightmares (which would be associated with REM sleep) and do not have any memory of the episodes the next day. Sleep terrors occur in 3% of children and 1% of adults. Although specific treatment for this disorder is seldom required, in rare cases it is necessary. Diazepam (Valium) in small doses at bedtime improves the condition and sometimes completely eliminates the attacks.

4-19. The answer is e. *(Cunningham, 21/e, pp 568–573.)* Hypertension in pregnancy is defined as blood pressure of 140/90 mmHg or greater on at least two separate occasions that are 6 h or more apart. The presence of edema is no longer used as a diagnostic criteria because it is so prevalent in normal pregnant women. A rise in systolic blood pressure of 30 mmHg and a rise in diastolic blood pressure of 15 mmHg is no longer used because women meeting this criteria are not likely to suffer adverse pregnancy outcomes if their absolute blood pressure is below 140/90 mmHg. In gestational hypertension, maternal blood pressure reaches 140/90 or greater for the first time during pregnancy, and proteinuria is not present. In preeclampsia, blood pressure increases to 140/90 after 20 weeks gestation and proteinuria is present (300 mg in 24 h or 1+ protein or greater on dipstick.) Eclampsia is present when women with preeclampsia develop seizures. Chronic hypertension exists when a woman has a blood pressure of 140/90 or greater prior to the pregnancy or before 20 weeks gestation. A woman with hypertension who develops preeclampsia is described as having chronic hypertension with superimposed preeclampsia.

4-20. The answer is a. *(Braunwald, 15/e, pp 2010–2011.)* The patient's multiple trigger points, associated sleep disturbance, and lack of joint or muscle findings make fibromyalgia a possible diagnosis. The diagnosis hinges on the multiple tender points. CBC and ESR are characteristically normal. Tricyclic antidepressants restore sleep; aspirin and other anti-inflammatory drugs are not helpful. Biofeedback and exercise programs have been partially successful. The clavicle, medial malleolus, and forehead are never trigger points for the process.

4-21. The answer is d. (*Behrman, 16/e, pp 632–633, 684–685. McMillan, 3/e, pp 2049–2053. Rudolph, 21/e, p 1196.*) This condition often worsens in adolescents. Although hereditary angioedema is relatively rare as a cause of edema, the recurrent episodes in late childhood, the normal laboratory results, and the family history make the other choices less likely. Hereditary angioedema, transmitted as an autosomal dominant trait, is due to inadequate function (due to either deficient quantity or quality) of an inhibitor of the first step in the complement cascade, which results in the excessive production of a vasoactive kinin. In addition to otherwise asymptomatic subcutaneous edema, edema can occur in the gastrointestinal tract and produce the symptoms mentioned in the question. Laryngeal edema with airway obstruction can also occur.

4-22. The answer is a. (*Tierney, 42/e, pp 181–183.*) **Otitis media with effusion** may follow an episode of acute respiratory tract infection or acute otitis media. Symptoms include hearing loss, ear fullness, ear pain, dizziness, and tinnitus. The eardrum appears retracted or scarred and a clear fluid is visible in the middle ear. Pain and fever are usually absent in otitis media with effusion. Treatment measures are aimed at facilitating drainage of the effusion, and antibiotics are generally not necessary.

4-23. The answer is d. (*Victor, p 73.*) Young adults who have self-administered MPTP in an effort to achieve an opiate high have developed progressive damage to the substantia nigra. The neurologic syndrome that results from this damage is indistinguishable from Parkinson's disease, except that it evolves over weeks or months rather than years. Affected persons exhibit rigidity, tremor, and bradykinesia. That a toxin can produce a syndrome indistinguishable from Parkinson's disease has increased speculation that some—perhaps many—persons with Parkinson's disease have had environmental exposure to a toxin that produced degeneration of the substantia nigra.

4-24. The answer is c. (*Schwartz, 7/e, pp 1639–1640.*) Acute adrenal insufficiency is classically manifested as changing mental status, increased temperature, cardiovascular collapse, hypoglycemia, and hyperkalemia. The diagnosis can be difficult to make and requires a high index of suspicion. Its clinical presentation is similar to that of sepsis; however, sepsis is generally associated with hyperglycemia and no significant change in potassium. The treatment for adrenal crisis is hydrocortisone 100 mg intravenously, volume resuscitation, and other supportive measures to treat any new or ongoing stress. Then, 200 to 400 mg hydrocortisone are administered over the next 24 h, followed by a taper of the steroid as tolerated.

4-25. The answer is c. (*Braunwald, 15/e, pp 823, 893.*) Erysipelas, the cellulitis described, is typical of infection caused by *S. pyogenes* group A β-hemolytic streptococci. There is often a preceding event such as a cut in the skin, dermatitis, or superficial fungal infection that precedes this rapidly spreading cellulitis. Anaerobic cellulitis is more often associated with underlying diabetes. *S. epidermidis* does not cause rapidly progressive cellulitis. *Staphylococcus aureus* can cause cellulitis that is difficult to distinguish from erysipelas, but it is usually more local and likely to produce furuncles, or abscesses.

4-26. The answer is b. (*Mishell, 3/e, pp 179–182.*) This patient presents with vaginismus, defined as involuntary painful spasm of the pelvic muscles and vaginal outlet. It is usually psychogenic. It should be differentiated from frigidity, which implies lack of sexual desire, and dyspareunia, which is defined as pelvic and/or back pain or other discomfort associated with sexual activity. Dyspareunia is frequently associated with pelvic pathology such as endometriosis, pelvic adhesions, or ovarian neoplasms. The pain of vaginismus may be psychogenic in origin, or may be caused by pelvic pathology such as adhesions, endometriosis, or leiomyomas. Treatment of vaginismus is primarily psychotherapeutic, as organic vulvar or pelvic causes (such as atrophy, Bartholin's gland cyst, or abscess) are very rare.

4-27. The answer is c. (*Hazzard, 4/e, pp 1156–1159.*) In addition to physical therapy, the best symptomatic treatment would be acetaminophen because it is frequently effective in providing pain relief and has an excellent safety profile in the elderly. Nonsteroidals should be avoided, at least initially, because they tend to cause gastrointestinal upset and impairment of renal function. Intraarticular steroids are indicated for large effusions in joints unresponsive to first-line therapy. Arthroplasty is highly effective in treating osteoarthritis of a single joint and is not contraindicated in the elderly. Such surgery is usually considered after attempts at physical therapy, education, and pain relief with pharmacotherapy.

4-28. The answer is d. (*Behrman, 16/e, pp 885–897. McMillan, 3/e, pp 1026–1039. Rudolph, 21/e, pp 949–959.*) The key to controlling tuberculosis in children and eradicating the disease is early detection and appropriate treatment of adult cases; the child, once infected, is at lifelong risk for the development of the disease and for infecting others unless given isoniazid prophylaxis. The usual source of the disease is an infected adult. Household contacts of a person with newly diagnosed active disease have a considerable risk of developing active tuberculosis, and the risk is greatest for infants and children. Therefore, when tuberculosis is diagnosed in a child, the immediate family and close contacts should be tested with tuberculin skin tests and chest radiographs and treated appropriately when indicated. Bronchoscopy would be indicated only in unusual circumstances. Three to eight weeks is required after exposure before hypersensitivity to tuberculin develops. This means that the tuberculin test must be repeated in exposed persons if there is a negative reaction at the time that contact with the source of infection is broken. TB skin tests are usually negative in infants of this age, even when active disease is ongoing. A logical preventive measure is the administration of isoniazid to the baby for 3 months when a Mantoux (purified protein derivative, PPD) can then be placed. Transmission of tuberculosis occurs when bacilli-laden, small-sized droplets are dispersed into the air by the cough or sneeze of an infected adult. Small children with primary pulmonary tuberculosis are not considered infectious to others, and they are not capable of coughing up and producing sputum. Sputum, when produced, is promptly swallowed, and for this reason specimens for microbial confirmation can be obtained by means of gastric lavage from smaller children.

4-29. The answer is b. (*Braunwald, 15/e, pp 2237–2239.*) This patient has widespread Paget's disease of bone. Excessive resorption of bone is followed by replacement of normal marrow with dense, trabecular, disorganized bone. Hearing loss and tinnitus are due to direct involvement of the ossicles of the inner ear. Plasma alkaline phosphatase levels represent increased bone turnover. Neither myeloma or metastatic bone disease would result in bony deformity such as skull enlargement. Alkaline phosphatase is a marker of bone formation and does not rise in pure lytic lesions such as multiple myeloma.

4-30. The answer is a. (*Braunwald, 15/e, pp 2105–2106.*) A hypertensive crisis in this young woman suggests a secondary cause of hypertension. In the setting of palpitations, apprehension, and hyperglycemia, pheochromocytoma should be considered. Pheochromocytomas are derived from the adrenal medulla. They are capable of producing and secreting catecholamines. Unexplained hypotension associated with surgery or trauma may also suggest the disease. Clinical symptoms are the result of catecholamine secretion. For example, the patient's hyperglycemia is a result of a catecholamine effect of insulin suppression and stimulation of hepatic glucose output. Hypercalcemia has been attributed to ectopic secretion of parathormone-related protein. Renal artery stenosis can cause severe hypertension but would not explain the systemic symptoms or laboratory abnormalities in this case.

4-31. The answer is b. *(Behrman, 16/e, pp 1279–1282. McMillan, 3/e, pp 570–571, 640. Rudolph, 21/e, pp 1277–1278.)* Recurrent pneumonias in an otherwise healthy child should indicate the potential for anatomic blockage of an airway. In the patient in this question, the findings on clinical examination suggest a foreign body in the airway. Inspiratory and expiratory films can be helpful. Routine inspiratory films are likely to appear normal or near normal (as outlined in the question). Expiratory films will identify air trapping behind the foreign body. It is uncommon for the foreign body to be visible on the plain radiograph; a high index of suspicion is necessary to make the diagnosis. Suspected foreign bodies in the airway are potentially diagnosed with fluoroscopy, but rigid bronchoscopy is not only diagnostic but also the treatment of choice for removal of the foreign body.

4-32. The answer is e. *(Hoskins, 2/e, pp 940–944.)* The survival of women who have ovarian carcinoma varies inversely with the amount of residual tumor left after the initial surgery. At the time of laparotomy, a maximum effort should be made to determine the sites of tumor spread and to excise all resectable tumor. Although the uterus and ovaries may appear grossly normal, there is a relatively high incidence of occult metastases to these organs; for this reason, they should be removed during the initial surgery. Ovarian cancer metastasizes outside the peritoneum via the pelvic or paraaortic lymphatics, and from there into the thorax and the remainder of the body.

4-33. The answer is c. *(Tierney, 42/e, pp 440–441.)* **Dissection of the aorta** occurs when the intima is interrupted so that blood enters the wall of the aorta and separates its layers, forming a second lumen. It is almost always fatal if left undiagnosed, but with prompt treatment most patients survive. Anything that weakens the media can lead to dissection, but hypertension is the most common risk factor. Aortic dissection is a major cause of morbidity and mortality in Marfan syndrome. Other etiologies of dissection include cystic medial necrosis (described in patients with bicuspid aortic valves), syphilis, Ehlers-Danlos syndrome, trauma, and bacterial infections. Patients often have murmurs due to aortic insufficiency. The treatment for dissection is to control the blood pressure and heart rate to prevent extension of the dissection. A **tracheal tug** is considered positive if the pulsating aorta is felt when the trachea is pulled upward.

4-34. The answer is c. (*Bradley, pp 1319–1323.*) The immediate concern is that the patient has bacterial meningitis, and she should be treated. A lumbar puncture and blood draw to obtain cultures should be done; however, it can take a few days for the results to come back, and it may be too late for the patient by then. Oral azithromycin is not the proper treatment for bacterial meningitis. Intravenous acyclovir would be used to treat herpes encephalitis.

4-35. The answer is d. (*Kaplan, 8/e, pp 456–491.*) Self-induced water intoxication should always be considered in the differential diagnosis of confusional states and seizures in schizophrenic patients. As many as 20% of patients with a diagnosis of schizophrenia drink excessive amounts of water. At least 4% of these patients suffer from chronic hyponatremia and recurrent acute water intoxication. Medications that cause excessive water retention, such as lithium and carbamazepine, can aggravate the symptomatology.

4-36. The answer is c. (*Cunningham, 21/e, pp 395–396.*) An estimate of the gestational age of a newborn can be made rapidly by a physical exam immediately following delivery. Important physical characteristics that are evaluated are the sole creases, breast nodules, scalp hair, earlobes, and scrotum. In newborns that are 39 weeks gestational age or more, the soles of the feet will be covered with creases, the diameter of the breast nodules will be at least 7 mm, the scalp hair will be coarse and silky, the earlobes will be thickened with cartilage, and the scrotum will be full with extensive rugae. In infants that are 36 weeks or less, there will be an anterior transverse sole crease only, the breast nodule diameter will be 2 mm, the scalp hair will be fine and fuzzy, the earlobes will be pliable and lack cartilage, and the scrotum will be small with few rugae. In infants of gestational age between 37 and 38 weeks, the soles of the feet will have occasional creases on the anterior two-thirds of the feet, the breast nodule diameter will be 4 mm, the scalp hair will be fine and fuzzy, the earlobes will have a small amount of cartilage, and the scrotum will have some but not extensive rugae.

4-37. The answer is b. (*Braunwald, 15/e, p 879.*) In the elderly or in patients with renal insufficiency, full doses of trimethoprim-sulfamethonazole frequently cause drug-induced interstitial nephritis and hyperkalemia (due to inhibition of the sodium-potassium transport system in the distal nephron). Levofloxacin is a very rare cause of renal dysfunction. In the setting of volume depletion, acyclovir may cause acute renal failure secondary to intratubular obstruction from crystal deposition. Crystals are absent from the urine in this case. Indinavir may crystallize and cause either nephrolithiasis or renal failure due to tubular obstruction.

4-38. The answer is b. (*Schwartz, 7/e, pp 194–195.*) Duodenal hematomas result from blunt abdominal trauma. They present as a high bowel obstruction with abdominal pain and occasionally a palpable right upper quadrant mass. An upper gastrointestinal series is almost always diagnostic with the classic coiled spring appearance of the second and third portions of the duodenum secondary to the crowding of the valvulae conniventes (circular folds) by the hematoma. Nonsurgical management is the mainstay of therapy because the vast majority of duodenal hematomas resolve spontaneously. Simple evacuation of the hematoma is the operative procedure of choice. However, bypass procedures and duodenal resection have been performed for this problem. In patients with duodenal obstruction from the superior mesenteric artery syndrome, the obstruction is usually the result of a marked weight loss and, in conjunction with this, loss of the retroperitoneal fat pad that elevates the superior mesenteric artery from the third and fourth portions of the duodenum. Nutritional repletion and replenishment of this fat pad will elevate the artery off the duodenum and relieve the obstruction.

4-39. The answer is a. (*Braunwald, 15/e, pp 727–733.*) The onset of multiple myeloma is usually insidious, with weakness and fatigue. Pain caused by bone involvement, anemia, renal insufficiency, and bacterial pneumonia often follow. This patient presented with fatigue and bone pain, then developed bacterial pneumonia probably secondary to *Streptococcus pneumoniae,* an encapsulated organism for which antibody to the polysaccharide capsule is not adequately produced by the myeloma patient. There is also evidence for renal insufficiency. Hypercalcemia is frequently seen in patients with multiple myeloma and may be life-threatening. Lymphoma typically presents with lymphadenopathy. Bone pain and renal insufficiency at the outset are uncommon; only the rare T cell lymphomas are commonly associated with hypercalcemia. Metastatic bronchogenic carcinoma can cause hypercalcemia but would rarely present with renal insufficiency and such severe anemia. Primary hyperparathyroidism is a common cause of hypercalcemia, but patients are usually minimally symptomatic. It does not cause severe anemia or increased incidence of infection.

4-40. The answer is e. *(Tierney, 42/e, pp 505–508.)* **Idiopathic thrombocytopenic purpura (ITP)** is an autoimmune disorder in which an IgG autoantibody binds to platelets. Destruction of the platelets takes place in the spleen, where macrophages bind to the antibody-coated platelets. Fifty percent of patients with ITP have no associated disease, but HIV infection, SLE, or a lymphoproliferative disorder should be considered. ITP is a disease of persons between the ages of 20 and 50 years and occurs in women more than men. There is no splenomegaly in ITP. The diagnosis is one of exclusion, but often megathrombocytes are seen on peripheral smear. **Evans syndrome** is ITP with coexistent autoimmune hemolytic anemia. **DIC** is a systemic coagulation disorder that can be accompanied by thrombocytopenia. It may be secondary to transfusion, infection, malignancy, trauma, or obstetric complications. **TTP** is unlikely since the patient does not have the pentad of symptoms seen in 40% of patients (**FAT R.N.** = **F**ever, **A**utoimmune hemolytic anemia, **T**hrombocytopenia, **R**enal disease, **N**eurologic disease). **HUS** presents with three of the five symptoms seen in TTP (**RAT** = **R**enal disease, **A**utoimmune hemolytic anemia, and **T**hrombocytopenia). Fever and neurologic disease are lacking. **Henoch-Schönlein purpura** occurs in children; patients present with **AGAR** = **A**bdominal pain, **G**lomerulonephritis, **A**rthralgia, and a **R**ash that is purpuric.

4-41. The answer is b. *(Cunningham, 21/e, pp 1283–1285, 1431–1435.)* Pruritic urticarial papules and plaques of pregnancy (PUPPP) is the most common dermatologic condition of pregnancy. It is more common in nulliparous women and occurs most often in the second and third trimesters of pregnancy. PUPPP is characterized by erythematous papules and plaques that are intensely pruritic and appear first on the abdomen. The lesions then commonly spread to the buttocks, thighs, and extremities with sparing of the face. Herpes gestationis is a blistering skin eruption that occurs more commonly in multiparous patients in the second or third trimester of pregnancy. The presence of vesicles and bullae help differentiate this skin condition from PUPPP. Prurigo gestationis is a very rare dermatosis of pregnancy that is characterized by small, pruritic excoriated lesions that occur between 25 and 30 weeks. The lesions first appear on the trunk and forearms and can spread throughout the body as well. In cases of intrahepatic cholestasis of pregnancy, bile acids are cleared incompletely and accumulate in the dermis, which causes intense itching. These patients develop pruritus in late pregnancy; there are no characteristic skin changes or rashes except in women who develop excoriations from scratching. Impetigo herpetiformis is a rare pustular eruption that forms along the margins of erythematous patches. This skin condition usually occurs in late pregnancy. The skin lesions usually begin at points of flexure and extend peripherally; mucous membranes are commonly involved. Patients with impetigo herpetiformis usually do not have intense pruritus, but more commonly have systemic symptoms of nausea, vomiting, diarrhea, chills, and fever.

4-42. The answer is e. (*Schwartz, 7/e, pp 487–493.*) Determination of CVP has been helpful in the overall hemodynamic assessment of the patient. This pressure can be affected by a variety of factors including those of cardiac, noncardiac, and artifactual origin. Venous tone, right ventricular compliance, intrathoracic pressure, and blood volume all influence CVP. Vasoconstrictor drugs, positive pressure, ventilation (with and without PEEP), mediastinal compression, and hypervolemia all increase CVP. Acute pulmonary embolism, when clinically significant, elevates CVP by causing right ventricular overload and increased right atrial pressure. Sepsis, on the other hand, decreases CVP through both the release of vasodilatory mediators and the loss of intravascular plasma volume due to increased capillary permeability. Trends in CVP measurement are more reliable than isolated readings.

4-43. The answer is c. (*Braunwald, 15/e, pp 2412–2414.*) The disease described involves motor neurons exclusively. Amyotrophic lateral sclerosis affects both upper and lower motor neurons. In this patient, there is upper and lower motor neuron involvement without sensory deficit. Lower

motor neuron signs include focal weakness, focal wasting, and fasciculations. Upper motor neuron signs include an extensor plantar response and
an increased tendon reflex in a weakened muscle. Peripheral neuropathy
and dementia do not occur in ALS. Primary muscle diseases produce weakness by affecting muscle fibers without interfering with the nerve itself or
the neuromuscular junction. Duchenne muscular dystrophy occurs at a
younger age and involves proximal muscle weakness and not motor neurons. Polymyositis is also primarily a muscle disease. Myasthenia gravis
would not cause hyperreflexia or Babinski reflex; it is a disease of muscle
weakness characterized by fatigability.

4-44 The answer is d. *(Behrman, 16/e, pp 1878–1879. McMillan, 3/e, pp
1973–1974. Rudolph, 21/e, pp 2293–2294, 2406.)* The child in the question
appears to have myotonic muscular dystrophy. An elevated creatine kinase
(especially in the preclinical phase) is often found and psychomotor retardation can be the presenting complaint (but may be identified only in retrospect). Ptosis, baldness, hypogonadism, facial immobility with distal
muscle wasting (in older children), and neonatal respiratory distress (in the
newborn period) are major features of this disorder. Cataracts are commonly seen, presenting either congenitally or at any point during childhood. The diagnosis is confirmed by identifying typical findings on muscle
biopsy. Seizures are not a feature of myotonic dystrophy. Enlarged gonads
are associated with fragile X syndrome, and hirsutism is found (among
other things) in children with congenital adrenal hyperplasia.

4-45. The answer is c. *(Greenfield, 2/e, pp 1137–1141.)* A markedly distended colon could have many causes in this 80-year-old man. The contrast study, however, reveals a classic apple core lesion in the distal colon,
which is diagnostic of colon cancer. No further diagnostic studies are
appropriate prior to relief of this large bowel obstruction. After medical
preparation (e.g., hydration, normalization of electrolytes), this patient
should undergo prompt surgical management of his mechanical obstruction; conservative management by resection and proximal colostomy
would generally be preferred in this elderly patient with an obstructed,
unprepared bowel.

4-46. The answer is d. *(Kaplan, 8/e, p 323.)* The patient's persecutory
delusions and disorganized thinking could suggest a psychotic disorder
such as schizophrenia or brief reactive psychosis, but fluctuations in con-

sciousness and disorientation are typically found in delirium. Memory, language, and sleep-wake cycle disturbances are also typical of delirium. Delusions, hallucinations, illusions, and misperceptions are also common. The causes of delirium are many and include metabolic encephalopathies (including fever and hypoxia, as in the patient in the question), intoxications with drugs and poisons; withdrawal syndromes; head trauma; epilepsy; neoplasms; vascular disorders; allergic reactions; and injuries caused by physical agents (heat, cold, radiation).

4-47. The answer is c. *(Braunwald, 15/e, p 560.)* The lesion described is characteristic of leukoplakia. This is a precancerous lesion that requires biopsy. Histologically, these lesions show hyperkeratosis, acanthosis, and atypia. There are homogeneous and nonhomogeneous types; the homogeneous are much more likely to undergo malignant transformation. Oropharyngeal *Candida* would be unlikely to occur in this patient and would appear as a more diffuse, lacy lesion of the buccal mucosa and oropharynx. The white plaque of thrush would rub off, leaving a slightly erythematous and inflamed mucosa underneath.

4-48. The answer is d. *(Braunwald, 15/e, pp 1917–1918.)* In the great majority of patients with urticaria, a cause is never found. Some do have underlying illnesses such as chronic infection, myeloproliferative disease, collagen vascular disease, or hyperthyroidism. There is no evidence for underlying disease in this patient.

4-49. The answer is d. *(Fleisher, 5/e, pp 732–735. Ransom, 2000, pp 511–515.)* The history, clinical picture, and ultrasound of the woman in the question are characteristic of hydatidiform mole. The most common initial symptoms include an enlarged-for-dates uterus and continuous or intermittent bleeding in the first two trimesters. Other symptoms include hypertension, proteinuria, and hyperthyroidism. Hydatidiform mole is 10 times as common in the Far East as in North America, and it occurs more frequently in women over 45 years of age. A tissue sample would show a villus with hydropic changes and no vessels. Grossly, these lesions appear as small, clear clusters of grapelike vesicles, the passage of which confirms the diagnosis.

4-50. The answer is d. *(Behrman, 16/e, pp 583–586, 1652–1653. McMillan, 3/e, pp 1555–1558, 1628–1629. Rudolph, 21/e, pp 260–270.)* The patient in the question may have a torsion of his testis that requires immediate attention. Another possibility would by epididymitis, especially if there is a possible antecedent history of sexual activity or urinary tract infection. Prehn's sign, although not totally reliable, is elicited by gently lifting the scrotum toward the symphysis. Relief of the pain points to epididymitis; its worsening, to torsion. Doppler ultrasound (or surgical consultation) is a logical first step in this man's evaluation, demonstrating absence of flow in torsion and increased flow in epididymitis. Alternatively, a radionuclide scan will show diminished uptake in torsion and increased uptake in epididymitis. Treatment for torsion is surgical exploration and detorsion and scrotal orchiopexy. Causative organisms for epididymitis include *Neisseria gonorrhoeae, Chlamydia trachomatis,* and other bacteria. Treatment with appropriate antibiotics and rest is indicated. However, treating this patient with antibiotics without first excluding testicular torsion is ill-advised; loss of the testis can be expected after 4 to 6 h of absent blood flow if the testis has torsioned. Strangulated hernia is associated with evidence of intestinal obstruction.

BLOCK 5

Answers

5-1. The answer is e. *(Tierney, 42/e, pp 1356–1357.)* **Botulism** bacillus is usually found in canned, smoked, or vacuum-packed foods. Patients present with dysphagia, dysphonia, visual disturbances, diplopia, ptosis, and fixed and dilated pupils. Patients with **anthrax** present with cough, dyspnea, and evidence of mediastinitis and pneumonia. Fried rice consumption is associated with **B. cereus** infection; patients present with a noninflammatory diarrhea. **Actinomyces** species are gram-positive organisms that may branch out into bacillary forms. Infection typically follows trauma, such as a dental extraction. **Listeria** is an intracellular pathogen with a predilection for causing illness in immunocompromised persons, including the elderly. Transmission is food-borne; implicated foods include coleslaws; soft cheeses, such as Mexican cheeses; pasteurized milk; undercooked hot dogs; and deli meats. Patients typically present with bacteremia and central nervous system infection.

5-2. The answer is b. *(Rowland, p 823.)* Most rhythmic to-and-fro movements of the eyes are called nystagmus. Nystagmus has a fast component in one direction and a slow component in the opposite direction. Nystagmus with a fast component to the right is called right-beating nystagmus. Phenytoin (Dilantin) may evoke nystagmus at levels of 20 to 30 mg/dL. The eye movements typically appear as a laterally beating nystagmus on gaze to either side; this type of nystagmus is called gaze-evoked. If the patient has nystagmus on looking directly forward, he or she is said to have nystagmus in the position of primary gaze. Therapeutic levels for phenytoin are usually 10 to 20 mg/dL, and some patients develop asymptomatic nystagmus even within that range. Ataxia, dysarthria, impaired judgement, and lethargy may also occur at toxic levels of phenytoin. Many other drugs also evoke nystagmus. Weakness of abduction of the left eye, or abducens palsy, is due either to injury to the sixth cranial nerve or to increased intracranial pressure. Impaired convergence can occur normally with age or may be a sign of injury to the midbrain. Papilledema is a sign of increased intracranial pressure. Impaired upward gaze may occur in many conditions, but would not be expected to occur with a toxic phenytoin level.

5-3. The answer is a. *(Schwartz, 7/e, pp 1459–1460.)* High-risk, critically ill patients with multisystem disease and cholecystitis experience a significant increase in morbidity and mortality following operative intervention. Tube cholecystostomy can be performed under local anesthesia in the operating room or via a percutaneous approach in the radiology suite. Open or laparoscopic procedures would carry the same general anesthetic risk whether done urgently or in a delayed (elective) fashion. Lithotripsy has no role in the treatment of acute cholecystitis.

5-4. The answer is c. *(Ebert, p 373.)* An extreme feeling of dislike for a part of the body in spite of a normal or nearly normal appearance is the main characteristic of body dysmorphic disorder. The fear of being ugly or repulsive is not decreased by reassurance and compliments and has almost a delusional quality. The social, academic, and occupational lives of individuals with this disorder are greatly affected, due to avoidance of social interactions for fear of embarrassment, the time spent in checking mirrors and seeking surgical treatment or cosmetic remedies, and the chronic emotional distress that accompanies the disorder.

5-5. The answer is b. *(Mishell, 3/e, pp 229–232.)* In patients with abnormal bleeding who are not responding to standard therapy, hysteroscopy should be performed. Hysteroscopy can rule out endometrial polyps or small fibroids, which, if present, can be resected. In patients with heavy abnormal bleeding who no longer desire fertility, an endometrial ablation can be performed. If a patient had completed childbearing and was having significant abnormal bleeding, a hysteroscopy rather than a hysterectomy would still be the procedure of choice to rule out easily treatable disease. Treatment with a GnRH agonist would only temporarily relieve symptoms.

5-6. The answer is b. *(Stobo, 23/e, pp 328–329.)* This obese patient on oral hypoglycemics has developed hyperglycemia and lethargy during an upper respiratory infection. Hyperosmolar nonketotic states that occur in type 2 diabetes can be fatal. When severe hyperglycemia and dehydration increase serum osmolarity above 380 mOsm/L, lethargy or coma occurs. Serum osmolarity is measured by the formula:

$$\frac{\text{Plasma glucose}}{18} + 2\,(\text{serum }Na^+ + K^+) + \frac{\text{blood urea nitrogen}}{2.8}$$

This patient's serum osmolality is as follows:

$$\frac{(900)}{18} + 2\,(138) + \frac{84}{2.8} = 50 + 276 + 30 = 356$$

Thus the serum osmolality is greater than 350 mOsm/kg. As can be seen from the equation, osmolarity depends mostly on the concentration of sodium. Serum osmolarity will rise significantly when dehydration prevents the dilution of serum sodium that might otherwise occur with hyperglycemia. Hyperosmolarity reflects both hyperglycemia and severe dehydration with hypernatremia. The serum bicarbonate is too high to be consistent with diabetic ketoacidosis. The hyponatremia is related to hyperglycemia. SIADH could not be diagnosed in this clinical setting. Patients with SIADH are not dehydrated but have an inappropriate excretion of ADH that leads to hyponatremia and water retention. The patient's diabetes likely went out of control due to infection. There is no clinical evidence for meningitis.

5-7. The answer is b. (*NCEP ATP III, pp 2486–2489.*) The National Cholesterol Education Program Adult Treatment Panel III includes lowering the LDL cholesterol to less than 100 in those with known coronary heart disease (secondary prevention). If dietary efforts are in place, a statin drug will likely be required. Gemfibrozil is used primarily for hypertriglyceridemia. ACE inhibitors have no significant effect on lipids.

5-8. The answer is e. (*Ebert, pp 468–469.*) There is nothing in the patient's history to suggest the presence of a personality disorder. The hallmark of a personality disorder is the presence of a constellation of behaviors or traits that cause significant impairment in social or occupational functioning or cause subjective distress. The patient in the question, on the contrary, reports a happy marriage and an ability to function well in social and occupational circumstances. While some persons in our society might object to his sexual behavior on moral grounds, such judgments are not a part of the diagnostic process.

5-9. The answer is e. (*Schwartz, 7/e, pp 1728–1729.*) A bypass procedure is the operation of choice for obstruction secondary to an annular pancreas. A Whipple procedure is too radical a therapy for this benign condition, and a partial resection of the annular pancreas often is complicated by fistula. Duodenojejunostomy is much more physiologic than gastrojejunostomy and does not require a vagotomy to prevent marginal ulceration; it is therefore the procedure of choice.

5-10. The answer is d. (*Tierney, 42/e, pp 280–282.*) The most frequent presenting clinical sign of **pulmonary embolus** (**PE**) is shortness of breath. Patients may also present with pleuritic chest pain, hemoptysis, and tachycardia. An excellent clue to the diagnosis of PE is deep venous thrombosis (DVT), but absence of signs of DVT does not exclude the diagnosis of PE. Embolus from a thrombus in the lower extremities (DVT) is the most common cause of PE. Common settings for PE include prolonged immobilization, use of oral contraceptives, obesity, recent surgery, burns, severe trauma, congestive heart failure, malignancy, pregnancy, sickle cell anemia, polycythemias, inherited deficiencies of the anticoagulating proteins (protein C, protein S, antithrombin III), and the Leiden factor V mutation. Chest radiograph in PE may be normal but may demonstrate a peripheral wedge-shaped density above the diaphragm (**Hampton's hump**), focal oligemia (**Westermark sign**), or abrupt occlusion of a vessel (**cutoff sign**). A loud S_2 is often heard in disorders that cause pulmonary hypertension, such as pulmonary embolism. The best next step in making the diagnosis would be to order a ventilation-perfusion (V/Q) scan. If the V/Q scan results are of low or indeterminate probability, the patient may need further studies, such as pulmonary arteriogram or venous ultrasonography of the lower extremity. The absence of D-dimer is strong evidence against thromboembolism. Helical (spiral) CT scans are comparable to V/Q scans and may be the first step in diagnosing pulmonary embolus.

5-11. The answer is d. (*Mishell, 3/e, pp 1011–1023.*) Conservative measures for treating dysmenorrhea include heating pads, mild analgesics, sedatives or antispasmodic drugs, and outdoor exercise. In patients with dysmenorrhea there is a significantly higher than normal concentration of prostaglandins in the endometrium and menstrual fluid. Prostaglandin synthase inhibitors such as indomethacin, naproxen, ibuprofen, and mefenamic acid are very effective in these patients. However, for patients with dysmenorrhea who are sexually active, oral contraceptives will provide needed protection from unwanted pregnancy and generally alleviate the dysmenorrhea. The OCPs minimize endometrial prostaglandin production during the concurrent administration of estrogen and progestin.

5-12. The answer is b. *(Beckmann, 4/e, pp 385–386, 393. Droegemueller, 3/e, pp 569, 740.)* This patient's history is most consistent with a diagnosis of urinary stress incontinence. Genuine stress incontinence is a condition of immediate involuntary loss of urine when intravesical pressure exceeds the maximum urethral pressure in the absence of detrusor activity. Patients with this condition complain of bursts of urine loss with physical activity or a cough, laugh, or sneeze. The cause of stress incontinence is structural, due to a cystocele or urethrocele. In cases of overflow incontinence, patients experience a continuous loss of a small amount of urine and associated symptoms of fullness and pressure. Overflow incontinence is usually due to obstruction or loss of neurologic control. Women with detrusor instability/dyssynergia have a loss of bladder inhibition and complain of urgency, frequency, and nocturia. Vesicovaginal fistulas are uncommon and usually occur as a complication of benign gynecologic procedures. Women with this complication usually present with a painless and continuous loss of urine from the vagina. Sometimes the uncontrolled loss of urine is not continuous but related to a change in position or posture. In the case of urinary tract infections, women usually present with symptoms of frequency, urgency, nocturia, dysuria, and hematuria.

5-13. The answer is e. *(Goldman, 21/e, p 164.)* S_1 consists of mitral valve closure followed by tricuspid closure. **Splitting of S_1** is seldom heard. In most cases, the valves close together and make a single sound, but if right ventricular contraction is delayed—as in the case of **right bundle branch block (RBBB)**—closure of the tricuspid valve occurs long after the mitral valve has closed and a split S_1 is heard.

5-14. The answer is e. *(Bradley, pp 1424–1425.)* This patient has a subacute to chronic progressive disease characterized by a combination of dementia, tremor, ataxia, and myoclonus. The EEG and MRI findings are typical of a spongiform encephalopathy. Multi-infarct dementia and subarachnoid hemorrhage would be expected to produce at least one very discrete event, and the imaging studies would be expected to show evidence of infarcts or other vascular abnormalities. Friedreich's disease may produce some dementia, but it is not a prominent part of the clinical deterioration. This patient is also much older than would be consistent with Friedreich's disease.

5-15. The answer is e. (*Sabiston, 15/e, pp 308–312.*) In the rapid-deceleration injuries associated with automobile crashes, the abdominal viscera tend to continue moving anteriorly after the body wall has been stopped. These organs exert great stress on the structures anchoring them to the retroperitoneum. Intestinal loops stretch and may tear their mesenteric attachments, injuring and thrombosing the superior mesenteric artery; kidneys and spleen may similarly shear their vascular pedicles. In these injuries, however, ordinarily the intraabdominal pressure does not rise excessively and diaphragmatic hernia is not likely. Diaphragmatic hernia is primarily associated with compression-type abdominal or thoracic injuries that increase intraabdominal or intrathoracic pressure sufficiently to tear the central portion of the diaphragm.

5-16. The answer is a. (*Behrman, 16/e, pp 728–729. McMillan, 3/e, pp 1490–1491, 2176–2179. Rudolph, 21/e, pp 842–844.*) The clinical presentation described supports the diagnosis of anaphylactoid purpura, a generalized, acute vasculitis of unknown cause involving small blood vessels. In this condition, the skin lesion, which is classic in character and distribution, is often accompanied by arthritis, usually of the large joints, and by gastrointestinal symptoms. Colicky abdominal pain, vomiting, and melena are common. Renal involvement occurs in a significant number of patients and is potentially the most serious manifestation of the disease. Although most children with this complication recover, some will develop chronic nephritis. Laboratory studies are not diagnostic. Serum complement and IgA levels can be normal or elevated. Coagulation studies and platelets are normal.

5-17. The answer is a. (*Kaplan, 8/e, pp 1000–1004.*) Tricyclic antidepressants such as clomipramine and amitriptyline and SSRIs such as paroxetine and sertraline, as well as MAOIs, can cause erectile dysfunction, delayed ejaculation, anorgasmia, and decreased libido. Bupropion, mirtazapine, trazodone, and nefazodone, in contrast, do not affect sexual functions in a negative way. Trazodone and nefazodone, however, have been implicated in cases of priapism and should not therefore be used as first-line medications in male patients.

5-18. The answer is c. (*Braunwald, 15/e, pp 1508–1510.*) Rhabdomyolysis-induced ARF may follow influenza. It is characterized by a creatinine disproportionately elevated compared to BUN (usual BUN-creatinine ratio ~ 10), hyperkalemia, hyperphosphatemia, and hyperuricemia, all due to release of intracellular muscle products. The high phosphorus causes hypocalcemia. All nonsteroidal agents may cause decreased renal function. Usually this is due to decreased blood flow—less commonly, to drug-induced nephritis. The laboratory abnormalities discussed are not seen in either situation. However, stopping the ibuprofen in this patient would be prudent. The absence of orthostatic hypotension makes the diagnosis of volume depletion very unlikely. Nothing on history, physical examination, or electrolyte abnormalities suggests obstruction. However, in a 76-year-old man, considering occult obstruction is always appropriate.

5-19. The answer is b. (*Braunwald, 15/e, pp 1414–1445.*) The diagnosis in this patient is suggested by the physical exam findings. The findings of poor excursion, flatness of percussion, and decreased fremitus on the right side are all consistent with a right-sided pleural effusion. A large right-sided effusion may shift the trachea to the left. Histoplasmosis would be one possible cause of such an effusion. A pneumothorax should result in hyperresonance of the affected side. Atelectasis on the right side would shift the trachea to the right. A consolidated pneumonia would characteristically result in increased fremitus, flatness to percussion, and bronchial breath sounds, and would not cause tracheal deviation.

5-20. The answer is c. (*Kaplan, 8/e, p 820.*) Cushing's syndrome due to exogenous administration of corticosteroids and more rarely to adrenocarcinoma or ectopic production of ACTH is often associated with psychiatric disturbances. Depression and mixed anxiety and depressive states are the most common psychiatric manifestations of the syndrome (from 35 to 68%, depending on the study). Since the affective symptoms are directly secondary to the administration of a substance (in this case steroids for the treatment of asthma), the patient's diagnosis would be a substance-induced mood disorder. Mania, psychosis, delirium, and cognitive disturbances also occur, but at a much lower rate. Depressive symptoms occur early in the disorder (in the prodromal period in 27% of cases). Most patients improve after the primary disorder is treated and serum cortisol decreases.

5-21. The answer is a. (*Schwartz, 7/e, p 458.*) Gastric aspiration is best treated by tracheal suctioning, oxygen, and positive-pressure ventilation.

Bronchoscopy is helpful if particulate matter is causing bronchial obstruction or if the vomitus is found to contain particulate material. Bronchial lavage is no longer recommended, and steroids have not been shown to be of value. Fluids should be given sparingly because hypervolemia will worsen the risk of pulmonary edema following aspiration. Tracheostomy may be indicated for long-term airway management in obtunded or otherwise severely debilitated patients; however, initial control of the airway should be by orotracheal intubation whenever possible. High positive end-expiratory pressure is not required unless respiratory failure develops.

5-22. The answer is d. *(Fuster, 10/e, pp 902–905.)* While the clinical picture itself could lead to these neurological symptoms, the only cardiovascular medication on this list likely to do so is lidocaine. Lidocaine is particularly likely to cause confusion in the elderly patient, for whom a lower dose of the drug should generally be given. Other potential adverse effects of lidocaine include tremor, convulsions, respiratory depression, bradycardia, and hypotension.

5-23. The answer is d. *(Rowland, pp 708–713.)* Motor neuron disease in the anterior horns of the spinal cord and damage to the corticospinal tracts or motor neurons contributing axons to the corticospinal tracts would account for these neurologic signs. Damage to the dorsal spinal root would be expected to produce sensory, rather than motor, deficits and would produce areflexia, rather than hyperreflexia, at the level of the injury. Damage to the ventral spinal roots would produce weakness and wasting, but no spasticity or hyperreflexia would develop. Purkinje cell damage would be expected to produce ataxia without substantial weakness. The arcuate fasciculus connects elements of the cerebral cortex not involved in the regulation of strength or motor tone.

5-24. The answer is a. *(Kaplan, 8/e, pp 508–509.)* Schizoaffective disorder is diagnosed when the required criteria for schizophrenia are met (delusions, hallucination, disorganized speech or behavior, and/or negative symptoms; duration of the disturbance, including prodromal and residual period, of at least 6 months with at least 1 month of active symptoms) and the patient experiences at some point in the course of the illness a major depressive episode or a manic episode. The man in the question meets all these criteria. Delusional disorder is not accompanied by decline in functions or significant affective symptoms. Individuals with schizoid personality disorder do not experience psychotic symptoms. Bipolar disorder is differentiated from schizoaffective disorder by the absence of periods of psychosis accompanied by prominent affective symptoms.

5-25. The answer is c. *(Tierney, 42/e, p 519.)* The patient most likely has **antiphospholipid syndrome.** Patients with this antibody are at risk for venous and arterial thrombotic events, probably due to antibody reactivity with platelets or endothelial cell phospholipids. Patients often have a history of miscarriages, leg ulcers, Raynaud's phenomenon, and livedo reticularis. Laboratory data often reveal a positive lupus anticoagulant, thrombocytopenia, a prolonged PTT (not corrected by adding normal plasma; a clotting factor deficiency would correct with normal plasma), elevated titers of anticardiolipin antibodies, and an abnormal dilute **Russell's viper venom. Takayasu's arteritis** (pulseless disease) is a granulomatous arteritis that affects women more than men. Patients are usually in their fourth decade of life. The disease typically affects the aorta and its major branches, including the arteries that supply the upper extremities. Patients have absent pulses in the upper arm and complain of arm claudication. **Livedo reticularis** is characterized by reddish or bluish mottling of the extremities and is usually idiopathic and requires no treatment. Livedo reticularis may be secondary to atheroembolism-induced emboli following an intraarterial procedure. **Libman-Sacks disease** is endocarditis in patients with SLE and may be associated with antiphospholipid antibodies.

5-26. The answer is e. *(Schwartz, 7/e, pp 812–826.)* With the exception of coarctation, in which no shunt (or cyanosis) exists, the anomalies listed cause a shunting of blood between the systemic and lower-pressure pulmonary circulation. Transposition of the great vessels is a right-to-left shunt that leads to cyanosis. Except where there is persistent congenital pulmonary hypertension, patent ductus arteriosus and atrial septal defects cause a shunting of oxygenated blood from the aorta and left atrium, respectively, back into the pulmonary artery and right atrium. These anomalies cause recirculation of oxygenated blood within the cardiopulmonary circuit but not cyanosis. When a ventricular septal defect is combined with pulmonary artery atresia (tetralogy of Fallot), the resulting undercirculation in the pulmonary system joins transposition as a cause of cyanosis. Other less common congenital lesions in which the pulmonary arterial blood flow is relatively decreased include tricuspid atresia, Ebstein's anomaly, and hypoplastic right ventricle.

5-27. The answer is d. *(Brewster, Surgery 109:447–454, 1991.)* The CT scan reveals a fractured ring of calcification in the abdominal aorta with significant density in the paraaortic area. The inferior mesenteric artery (IMA) is always at risk in patients with the changes in the vessel wall characteristic of abdominal aneurysms, but particularly so in the presence of rupture and retroperitoneal dissection of blood under systemic arterial pressures. The incidence of ischemic colitis following abdominal aortic resection is about 2%. Blood flow to the left colon normally derives from the IMA with collateral flow from the middle and inferior hemorrhoidal vessels. The superior mesenteric artery (SMA) may also contribute via the marginal artery of Drummond. If the SMA is stenotic or occluded, flow to the left colon will be primarily dependent on an intact IMA. The IMA is usually ligated at the time of aneurysmorrhaphy. Patients at highest risk for diminished flow through collateral vessels are those with a history of visceral angina, those found to have a patent IMA at the time of operation, those who have suffered an episode of hypotension following rupture of an aneurysm, those in whom preoperative angiograms reveal occlusion of the SMA, and those in whom Doppler flow signals along the mesenteric border cease following occlusion of the IMA. Bowel ischemia recognized at the time of operation should be treated by reimplantation of the IMA into the graft to restore flow.

5-28. The answer is b. *(Kaplan, 8/e, p 576.)* Excessive motor activity, usually with intrusive and annoying qualities, poor sustained attention, difficulties inhibiting impulsive behaviors in social situations and on cognitive tasks, and difficulties with peers are the main characteristics of ADHD, combined type. Symptoms must be present in two or more settings (in this case, home and school) and must cause significant impairment.

5-29. The answer is c. *(Behrman, 16/e, p 460. McMillan, 3/e, p 477.)* Most medications are secreted to some extent in breast milk. Some lipid-soluble medications may be concentrated in breast milk. Although the list of contraindicated medications is short, caution should always be exercised when giving a medication to a breast-feeding woman. Medications that are clearly contraindicated include lithium, cyclosporin, antineoplastic agents, illicit drugs including cocaine and heroin, ergotamines, and bromocriptine (which supresses lactation). Although some suggest that oral contraceptives may have a negative impact on milk production, the association has not been proven conclusively. In general, antibiotics are safe, with only a few exceptions. While sedatives and narcotic pain medications are probably safe, the infant must be observed carefully for sedation. All of the medications listed in the question are considered safe, except for lithium.

5-30. The answer is b. (*Droegemueller, 3/e, pp 625–635. Beckmann, 4/e, pp 370–371.*) Bacterial vaginosis is a condition is which there is an overgrowth of anaerobic bacteria in the vagina that replaces the normal lactobacillus. Women with this type of vaginitis complain of an unpleasant vaginal odor that is described as musty or fishy and a thin, gray-white vaginal discharge that is adherent to the vaginal walls. Vulvar irritation and pruritus are rarely present. To confirm the diagnosis of bacterial vaginosis, a wet smear is done. To perform a wet smear, saline is mixed with the vaginal discharge and clumps of bacteria and clue cells are identified. Clue cells are vaginal epithelial cells with clusters of bacteria adherent to their surfaces. In addition, a whiff test can be performed by mixing potassium hydroxide with the vaginal discharge. In cases of bacterial vaginosis, an amine-like odor will be detected. The treatment of choice for bacterial vaginosis is metronidazole (Flagyl) 500 mg given twice daily for 7 days. In cases of a normal or physiologic discharge, vaginal secretions are white, curdy, and odorless. In addition, normal vaginal secretions do not adhere to the vaginal side walls. In cases of candidiasis, patients commonly complain of vulvar burning, pain, pruritus, and erythema. The vaginal discharge tends to be white, highly viscous, granular, and adherent to the vaginal walls. A wet smear with potassium hydroxide can confirm the diagnosis by the identification of hyphae. Treatment of candidiasis can achieved with the administration of topical imidazoles or triazoles or the oral medication Diflucan. *Trichomonas* vaginitis is the most common nonviral, nonchlamydial sexually transmitted disease of women. It is caused by the anaerobic, flagellated protozoan *T. vaginalis.* Women with *Trichomonas* vaginitis commonly complain of a copious vaginal discharge that may be white, yellow, green, or gray and that has an unpleasant odor. Some women complain of vulvar pruritus, which is primarily confined to the vestibule and labia minora. On physical exam, the vulva and vagina frequently appear red and swollen. Only a small percentage of women possess the classically described strawberry cervix. Diagnosis of trichomoniasis is confirmed with a wet saline smear. Under the microscope, the *Trichomonas* organisms can be visualized under high power; these organisms are unicellular protozoans that are spherical in shape with three to five flagella extending from one end. The recommended treatment for trichomoniasis is a one-time dose of 2 g metronidazole. *Chlamydia trachomatis* is an intracellular parasite that can cause an infection that may be manifested as cervicitis, urethritis, or salpingitis. Patients with mild cases may be asymptomatic. On physical exam, women with chlamydial infections may demonstrate a mucopurulent cervicitis. The diagnosis of chlamydia is suspected on clinical exam and confirmed with cervical cultures. Treatment for a chlamydial cervicitis is with oral azithromycin, 1 g, or doxycycline 100 mg twice daily for 7 days.

5-31. The answer is b. (*Braunwald, p 2459.*) Gastric disturbances are a common side effect of corticosteroid use. Ranitidine is an appropriate prophylactic treatment. Patients with high cholesterol should be given a heart-healthy diet. Neurological checks every hour, central venous line, and stat head CT for change in mental status are all things that should be done for unstable trauma patients with a cranial component.

5-32. The answer is c. (*Tierney, 42/e, p 445.*) The patient described has a **Hollenhorst plaque.** A Hollenhorst plaque or cholesterol embolus represents an arterial embolus that originates from an atheromatous plaque in a more proximal vessel, usually the internal carotid. It is a sign of severe atherosclerosis. These plaques are bright, refractile, and yellow. They appear to migrate down the vessel; carefully massaging the eyeball can actually facilitate migration.

5-33. The answer is d. (*Behrman, 16/e, pp 1176–1178. McMillan, 3/e, pp 1685–1686. Rudolph, 21/e, pp 1357–1363.*) Recurrent abdominal pain is a common complaint occurring in at least 10% of school-aged children. In children older than 2 years, less than 10% of cases have an identifiable organic cause. Management of these children is difficult and frustrating for the physician and the family. Excessive testing and treatments are contraindicated. A thorough history and physical examination, including growth parameters, are frequently helpful in separating organic from nonorganic causes of abdominal pain. Any signs or symptoms of organic causes should be pursued. If nothing in the history or physical examination is found, as is likely in the case described, reassurance of the children and family members is indicated. Close follow-up for new or changing symptoms as well as further reassurance to the family is important.

5-34. The answer is c. *(Tierney, 42/e, pp 1123–1125.)* Ninety percent of the adrenal gland must be destroyed for **Addison's disease** (hypoadrenalism) to develop; glucocorticoids, mineralocorticoids, and androgens are affected. Etiologies include tuberculosis, malignancy, sarcoidosis, trauma, histoplasmosis, hemochromatosis, amyloidosis, sepsis, cytomegalovirus infection, and medications (ketoconazole, rifampin, anticoagulants, and anticonvulsants). Patients without a clear etiology have idiopathic hypoadrenalism. Symptoms include weakness, hypotension, anorexia, weight loss, and hyperpigmentation of the skin. Patients may have hyponatremia, hyperkalemia, and eosinophilia. Adults with **craniopharyngioma** present with headache, visual problems, papilledema, personality changes, and hypopituitarism. **Sheehan syndrome** is postpartum hemorrhage and necrosis of the pituitary gland. **Empty sella syndrome** occurs when CSF fills the sella space and flattens the pituitary gland, which continues to function normally. The disorder is seen in obese, hypertensive, multiparous women. Insulinoma causes hypoglycemia, which is often a feature of hypoadrenalism. **Schmidt syndrome** is the combination of Hashimoto's thyroiditis with Addison's disease. **Pituitary apoplexy** occurs in <5% of patients with a pituitary macroadenoma (>1 cm); patients complain of headache, neck stiffness, fever, and visual disturbance and may present with acute adrenal insufficiency.

5-35. The answer is c. *(Behrman, 16/e, pp 751–757. McMillan, 3/e, pp 413–416, 855–883. Rudolph, 21/e, pp 970–972, 977–979.)* Unsuspected bacteremia due to *Haemophilus influenzae* type B (now rare), *Neisseria menigitidis,* or *Streptococcus pneumoniae* should be considered before prescribing treatment for otitis media in a young, febrile, toxic-appearing infant. Blood culture should be performed before antibiotic therapy is initiated, and examination of the cerebrospinal fluid is indicated if meningitis is suspected. The classic signs of meningitis are found with increasing reliability in children over the age of 6 months. Nevertheless, a febrile, irritable, inconsolable infant with an altered state of alertness deserves a lumbar puncture even in the absence of meningeal signs. A petechial rash, characteristically associated with meningococcal infection, has been known to occur with other bacterial infections as well. Organisms may be identified on smear of these lesions.

A fever accompanied by inability to flex rather than rotate the neck immediately suggests meningitis. An indolent clinical course does not rule out bacterial meningitis. A lumbar puncture is of prime diagnostic importance in determining the presence of bacterial meningitis, which requires immediate antibiotic therapy. A delay in treatment can lead to complications such as cerebrovascular thrombosis, obstructive hydrocephalus, cerebritis with seizures or acute increased intracranial pressure, coma, or death. In the described patient, lumbar puncture is warranted because of the change in his clinical status.

5-36. The answer is c. *(Behrman, 16/e, pp 1418–1420. McMillan, 3/e, pp 1431–1432. Rudolph, 21/e, pp 1452–1453.)* The child described in the question, who has no cyanosis or murmur, no cardiac or pulmonary vascular abnormalities by chest x-ray, and no evidence of structural anomalies by echocardiogram, is unlikely to have an underlying gross anatomic defect. The electrocardiographic pattern in the figure shows the configuration of preexcitation, the pattern seen in the Wolff-Parkinson-White syndrome (WPW). These patients have an aberrant atrioventricular conduction pathway, which causes the early ventricular depolarization appearing on the electrocardiogram as a shortened PR interval. The initial slow ventricular depolarization wave is referred to as the *delta wave.* Seventy percent of patients with WPW have single or repeated episodes of paroxysmal supraventricular tachycardia, which can cause the symptoms described in the question. The preexcitation electrocardiographic pattern and WPW can occur in Ebstein malformation, but this is unlikely in the absence of cyanosis and with a normal echocardiogram. If ventricular tachycardia were present, the symptoms would likely be more profound. Active play and exposure to over-the-counter medications containing sympathomimetics in a healthy 4-year-old child can cause symptoms such as those described in the question in children with WPW by precipitating paroxysmal supraventricular tachycardia.

5-37. The answer is d. *(Bradley, pp 1556–1557.)* Normal-pressure hydrocephalus (NPH) is a chronic, communicating form of hydrocephalus affecting elderly adults. The cause is unknown, but it may relate to prior episodes of trauma, infection, or subarachnoid hemorrhage. The clinical picture typically includes a triad of gait disturbance, dementia, and incontinence. The gait disorder may be difficult to distinguish from that of Parkinson's disease, and has been labeled an apraxic gait as patients often have difficulty even lifting their feet off the floor, though they have no weakness and may perform motor tasks well with the legs when seated. CT or MRI in these patients usually shows enlargement of the temporal and frontal horns of the lateral ventricles out of proportion to the degree of cortical atrophy. There may also be a squaring off or blunted appearance of the frontal horns, and increased signal on T2-weighted images may be seen in the periventricular regions, consistent with the presence of fluid related to transependymal flow of CSF.

5-38. The answer is d. (*Rock, 8/e, pp 121–122.*) The clinical history presented in this question is classic for a ruptured tubal pregnancy accompanied by hemoperitoneum. Because pregnancy tests are negative in almost 50% of cases, they are of little practical value in an emergency. Dilation and curettage would not permit rapid enough diagnosis, and the results obtained by this procedure are variable. Posterior colpotomy requires an operating room, surgical anesthesia, and an experienced operator with a scrubbed and gowned associate. Refined optic and electronic systems have improved the accuracy of laparoscopy, but this new equipment is not always available, and the procedure requires an operating room and, usually, surgical anesthesia. Culdocentesis is a rapid, nonsurgical method to confirm the presence of unclotted intraabdominal blood from a ruptured tubal pregnancy. Culdocentesis, however, is also not perfect, and a negative culdocentesis should not be used as the sole criterion for whether or not to operate on a patient.

5-39. The answer is a. (*Schwartz, 7/e, pp 1679–1707.*) The patient described is exhibiting classic signs and symptoms of hyperparathyroidism. In addition, if a history is obtainable, frequently the patient will relate a history of renal calculi and bone pain—the syndrome characterized as "groans, stones, and bones." Acute management of the hypercalcemic state includes vigorous hydration to restore intravascular volume, which is invariably diminished. This will establish renal perfusion and thus promote urinary calcium excretion. Thiazide diuretics are contraindicated because they frequently cause patients to become hypercalcemic. Instead, diuresis should be promoted with the use of loop diuretics such as furosemide

(Lasix). The use of intravenous phosphorus infusion is no longer recommended because precipitation in the lungs, heart, or kidney can lead to serious morbidity. Mithramycin is an antineoplastic agent that in low doses inhibits bone resorption and thus diminishes serum calcium levels; it is used only when other maneuvers fail to decrease the calcium level. Calcitonin is useful at times. Bisphosphonates are newer agents particularly useful for lowering calcium levels in resistant cases, such as those associated with humoral malignancy. Emergency neck exploration is seldom warranted. In unprepared patients, the morbidity is unacceptably high.

5-40. The answer is d. (*Sabiston, 15/e, pp 1277–1278.*) A subperichondrial hematoma in the pinna of the ear may lead to avascular necrosis of the cartilage with shriveling of the pinna and fibrosis and calcification of the hematoma. The result is the deformity known as cauliflower ear. Appropriate treatment consists of evacuation of the hematoma by incision and tight packing of the skin and perichondrium onto the cartilage with a pressure dressing. Needle aspiration does not effect adequate drainage. Ice packs may be helpful early, but are not sufficient to prevent the deformity; antibiotics are not indicated for this lesion. Since the hematoma is subperichondrial, excision of the hematoma would remove the perichondrium and lead to cartilage deformities.

5-41. The answer is a. (*Tierney, 42/e, p 796.*) The patient is describing **pseudoclaudication,** which is characteristic of lumbar spinal stenosis. This arises from compression of the exiting nerve roots by a disk, osteophyte, or narrow canal. The leg pain is most pronounced when walking downhill or descending stairs and takes several minutes of sitting or flexing forward before resolution. Often patients who continue to walk with pain will stoop over to relieve the symptoms (**stoop sign**). **Claudication** is seen in peripheral vascular disease, but the pain that occurs with walking resolves immediately upon stopping or standing without sitting. Peripheral pulses may be compromised. **Diffuse idiopathic skeletal hyperostosis** (**DISH**) causes calcification of the longitudinal ligaments of the spine and is usually found in patients with diabetes mellitus.

5-42. The answer is a. (*Braunwald, p 174.*) The fact that vision is preserved excludes optic neuritis and cavernous sinus thrombosis. Optic neuritis will produce pain in the affected eye and may be associated with a normal optic disc, but visual acuity should be deficient and an afferent pupillary defect should be apparent. Cavernous sinus thrombosis usually produces proptosis and pain, but impaired venous drainage from the eye should interfere with acuity, and the retina should appear profoundly disturbed. With a diphtheritic polyneuropathy, an ophthalmoplegia may develop, but this would not be limited to one eye and is not usually associated with facial trauma. Transverse sinus thrombosis may produce cerebrocortical dysfunction or stroke, but ophthalmoplegia would not be a manifestation of this problem.

5-43. The answer is d. *(Ebert, p 570.)* Children with conduct disorder display a persistent disregard for rules and other people's rights that lasts at least 1 year. Aggression toward people and animals, destruction of property, deceit and illegal activities, and frequent truancy from school are the main characteristics of the disorder. Approximately one-third of children diagnosed with conduct disorder proceed to become delinquent adolescents, and many are diagnosed with antisocial personality disorder in adulthood. Patients with antisocial personality disorder display a pervasive pattern of disregard for and violation of the rights of others since the age of 15 years, with evidence of a conduct disorder before age 15. Substance abuse is just one facet of conduct disorder. Children with oppositional defiant disorder are problematic and rebellious but do not routinely engage in aggressive, destructive, or illegal activities. Also, they do not present with the lack of empathy for others and the disregard for other people's rights that are typical of conduct disorder.

5-44. The answer is c. *(Behrman, 16/e, pp 1231–1233. McMillan, 3/e, pp 177, 217–218, 222. Rudolph, 21/e, pp 189–191.)* Diaphragmatic hernia occurs with the transmittal of abdominal contents across a congenital or traumatic defect in the diaphragm. In the newborn, this condition results in profound respiratory distress with significant mortality. Prenatal diagnosis is common and, when found, necessitates that the birth take place at a tertiary level center. In the neonate, respiratory failure in the first hours of life, a scaphoid abdomen, and presence of bowel sounds in the chest are common findings. Intensive respiratory support including mechanical ventilation and extracorporeal membrane oxygenation (ECMO) has increased survival. Mortality can be as high as 50% despite aggressive treatment.

5-45. The answer is c. *(Tierney, 42/e, pp 976–977.)* **Shy-Drager syndrome** (also called multiple system atrophy or MSA) is parkinsonism associated with autonomic dysfunction; patients may present with anhidrosis, disturbance of sphincter control, impotence, and orthostatic hypotension. Patients typically have signs of LMN involvement (everything is down or low, meaning flaccid paralysis, diminished reflexes, and flexor Babinski reflex). **Parkinson's disease** (**PD**) is a triad of resting asymmetric tremor, rigidity (cogwheel in nature), and bradykinesia. Patients have difficulty getting out of a chair, and gait, which is slow at first, becomes faster (festination) with ambulation. The **get-up-and-go test** (patient gets out of a chair, walks 10 ft, turns around, and returns to chair in under 15 s) is a good test for assessing gait and will be abnormal in patients with parkinsonism. PD is an idiopathic progressive disease in which there is **Lewy body inclusion** and degeneration of neurons in the substantia nigra. **Benign essential tremor** is also called senile tremor or familial tremor (autosomal dominant) and is reduced by alcohol use. **Cerebellar tremor** occurs with intention and is absent at rest. Patients usually have other signs of cerebellar disease, such as ataxia. **Progressive supranuclear palsy** is a disorder of bradykinesia and rigidity with dementia and loss of voluntary control of eye movements. **Creutzfeldt-Jakob disease** is accompanied by parkinsonian features, but patients typically have dementia and myoclonic jerky movements.

5-46. The answer is c. (*Schwartz, 7/e, pp 494–496.*) Because of the ease with which carbon dioxide diffuses across the alveolar membranes, $PaCO_2$ is a highly reliable indicator of alveolar ventilation. In this postoperative patient with respiratory acidosis and hypoxemia, the hypercarbia is diagnostic of alveolar hypoventilation. Acute hypoxemia can occur with pulmonary embolism, pulmonary edema, and significant atelectasis, but in all those situations the $PaCO_2$ should be normal or reduced as the patient hyperventilates to improve oxygenation. The absorption of gas from the peritoneal cavity may transiently affect the $PaCO_2$, but should have no effect on oxygenation.

5-47. The answer is d. (*Cunningham, 21/e, pp 180, 189–190, 1275–1281.*) This patient's history and physical exam are consistent with an intestinal obstruction. An intestinal obstruction must be ruled out because, if it goes undiagnosed and untreated, it can result in a bowel perforation. This patient has a history of a previous abdominal surgery, which places her at risk for adhesions. Beginning in the second trimester, the gravid uterus can push on these adhesions and result in a bowel strangulation. Common symptoms of intestinal obstruction include colicky abdominal pain, nausea, and emesis. Signs of a bowel obstruction include abdominal tenderness and decreased bowel sounds. Fever and an elevated white blood cell count are present with bowel strangulation and necrosis. This patient has a mild leukocytosis, which is also characteristic of normal pregnancy. In order to rule out an intestinal obstruction, an upright or lateral decubitus abdominal x-ray should be done to identify the presence of distended loops of bowel and air-fluid levels, which confirm the diagnosis. Treatment consists of bowel rest, intravenous hydration, and nasogastric suction; patients who do not respond to conservative therapy may require surgery. Bowel stimulants such as laxatives or enemas should not be administered. Pregnant women are predisposed to constipation secondary to decreased bowel motility induced by elevated levels of progesterone. The symptoms of nausea and emesis in this patient and the presence of a low-grade fever prompt further workup because her presentation is not consistent with uncomplicated constipation. In pregnancy, constipation can be treated with hydration, increased fiber in the diet, and the use of stool softeners. The patient's sudden onset of emesis and abdominal pain is not consistent with the normal presentation of hyperemesis gravidarum. Hyperemesis typically has an onset in the early part of the first trimester and usually resolves by 16 weeks. It is characterized by intractable vomiting causing severe weight loss, dehydration, and electrolyte imbalance. The ingestion of spicy foods during pregnancy can cause or exacerbate gastric reflux or "heartburn", but would not cause the severity of the symptoms described in this patient's presentation. Dyspepsia during pregnancy can be treated with antacids. The patient with gastric reflux in pregnancy should also be counseled to eat smaller, more frequent meals and bland food.

5-48. The answer is a. (*Shuaib, p 33.*) The head CT scan is the mainstay of emergency department management of acute stroke. It is crucial to exclude intracranial hemorrhage prior to the potential administration of intravenous thrombolytic agents. A cerebral angiogram may play a role in the management of the acute stroke patient, particularly if there is evidence of cerebral or subarachnoid hemorrhage, or if there exists a possibility of performing intraarterial thrombolysis, but CT scan is required first. T2-weighted MRI may also show ischemic and hemorrhagic injury, but infarction may not appear this quickly on MRI and hemorrhage may also be missed. MRI is also not as widely available as CT. In the absence of evidence of trauma at the time of the patient's fall, C-spine MRI and skull x-rays play no role in management.

5-49. The answer is c. (*Schwartz, 7/e, pp 966–967.*) Acute mesenteric ischemia may be difficult to diagnose. The condition should be suspected in patients with either systemic manifestations of arteriosclerotic vascular disease or low cardiac output states associated with a sudden development of abdominal pain that is out of proportion to the physical findings. Lactic acidosis and an elevated hematocrit reflecting hemoconcentration are common laboratory findings. Abdominal films show a nonspecific ileus pattern. The cause may be embolic occlusion or thrombosis of the superior mesenteric artery, primary mesenteric venous occlusion, or nonocclusive mesenteric ischemia secondary to low cardiac output states. A mortality of 65 to 100% is reported. The majority of affected patients are at high operative risk, but, since early diagnosis followed by revascularization or resectional surgery or both is the only hope for survival, celiotomy must be performed once the diagnosis of arterial occlusion or bowel infarction has been made. Initial treatment of nonocclusive mesenteric ischemia includes measures to increase cardiac output and blood pressure and the direct intraarterial infusion of vasodilators such as papaverine into the superior mesenteric system. This patient is at risk for both occlusive and nonocclusive mesenteric ischemic disease. If his clinical status permits, angiographic studies should be performed before the operation to establish the diagnosis and to determine whether embolectomy, revascularization, or nonsurgical management is indicated as initial treatment.

5-50. The answer is a. (*Kaplan, 8/e, p 999.*) Neuroleptic medications can produce hyperprolactinemia even at very low doses and are the most common cause of galactorrhea in psychiatric patients. Hyperprolactinemia with neuroleptic use is secondary to the blockade of dopamine receptors with these drugs. (Dopamine normally inhibits prolactin, and with dopamine's blockade, hyperprolactinemia can result.) Amenorrhea and galactorrhea are the main symptoms of hyperprolactinemia in women, and impotence is the main symptom in men, although men can also develop gynecomastia and galactorrhea. Other causes of hyperprolactinemia include severe systemic illness such as cirrhosis or renal failure, pituitary tumors, idiopathic causes, and pregnancy.

BLOCK 6

Answers

6-1. The answer is c. *(Cunningham, 21/e, pp 209, 241, 1011–1012, 1019.)* Alcohol is a potent teratogen. Fetal alcohol syndrome is the most common cause of mental retardation in the United States and consists of a constellation of fetal defects including craniofacial anomalies, growth restriction, behavioral disturbances, brain defects, cardiac defects, and spinal defects. Alcohol use in pregnancy has a prevalence of 1 to 2%, and the incidence of fetal alcohol syndrome is approximately 6 in 10,000 births. No safe threshold for alcohol use during pregnancy has been established. Fetal injury can occur with as little as one drink per day, but women who engage in binge drinking are at the greatest risk. There is no way to diagnose fetal alcohol syndrome prenatally. There are many potential teratogens in cigarette smoke, including nicotine, carbon monoxide, cadmium, lead, and hydrocarbons. Smoking has been shown to cause fetal growth restriction and to be related to increased incidences of subfertility, spontaneous abortions, placenta previa, abruption, and preterm delivery. The mechanisms for these adverse effects include increased fetal carboxyhemoglobin levels, reduced uteroplacental blood flow, and fetal hypoxia. Most studies do not indicate that tobacco use is related to an increased risk of congenital malformations. Alcohol consumption in pregnancy, not tobacco use, is a common cause of mental retardation and developmental day. However, tobacco use has been associated with attention deficit hyperactivity disorder and behavioral and learning problems.

6-2. The answer is c. *(Behrman, 16/e, pp 790–792. McMillan, 3/e, p 587.)* Mammalian bites should be promptly and thoroughly scrubbed with soap and water and debrided. The decision to suture depends on the location, age, and nature of the wound. Antibiotic prophylaxis should be considered in cat, human, or monkey bites. Only 4% of dog bites become infected (and do not necessarily need antibiotic prophylaxis), compared with 35% of cat bites and 50% of monkey bites (which require antibiotics in most cases). Cat bites are usually deep punctures. Human bites almost invariably become infected. The etiologies of these infections are polymicrobial. *Pasteurella multocida* is a common organism in infected cat and dog bites. Infected human bites tend to have positive cultures for *Streptococcus viridans, Staphylococcus aureus,* and *Bacteroides* spp. Treatment with oral amoxicillin-clavulanate or erythromycin is recommended. Antibiotic prophylaxis is recommended for any bite sustained by an infant, a diabetic, or an immunocompromised patient because of the higher risk of infection in these persons. Since the child is fully immunized, tetanus boosters are not required. Similarly, as the dog was provoked and was fully immunized, rabies should not be a concern.

6-3. The answer is d. *(Sabiston, 15/e, p 124.)* Allergic and febrile reactions occur in about 1% of all transfusions. Hemolytic transfusion reactions are much less common (0.2%), with fatal reactions in 1 of 100,000 transfusions. Hemolytic transfusion reactions are due to the reaction of recipient antibodies against transfused antigens. These reactions can be both immediate and delayed. Symptoms of a hemolytic transfusion reaction include fever, chills, and pain and heat at the infusion site, as well as respiratory distress, anxiety, hypotension, and oliguria. During surgery a hemolytic transfusion reaction can manifest as abnormal bleeding.

6-4. The answer is d. *(Braunwald, 15/e, pp 2257–2261.)* Hemochromatosis is a disorder of iron storage that results in deposition of iron in parenchymal cells. The liver is usually enlarged, and excessive skin pigmentation is present in 90% of symptomatic patients at the time of diagnosis. Diabetes occurs secondary to direct damage of the pancreas by iron deposition. Arthropathy develops in 25 to 50% of cases. Other diagnoses listed could not explain all the manifestations of this patient's disease process. Addison's disease can cause weight loss and hyperpigmentation but does not affect the liver or joints; it is associated with hypoglycemia rather than diabetes mellitus.

6-5. The answer is b. *(Behrman, 16/e, p 91. McMillan, 3/e, p 622. Rudolph, 21/e, pp 364–365.)* Poisoning with tricyclic antidepressants is a leading reason for admissions to pediatric intensive care units and a leading cause of fatal drug overdose in adolescents. These preparations produce a variety of pharmacologic effects, including inhibition of muscarinic/cholinergic receptors, blockade of norepinephrine and serotonin uptake, and depression of sodium channels responsible for cardiac cell membrane depolarization. The toxic-to-therapeutic ratio is low. Young children often ingest poisons and drugs during times of household disruption. Visitors' handbags are a great temptation for the inquisitive toddler.

6-6. The answer is a. *(Kaplan, 8/e, p 642.)* Pain disorder is defined as the presence of pain that is the predominant focus of clinical attention. Psychological factors play an important role in the disorder. The primary symptom is pain, in one or more sites, that is not fully accounted for by a nonpsychiatric medical or neurological condition. The symptoms of pain are associated with emotional distress and functional impairment.

6-7. The answer is d. *(Sabiston, 15/e, pp 307–309.)* The preeminent concern in treatment of rib fractures is the prevention of pulmonary complications (atelectasis and pneumonia), particularly for patients with preexisting pulmonary disease, who are in danger of progressing to respiratory failure. Attempts to relieve pain by immobilization or splinting, such as strapping the chest, merely compound the problem of inadequate ventilation. Tube thoracostomy is indicated only if pneumothorax is diagnosed. Mild pain may be controlled with oral analgesics, and patients with minor fracture injuries, if they can be closely monitored, may be managed at home with appropriate instructions for coughing and deep breathing. Patients with significant fractures or severe pain should be hospitalized. Rib fractures in the elderly are particularly treacherous. Intercostal nerve blocks often provide prolonged periods of pain relief and, together with appropriate pulmonary physiotherapy, will inhibit development of respiratory complications. Rib fractures are often associated with either intrathoracic or intraabdominal injuries. In particular, fractures of the left chest wall should arouse suspicion of splenic trauma. In equivocal cases, peritoneal lavage will often be diagnostic. Rib fractures heal spontaneously, without need for surgical fixation.

6-8. The answer is e. *(Braunwald, 15/e, p 1293.)* PVCs are common in patients with and without heart disease, and are detected in 60% of adult males on Holter monitoring. Occasional unifocal PVCs do not suggest any of the underlying diseases described.

6-9. The answer is e. *(Kaplan, 8/e, p 1141.)* Prader-Willi syndrome is a genetic disorder caused by a defect of the long arm of chromosome 15. Characteristically, children are underweight in infancy. In early childhood, due to a hypothalamic dysfunction, they start eating voraciously and quickly become grossly overweight. Individuals with this syndrome have characteristic facial features and present with a variety of neurologic and neuropsychiatric symptoms including autonomic dysregulation; muscle weakness; hypotonia; mild to moderate mental retardation; temper tantrums; violent outbursts; perseveration; skin picking; and a tendency to be argumentative, oppositional, and rigid.

6-10. The answer is a. (*ACOG, Technical Bulletin 207.*) A fetal heart rate tracing indicating tachycardia, decreased or absent variability, and persistent late decelerations is indicative of fetal metabolic acidosis and hypoxia. Prompt intervention and delivery is indicated. There is no indication for administering $MgSO_4$ since the patient is not preeclamptic; her blood pressure is not elevated. Since imminent delivery of the fetus is indicated by the nonreassuring fetal heart rate pattern, there is no role for administering cervical ripening agents or Pitocin.

6-11. The answer is c. (*Gleicher, 3/e, pp 647–652.*) Spectinomycin is the treatment of choice for pregnant women who have asymptomatic *N. gonorrhoeae* infections and who are allergic to penicillin. Erythromycin is another drug that is effective in treating asymptomatic gonorrhea. Although tetracycline is an effective alternative to penicillin, its use is generally contraindicated in pregnancy. Administration of chloramphenicol is not recommended to treat women, pregnant or not, who have cervical gonorrhea, and the use of ampicillin or penicillin analogues is contraindicated for penicillin-allergic patients.

6-12. The answer is c. (*Tierney, 42/e, pp 480–483.*) Patients with hemoglobin SC disease and children with sickle cell disease are at risk for **splenic sequestration crisis** when blood is trapped in the spleen (leading to further splenic enlargement and anemia). **Splenic infarction** is not associated with anemia or sudden splenomegaly; patients often have a left upper quadrant rub on physical examination. Episodes of **vasoocclusive crisis** (pain crises) are not associated with increased hemolysis, anemia, or splenomegaly.

6-13. The answer is e. (*Ebert, p 514.*) Huntington's disease is a progressive neurodegenerative disorder, inherited as an autosomal dominant trait, that usually manifests between 35 and 40 years of age. Affected individuals present with a progressive dementia, choreoathetoid movements, and, often, psychiatric symptoms. Computed tomography (CT) scan and nuclear magnetic resonance imaging (MRI) demonstrate gross atrophy of the putamen and the caudate.

6-14. The answer is d. (*Greenfield, 2/e, pp 1092–1093.*) As classically described, Olgilvie syndrome was associated with the rare occurrence of malignant infiltration of the colonic sympathetic nerve supply in the region of the celiac plexus. The eponym is now applied to the condition in which massive cecal and colonic dilation is seen in the absence of mechanical obstruction. Other terms used to describe this condition are acute colonic pseudo-obstruction, colonic ileus, and functional colonic obstruction. It tends to occur in elderly patients in the setting of cardiopulmonary insufficiency, in other systemic disorders that require prolonged bed rest, and in the postoperative state. The diagnosis of Olgilvie syndrome cannot be confirmed until mechanical obstruction of the distal colon is excluded by colonoscopy or contrast enema. Anticholinergic agents and narcotics need to be discontinued, but any delay in decompressing the dilated cecum is inappropriate since colonic ischemia and perforation become a distinct hazard as the cecum reaches this degree of dilation. Cautious endoscopic colonic decompression has been demonstrated recently to be a safe and effective form of treatment. Endoscopy should be combined with rectal tube placement, correction of metabolic abnormalities, and discontinuation of medications that diminish gastrointestinal motility. The high complication rate in this population notwithstanding, a direct surgical approach to decompression becomes necessary when colonoscopic decompression fails; a perforated cecum is a catastrophic event in such patients.

6-15. The answer is a. (*Behrman, 16/e, pp 525–526. McMillan, 3/e, pp 240–245, 362–363. Rudolph, 21/e, pp 192–193.*) An infant of 2100 g at 38 weeks would be considered small for gestational age (SGA), a not uncommon consequence of maternal toxemia. Pregnancy-induced hypertension can produce a decrease in uteroplacental blood flow and areas of placental infarction. This can result in fetal nutritional deprivation and intermittent fetal hypoxemia, with a decrease in glycogen storage and a relative erythrocytosis, respectively. Hence, neonatal hypoglycemia and polycythemia are common clinical findings in these infants. A blood glucose level of 30 mg/dL in a full-term infant, however, is probably normal during the first postnatal day, and an infant is very unlikely to have a convulsion as a result of a level of 38 mg. Serum calcium levels usually decline during the first 2 to 3 postnatal days, but will only be considered abnormally low in a term infant when they fall below 7.5 to 8 mg/dL. Neonatal hypermagnesemia is common in an infant whose mother has received $MgSO_4$ therapy, but is usually asymptomatic or produces decreased muscle tone or floppiness. A persistent venous hematocrit of greater than 65% in a neonate is regarded as polycythemia and will be accompanied by an increase in blood viscosity. Manifestations of the "hyperviscosity syndrome" include tremulousness or jitteriness that can progress to seizure activity because of sludging of blood in the cerebral microcirculation or frank thrombus formation, renal vein thrombosis, necrotizing enterocolitis, and tachypnea. Therapy by partial exchange transfusion with albumin is probably more likely to be useful if performed prophylactically before significant symptoms have developed.

6-16. The answer is a. (*Victor, p 1484.*) Dermatomyositis occurs as a para-neoplastic syndrome in about 15% of cases overall. Among those over age 40, the proportion of paraneoplastic cases increases to 40% for women and 66% for men. Tumors underlying dermatomyositis may develop in the lungs, ovaries, gastrointestinal tract, breasts, or other organs, but the CNS is generally not the site of a tumor associated with dermatomyositis. Because of the higher probability of malignancy in adults with dermatomyositis, patients diagnosed with this inflammatory disease should routinely undergo a variety of diagnostic studies, including rectal and breast examinations, periodic screens for occult blood in the stool, and hemograms. Sputum cytologies and chest x-rays, as well as urine cytologic studies, are recommended by some physicians. Both PML and MS are strictly CNS diseases. Trichinosis is a parasitic disease that involves skeletal muscle and may produce substantial weakness but is not associated with any tumors.

6-17. The answer is b. (*Braunwald, 15/e, pp 70–71.*) This headache is most consistent with a type of neurovascular headache called cluster headache. These occur most often in young men; have a characteristic periodicity, or cluster; and cause lacrimation, nasal stuffiness, and sometimes conjunctival inflammation. Migraines tend not to come and go in this manner, are more throbbing, and are more likely to be associated with nausea and vomiting. Sinusitis is usually bilateral with associated fever and purulent discharge. Tension headaches are usually described as bandlike, without lacrimation or nasal congestion.

6-18. The answer is e. *(Behrman, 16/e, pp 204–210, 743–744, 799–801, 1248–1250, 1479–1483. McMillan, 3/e, pp 1450–1451. Rudolph, 21/e, pp 1531–1534.)* Fever, cough, and tachypnea in a patient with sickle cell anemia can be manifestations of pneumonia, pulmonary thromboemboli, or sepsis. Aside from being relatively common in patients with sickle cell anemia, these diseases can be rapidly progressive and quickly fatal. It is, therefore, important for the patient to be evaluated and treated on an emergency basis. The treatment requires hospitalization because it will almost certainly include systemic antibiotics, intravenous fluids, oxygen, and, perhaps, blood transfusion.

In order to see cyanosis, there must be about 5 g of unoxygenated hemoglobin in the skin capillaries. In anemia this may not be possible, as the total hemoglobin level can be beneath that. In addition, dark skin pigmentation and poor lighting contribute to making cyanosis an unreliable negative sign. With anemia and pulmonary disease, it should be assumed that the patient has impaired oxygenation.

The low pH in the arterial blood can be called acidemia. In this context, it is likely that the hydrogen ions come from lactic acid produced by anaerobic metabolism in tissues with inadequate oxygen delivery. Inadequate oxygenation is caused by the low PO_2, the low oxygen-carrying capacity of the blood (Hb 5 g/dL), and circulatory inadequacy due to the sickling itself and to the vascular disease it produces. The low PCO_2 reflects the hyperventilation, which is secondary to the respiratory difficulty, and to the anemia, and is also respiratory compensation for the metabolic acidosis.

Administration of 100% oxygen will rapidly raise alveolar oxygen concentration and, in the absence of substantial right-to-left shunting of blood, will fully saturate the arterial hemoglobin. It will also dissolve 0.003 mL of oxygen per mmHg of oxygen partial pressure in each deciliter of blood. This will serve to decrease the tissue hypoxia and increase the concentration of mixed venous oxygen, which may decrease the amount of sickling. The other choices are all undesirable or contraindicated.

6-19. The answer is a. *(Tierney, 42/e, p 218.)* **Massive life-threatening hemoptysis is >100 mL of blood in 24 h.** The most common cause for nonmassive hemoptysis (<30 mL/day) in smokers and nonsmoking patients with a normal chest radiograph is bronchitis. Chronic bronchitis is characterized by excessive secretions manifested by a productive cough, often purulent or bloody, for 3 months or more for 2 consecutive years in the absence of any other disease to explain the symptoms. Patients are often obese and cyanotic (**blue bloater**). The mnemonic is **BBB = B**ronchitis/**B**lue **B**loater.

6-20. The answer is e. (*Kaplan, 8/e, p 546.*) This patient is presenting with a major depression with psychotic features. For over 2 weeks (the minimum for the diagnosis), the patient has been complaining of anhedonia, crying, anergia, decreased concentration, 25-lb weight loss, and insomnia with early morning awakening. She also has somatic delusions that are mood congruent and an auditory hallucination. The presence of psychotic phenomena that follow a clear mood disorder picture makes the diagnosis of major depression with psychotic features the most likely.

6-21. The answer is d. (*Cunningham, 21/e, p 1236.*) Noninvasive modalities are currently the preferred tests for diagnosing venous thromboemboli. Venography is still the gold standard, but it is not commonly used because it is cumbersome to perform and expensive and has serious complications. Real-time ultrasonography or color Doppler ultrasound is the procedure of choice to detect proximal deep vein thrombosis. MRI and CT scanning are used in specific cases when ultrasound findings are equivocal.

6-22. The answer is c. (*Braunwald, 15/e, pp 2423, 2430, 2507.*) This patient presents with an acute symmetrical polyneuropathy characteristic of Guillain-Barré syndrome. This is a demyelinating polyneuropathy that is often preceded by a viral illness. Characteristically, there is little sensory involvement, and about 30% of patients require ventilatory assistance. Dermatomyositis usually presents insidiously with proximal muscle weakness. Myasthenia gravis also presents insidiously with muscle weakness worsened by repetitive use. Diplopia, ptosis, and facial weakness are common first complaints. Multiple sclerosis causes demyelinating lesions disseminated in time and space and would not occur in this acute, symmetrical manner. Diabetes mellitus can cause a variety of neuropathies, but would not be rapidly progressive as in this patient.

6-23. The answer is b. (*Braunwald, 15/e, pp 2259–2260.*) Patients with hemochromatosis and cirrhosis have a very high incidence of hepatocellular carcinoma. The incidence of this complication is 30% and increases with age. Weight loss and abdominal pain suggest hepatoma in this patient. A CT scan or ultrasound would be indicated. The picture of right upper quadrant pain and elevated alkaline phosphatase would not suggest acute hepatitis (which causes an elevation of the transaminases) or worsening of the cirrhosis caused by hemochromatosis. Primary biliary cirrhosis can cause an obstructive biliary disease, but would be much less likely in this patient.

6-24. The answer is d. *E* *(Schwartz, 7/e, pp 1697–1707.)* This patient's presentation and films are consistent with primary hyperparathyroidism. The elevated parathormone level (PTH) confirms the diagnosis. Her chest film demonstrates marked osteopenia, and the hand films are classic for this disease, with severe demineralization and periosteal bone resorption most prominent in the middle phalanges. The films show no evidence of malignant lesions or mediastinal adenopathy consistent with sarcoidosis, and an elevated PTH level is not found in Paget's disease or vitamin D intoxication.

Treatment for primary hyperparathyroidism in this setting is resection of the diseased parathyroid glands after initial correction of the severe hypercalcemia. Neck exploration will yield a single parathyroid adenoma in about 85% of cases. Two adenomas are found less often (approximately 5% of cases) and hyperplasia of all four glands occurs in about 10 to 15% of patients. If hyperplasia is found, treatment includes resection of three and one-half glands. The remnant of the fourth gland can be identified with a metal clip in case reexploration becomes necessary. Alternatively, all four glands can be removed with autotransplantation of a small piece of parathyroid tissue into the forearm or sternocleidomastoid muscle. Subsequent hyperfunction, should it develop, can then be treated by removal of this tissue. A patient with osteopenia this severe will need calcium supplementation postoperatively. Vitamin D supplementation may also be necessary if hypocalcemia develops and persists despite treatment with oral calcium.

6-25. The answer is a. *(Behrman, 16/e, pp 1147–1150. McMillan, 3/e, pp 1195, 1642–1655, 1702–1704. Rudolph, 21/e, pp 1105–1106, 1405–1408, 1433–1434, 1450–1451.)* The presence of nocturnal abdominal pain and gastrointestinal bleeding and a positive family history support a diagnosis of peptic ulcer disease. Pain is the most common symptom. Symptoms often persist for several years before diagnosis. The increased incidence of peptic ulcer disease in families (25 to 50%) and concordance in monozygotic twins suggest a genetic basis for the disease. Antibiotic treatment for *Helicobacter pylori* in patients not responding to conventional therapy can cure this disease in some patients. Appendicitis and intussusception are acute events. Pinworms produce perianal pruritus but do not commonly cause abdominal pain or other serious problems. Meckel diverticulum causes painless rectal bleeding, usually during early childhood.

6-26. The answer is c. *(Braunwald, 15/e, p 1509.)* While all of these signs and symptoms can occur in acute pulmonary embolus, tachypnea is by far the most common. Tachypnea occurs in more than 90% of patients with pulmonary embolus. Pleuritic chest pain occurs in about half of patients and is less common in the elderly and those with underlying heart disease. Hemoptysis and wheezing occur in less than half of patients. A right-sided S_3 is associated with large emboli that result in acute pulmonary hypertension.

6-27. The answer is d. *(Victor, pp 356–360.)* Anticoagulation with warfarin or heparin and thrombolysis with r-TPA or urokinase are contraindicated in anyone with an intracranial hemorrhage. Focal seizures that secondarily generalize after an intracerebral or subarachnoid hemorrhage occur frequently and are appropriately treated with an antiepileptic drug, such as phenytoin (Dilantin). Lamotrigine is an anticonvulsant, but would be a very poor choice in this case because this patient needs a drug that will be immediately therapeutic. Lamotrigine must be slowly titrated over many weeks when first started, because of the risk of severe rash.

6-28. The answer is d. *(ACOG, Committee Opinion 260. Cunningham, 21/e, pp 398–399.)* The American Academy of Pediatrics and the American College of Obstetrics and Gynecology do not recommend that routine circumcision procedures be performed on newborn male infants. It is generally agreed that circumcision results in a decreased incidence of penile cancer, but there are no well-designed studies that indicate that circumcision results in a decreased incidence of urinary tract infections in babies or a decreased incidence of sexually transmitted diseases. When performed by an experienced person on a healthy, stable infant, circumcisions are generally safe procedures, although potential complications include infection and bleeding. Parents should discuss the risks and benefits of the procedure and obtain informed consent.

6-29. The answer is b. *(Braunwald, 15/e, pp 1258–1259.)* Normally, the second heart sound (S_2) is composed of aortic closure followed by pulmonic closure. Because inspiration increases blood return to the right side of the heart, pulmonic closure is delayed, which results in normal splitting of S_2 during inspiration. Paradoxical splitting of S_2, however, refers to splitting of S_2 that is narrowed instead of widened with inspiration consequent to a delayed aortic closure. Paradoxical splitting can result from any electrical or mechanical event that delays left ventricular systole. Thus, aortic stenosis and hypertension, which increase resistance to systolic ejection of blood, delay closure of the aortic valve. Acute ischemia from angina or acute myocardial infarction also can delay ejection of blood from the left ventricle. The most common cause of paradoxical splitting—left bundle branch block—delays electrical activation of the left ventricle. Right bundle branch block results in a wide splitting of S_2 that widens further during inspiration. An S_3 is typically heard with congestive heart failure, an S_4 with hypertension, an opening snap with mitral stenosis, and a midsystolic click with mitral valve prolapse.

6-30. The answer is c. *(Kaplan, 8/e, p 332.)* HIV dementia is the most frequent neurological complication of HIV infection and can be the first symptom of the infection. It is due to a direct effect of the virus on the brain and is always accompanied by some brain atrophy. HIV dementia presents with the combination of cognitive impairment, motor deficits, and behavioral changes typical of a subcortical dementia. Common features include impaired attention and concentration, psychomotor slowing, forgetfulness, slow reaction time, and mood changes.

6-31. The answer is e. *(Greenberg, 5/e, p 12.)* This is a typical example of alcohol withdrawal seizure. The greatest risk for alcohol withdrawal seizures occurs within the first day after drinking cessation, in contrast to delirium tremens, which usually occurs within 2 to 4 days of drinking cessation. There is no evidence of an autoimmune process in this patient. Rasmussen encephalitis is an example of a seizure disorder thought to be of autoimmune etiology. There are many examples of genetically transmitted epilepsies, which usually present during childhood. Infections such as meningitis, brain abscess, or encephalitis can cause seizures. Signs of these include meningeal signs, fever, and MRI findings. If this patient had a brain tumor, you might expect a history of headache due to increased intracranial pressure. Additionally, the exam and MRI would likely be abnormal.

6-32. The answer is a. *(Braunwald, 15/e, pp 1984–1986.)* Carpal tunnel syndrome results from median nerve entrapment and is usually due to excessive use of the wrist. The process has been associated with thickening of connective tissue as in acromegaly, or with deposition of amyloid. It also occurs in hypothyroidism, rheumatoid arthritis, and diabetes mellitus. As in this patient, numbness occurs in the distribution of the median nerve. Later in the process, atrophy of the abductor pollicis brevis becomes apparent. The Tinel sign (parasthesia induced in the median nerve distribution by a reflex hammer hitting on the volar aspect of the wrist) is very characteristic. De Quervain's tenosynovitis causes focal wrist pain on the radial aspect of the hand and is due to inflammation of the tendon sheath of the abductor pollicis longus. It should not produce a postive Tinel sign. Amyotrophic lateral sclerosis may present with distal muscle weakness that is diffuse and not focal. Diffuse atrophy and muscle fasiculations would be prominent. Rheumatoid arthritis would not produce these symptoms unless inflammation of the wrist was causing median nerve entrapment in the carpal tunnel.

6-33. The answer is d. (*Greenfield, 2/e, pp 317–331.*) Gunshot wounds to the lower chest are often associated with intraabdominal injuries. The diaphragm can rise to the level of T4 during maximal expiration. Therefore, any patient with a gunshot wound below the level of T4 should be subjected to abdominal exploration. Exploratory thoracotomy is not indicated because most parenchymal lung injuries will stop bleeding and heal spontaneously with the use of tube thoracostomy alone. Indication for thoracic exploration for bleeding is usually in the range of 100 to 150 mL/h over several hours. Peritoneal lavage is not indicated even when the abdominal examination is unremarkable. As many as 25% of patients with negative physical findings and negative peritoneal lavage will have significant intraabdominal injuries in this setting. These injuries include damage to the colon, kidney, pancreas, aorta, and diaphragm. Local wound exploration is not recommended because the determination of diaphragmatic injury with this technique is unreliable.

6-34. The answer is c. (*Kaplan, 8/e, p 958.*) The patient has neuroleptic malignant syndrome (NMS), a life-threatening complication of antipsychotic treatment. The symptoms include muscular rigidity and dystonia, akinesia, mutism, obtundation, and agitation. The autonomic symptoms include high fever, sweating, and increased blood pressure and heart rate. Mortality rates are reported to be 10 to 20%. In addition to supportive medical treatment, the most commonly used medications for the condition are dantrolene (Dantrium) and bromocriptine (Parlodel), although amantadine is sometimes used. Bromocriptine and amantadine possess direct dopamine receptor agonist effects and may serve to overcome the antipsychotic-induced dopamine receptor blockade. Dantrolene is a direct muscle relaxant.

6-35. The answer is a. *(Behrman, 16/e, pp 817–820, 946–955, 961–962, 973–977. McMillan 3/e, pp 704, 1127–1130, 1134–1142. Rudolph, 21/e, pp 1042–1045, 1053–1058, 1075–1079, 1223.)* In addition to the findings described, mumps typically swells to the opposite side in a day or so after symptoms appear on the first side. Other findings include redness and swelling at the opening of Stensen's duct, edema and swelling in the pharynx, and displacement of the uvula on the affected side. A rash would not be expected. Measles presents in a child with a several-day history of malaise, fever, cough, coryza, and conjunctivitis followed by the typical, widespread, erythematous, maculopapular rash. Koplik spots, white pinpoint lesions on a bright red buccal mucosa often in the area opposite his lower molars, appear transiently and are pathognomonic. Symptoms of rubella, usually a mild disease, include a diffuse maculopapular rash that lasts for 3 days, marked enlargement of the posterior cervical and occipital lymph nodes, low-grade fever, mild sore throat, and, occasionally, conjunctivitis, arthralgia, or arthritis. Signs and symptoms of varicella include a prodrome of fever, anorexia, headache, and mild abdominal pain, followed 24 to 48 h later by the typical clear, fluid-filled vesicles (dewdrop on a rose petal). The rash of varicella typically starts on the scalp, face, or trunk. The lesions are pruritic and appear in crops over the next several days, with old lesions crusting over as new lesions develop. Herpangina causes sudden (usually high) fever, headache, backache, and, frequently, vomiting. Oral lesions are vesicles or ulcers usually found on the anterior tonsillar pillars, but can occur nearly anywhere in the mouth. They are caused by an enterovirus for which vaccination is not available.

6-36. The answer is d. *(Braunwald, 15/e, pp 85–87.)* The patient presents with symptoms consistent with acute mechanical low back pain. Even patients with lumbar disc herniation and sciatica improve with nonoperative care, and imaging studies do not affect initial management. Activity as tolerated with optional 2 days of bed rest is recommended along with adequate pain control and reassurance. Active therapy to restore range of motion and function may be appropriate after pain and spasm are relieved.

6-37. The answer is d. (*Droegemueller, 3/e, pp 569, 590–591. Beckmann, 4/e, p 389.*) This patient's presentation is most consistent with urge incontinence. Urge incontinence is the involuntary loss of urine associated with a strong desire to void. Most urge incontinence is caused by detrusor or bladder dyssynergia in which there is an involuntary contraction of the bladder during distension with urine. The management of urge incontinence includes bladder training, biofeedback, or medical therapy. Treatment with anticholinergic drugs (oxybutynin chloride), β-sympathomimetic agonists (metaproterenol sulfate), Valium, antidepressants (imipramine hydrochloride), and dopamine agonists (Parlodel) has been successful. These pharmacologic agents will relax the detrusor muscle. In postmenopausal women who are not on estrogen replacement therapy, estrogen therapy may improve urinary control. Kegel exercises may strengthen the pelvic musculature and improve bladder control in women with stress urinary incontinence.

6-38. The answer is e. (*Patten, p 375.*) This woman probably has trigeminal neuralgia (tic douloureux). The treatment options for this facial pain disorder include carbamazepine (Tegretol). Although carbamazepine is a potent antiepileptic medication, other antiepileptic medications, such as phenobarbital and divalproex sodium (Depakote), are usually ineffective in blunting the pain. Phenytoin (Dilantin) is another antiepileptic useful in the management of trigeminal neuralgia, and recently gabapentin (Neurontin) has had some success as well. Analgesics and anti-inflammatory drugs, such as indomethacin (Indocin), are notably ineffective in managing this disorder.

6-39. The answer is b. (*Kaplan, 8/e, p 531.*) According to *DSM-IV* criteria, patients developing a mood disorder after using a substance (either illicit or prescribed) are diagnosed with a substance-induced mood disorder. The diagnosis of major depression cannot be made in the presence of either substance use or a general medical condition that might be the cause of the mood disorder. Prednisone is a common culprit in causing mood disorders ranging from depression to mania to psychosis.

6-40. The answer is e. (*Schwartz, 7/e, pp 1804–1807.*) If a rupture of the urethra is suspected, a retrograde urethrogram should be obtained before any attempts are made to place a Foley catheter, as efforts to do so may result in the creation of multiple false passages or conversion of a partial laceration into complete rupture. Previously, treatment had included attempts to realign the urethra immediately through the placement of interlocking sounds and traction using either a catheter passed over the sounds or perineal traction sutures through the bladder neck. Preferred treatment currently avoids both dissection into the pelvic hematoma surrounding the disruption and manipulation of the urethra; instead, only a suprapubic tube is placed immediately, with delayed reconstruction after 3 to 6 months, at which time the hematoma will have resolved and the prostate will have descended into the proximity of the urogenital diaphragm. Percutaneous nephrostomy has no role in the management of this problem.

6-41. The answer is d. (*Stein, 5/e, p 1861.*) Episodic hypoglycemia at night is followed by rebound hyperglycemia. This condition, called the Somogyi phenomenon, develops in response to excessive insulin administration. An adrenergic response to hypoglycemia results in increased glycogenolysis, gluconeogenesis, and diminished glucose uptake by peripheral tissues. After hypoglycemia is documented, the insulin dosages are slowly reduced.

6-42. The answer is d. (*Kaplan, 8/e, p 1089.*) Serotonin syndrome is characterized by abdominal pain, diarrhea, excessive sweating, fever, tachycardia, elevated blood pressure, alteration of mental status including delirium, myoclonus, increased motor activity, and mood changes. In the most severe cases, hyperpyrexia, shock, and death can occur. This syndrome is due to an overactivation of serotoninergic receptors by an excess of serotonin. Serotonin syndrome can develop whenever two serotoninergic medications are combined or during the coadministration of an MAO inhibitor and an SSRI or a tricyclic antidepressant. For this reason, when switching from a TCA or an SSRI to an MAO inhibitor, a washout period of 2 weeks is recommended (5 weeks for fluoxetine, given its long half-life).

6-43. The answer is e. (*Victor, pp 1211–1212.*) This woman was at risk for Wernicke's encephalopathy. She should have received supplemental thiamine for at least 3 days, even though this would not have prevented the cognitive deterioration that she exhibited. There was no indication for using a neuroleptic (e.g., haloperidol, chlorpromazine, or prochlorperazine), even though her alcohol and benzodiazepine use placed her at risk for developing a withdrawal psychosis. The anticholinergic trihexyphenidyl would not be appropriate as either a neuroleptic or an antiepileptic.

6-44. The answer is c. *(Kaplan, 8/e, p 821.)* Huntington's disease is a neurodegenerative disorder characterized by choreic movements of the face, limbs, and trunk; progressive dementia; and psychiatric symptoms. Deficits in sustained attention, memory retrieval, procedural memory (ability to acquire new skills), and visuospatial skills are predominant and early manifestations of the disorder. Language skills are usually preserved until the late stages of the disease. Personality changes and mood disturbances, including depression and mania, are frequent and can predate the onset of the dementia and the movement disorder. Neuroimaging reveals atrophy of the caudate and the putamen.

6-45. The answer is d. *(Tierney, 42/e, pp 891–893.)* The patient with edema, proteinuria, hypoalbuminemia, and hyperlipidemia has **nephrotic syndrome** secondary to HIV disease. Hyperlipidemia occurs because of increased hepatic protein synthesis and reduced lipoprotein clearance from the blood by lipoprotein lipase. Patients have elevations of low-density lipoprotein (LDL), very-low-density lipoprotein (VLDL), and triglycerides (TGL). High-density lipoprotein (HDL) may be normal or decreased. Dietary cholesterol should be limited in these patients (<300 mg/day); pharmacological therapy is often required. The severity of **edema** is characterized by a grading system, which is as follows:

1+: Slight pitting edema (2 mm deep) with no distortion on release of finger
2+: A 4-mm-deep pit whose detectable distortion disappears in 10 to 15 s
3+: A 6-mm-deep pit that lasts more than 1 min on release of finger
4+: An 8-mm-deep pit that lasts 2 to 5 min on release of finger

6-46. The answer is c. *(Behrman, 16/e, pp 1660–1663, McMillan, 3/e, pp 560–561.)* The symptoms listed are those of vulvovaginitis, with nonspecific (or chemical) vulvovaginitis accounting for 70% of all pediatric vulvovaginitis cases. The discharge in nonspecific vulvovaginitis is usually brown or green and with a fetid odor. The burning with urination occurs because of contact between raw skin and urine. Further history in this case might reveal use of tight-fitting clothing (including rubber pants), prolonged bubble baths with contamination of the vagina with soap products, use of perfumed lotions in the vaginal area, or improper toilet habits (wiping of fecal material toward rather than away from vagina). Attention to these causative conditions usually results in resolution of the symptoms. The finding of a normal hymen points away from sexual abuse. Pinworms can infest the vagina, but symptoms usually include significant itching of the rectum and vagina. Pediculosis pubis requires pubic hair and, thus, is usually not seen before adolescence. Giardiasis can result in vaginal discharge, but associated symptoms usually include diarrhea and malabsorption syndrome as well. In a sexually active adolescent (or in a sexually abused younger child) a variety of infectious agents such as candida, *Chlamydia trachomatis, Trichomonas vaginalis, Gardnerella vaginalis,* and *Neisseria gonorrhoeae* would be higher on the differential.

6-47. The answer is c. (*Victor, pp 1206–1212.*) Wernicke's encephalopathy is a potentially fatal consequence of thiamine deficiency, a problem for which this woman was at risk by virtue of being an alcoholic. When she came to the emergency room, intravenous fluids were started that probably contained glucose. The stress of a large glucose load will abruptly deplete the CNS of the little thiamine it has available and will precipitate the sort of deterioration evident in this woman. Features characteristic of a Wernicke's encephalopathy include deteriorating level of consciousness, autonomic disturbances, ocular motor problems, and gait difficulty. Autonomic disturbances may include lethal hypotension or profound hypothermia. Hemorrhagic necrosis in periventricular gray matter will be evident in this woman's brain if she dies. The mamillary bodies are especially likely to be extensively damaged.

6-48. The answer is c. (*Speroff, 6/e, pp 562–563.*) The only medications that have been shown in randomized, double-blind, placebo-controlled trials to be consistently effective in treating the emotional symptoms of PMS are the selective serotonin reuptake inhibitors. Such antidepressants include fluoxetine, sertraline, and paroxetine. Some women can be effectively treated by limiting use of the medication to the luteal phase.

6-49. The answer is b. (*Braunwald, 15/e, pp 274–275.*) Inappropriate secretion of antidiuretic hormone is a diagnosis of exclusion, but a chest x-ray might reveal a lung mass. This syndrome may be idiopathic, associated with certain pulmonary and intracranial pathologies, due to endocrine disorders (e.g., hypothyroidism), or drug-induced (e.g., many psychotropic agents). Significant volume depletion is excluded by the absence of orthostatic hypotension. As one can excrete 20% of the glomerular filtration rate, one would have to ingest more than 20 L/day to become hyponatremic. Cirrhosis is very unlikely in the absence of ascites and edema.

6-50. The answer is c. *(Behrman, 16/e, pp 1635–1637. McMillan, 3/e, pp 341–342, 1558–1559. Rudolph, 21/e, pp 1737–1738.)* Prune belly syndrome, a malformation that occurs mostly in males, is characterized by a lax, wrinkled abdominal wall, a dilated urinary tract, and intra-abdominal testes. There are additional urinary tract abnormalities including significant renal dysfunction or dysplasia. Oligohydramnios and commonly associated pulmonary complications, such as pulmonary hypoplasia and pneumothorax, are seen frequently. Congenital hip dislocation, clubfeet, and intestinal malrotation with possible secondary volvulus can occur. There does not appear to be a genetic predisposition to prune belly syndrome.

BLOCK 7

Answers

7-1. The answer is c. *(Kaplan, 8/e, p 880. Ebert, p 337.)* Hyperventilation causes hypocapnia and respiratory alkalosis, which in turn lead to decreased cerebral blood flow and a decrease in ionized serum calcium. Dizziness, derealization, and light-headedness are due to the cerebral vasoconstriction, while circumoral tingling, carpopedal spasm, and paresthesias are symptoms of hypocalcemia. Hyperventilation is a central feature of panic disorder and acute anxiety attacks, though more symptoms are required (beyond just hyperventilation) to make those diagnoses. Panic disorder is characterized by recurring, spontaneous, unexpected anxiety attacks with rapid onset and short duration. The symptoms of an attack climb to maximum intensity within 10 min, but can peak within a few seconds. Typical symptoms include shortness of breath, tachypnea, tachycardia, tremor, dizziness, hot or cold sensations, chest discomfort, and feelings of depersonalization or derealization. A minimum of four symptoms is required to meet the diagnosis of panic attack. Generalized anxiety disorder is characterized by excessive anxiety and worry occurring more days than not for at least 6 months about a number of events or activities. The anxiety and worry are associated with three or more of six symptoms: (1) restlessness or feeling keyed up or on edge, (2) becoming easily fatigued, (3) difficulty concentrating, (4) irritability, (5) muscle tension, (6) sleep disturbance. Anxiety disorder not otherwise specified is characterized by similar constellations of symptoms with one of the other *DSM-IV* diagnoses (panic disorder, phobia, GAD, PTSD, etc.). There are insufficient criteria to meet any one of the diagnoses, but perhaps a number of symptoms for several. Anxiety disorder secondary to a general medical condition is characterized by symptoms of anxiety, but these symptoms must be related to (and caused by) a medical illness, such as hyperthyroidism, angina, hypoglycemia, etc.

7-2. The answer is a. *(Greenfield, 2/e, pp 96–97.)* In a heparinized patient with significant life-threatening hemorrhage, immediate reversal of heparin anticoagulation is indicated. Protamine sulfate is a specific antidote to heparin and should be given at 1 mg for each 100 U heparin if hemorrhage begins shortly after a bolus of heparin. For a patient in whom heparin therapy is ongoing, the dose should be based on the half-life of heparin (90 min). Since protamine is also an anticoagulant, only half the calculated circulating heparin should be reversed. The protaminization should be followed by placement of a percutaneous vena caval filter (Greenfield filter). In this critically ill patient, exploration of the retroperitoneal space would be surgically challenging and meddlesome.

7-3. The answer is c. (*Rowland, p 156.*) The patient has progressive multifocal leukoencephalopathy. It is caused by the JC virus, which is a double-stranded DNA virus. The prognosis is poor, but HAART has been known to be effective in improving survival. JC virus is ubiquitous and may be transmitted through respiratory secretions. Cranial radiation is used to treat malignancies. Amphotericin B is used to treat fungal infections. Intravenous acyclovir is not effective against JC virus, but is used to treat herpes simplex virus encephalitis. Intravenous ceftriaxone is used to treat bacterial meningitis.

7-4. The answer is b. (*Tierney, 42/e, pp 537–540.*) **Mallory-Weiss tears** are longitudinal tears in the mucosa of the gastroesophageal junction due to prolonged and violent retching or vomiting. A bleeding **peptic ulcer** or **gastritis** can cause hematemesis, but usually, if the blood has been retained in the stomach, the digestive processes change the hemoglobin to a brown or black pigment commonly referred to as coffee ground emesis. **Esophageal varices** may cause gastrointestinal bleeding, but this patient has no history of alcoholism and no past history of liver disease. **Boerhaave syndrome** is a transmural tear of the esophagus that causes gastric contents to escape into the mediastinum, leading to severe mediastinal complications. **Dieulafoy lesion** is a large submucosal artery, which may rupture and cause massive bleeding.

7-5. The answer is c. (*Kaplan, 8/e, pp 504–508.*) Schizophreniform disorder and chronic schizophrenia differ only in the duration of the symptoms and the fact that the impaired social or occupational functioning associated with chronic schizophrenia is not required to diagnose schizophreniform disorder. As with schizophrenia, schizophreniform disorder is characterized by the presence of delusions, hallucinations, disorganized thoughts and speech, and negative symptoms. The total duration of the illness, including prodromal and residual phases, is at least 1 month and less than

6 months. Approximately one-third of patients diagnosed with schizophreniform disorder experience a full recovery, while the rest progress to schizophrenia and schizoaffective disorder.

Depending on the predominance of particular symptoms, four subtypes of schizophrenia are recognized: paranoid, disorganized, catatonic, and residual. The man in the question presents with the classical symptoms of paranoid schizophrenia. This subtype of schizophrenia is characterized by prominent hallucinations and delusional ideations with a relative preservation of affect and cognitive functions. Delusions are usually grandiose or persecutory or both, organized around a central coherent theme. Hallucinations, usually auditory, are frequent and related to the delusional theme. Anxiety, anger, argumentativeness, and aloofness are often present. Paranoid schizophrenia tends to develop later in life and it is associated with a better prognosis.

7-6. The answer is c. (*Reece, 2/e, pp 1142–1145.*) The most probable diagnosis in this case is acute pancreatitis. The pain caused by a myoma in degeneration is more localized to the uterine wall. Low-grade fever and mild leukocytosis may appear with a degenerating myoma, but liver function tests are usually normal. The other obstetric cause of epigastric pain, severe preeclamptic toxemia (PET), may exhibit disturbed liver function [sometimes associated with the HELLP syndrome (hemolysis, elevated liver enzymes, low platelets)], but this patient has only mild elevation of blood pressure and no proteinuria. Acute appendicitis in pregnancy is one of the more common nonobstetric causes of abdominal pain. Symptoms of acute appendicitis in pregnancy are similar to those in nonpregnant patients, but the pain is more vague and poorly localized and the point of maximal tenderness moves to the right upper quadrant with advancing gestation. Liver function tests are normal with acute appendicitis. Acute cholecystitis may cause fever, leukocytosis, and pain of the right upper quadrant with abnormal liver function tests, but amylase levels would be elevated only mildly, if at all, and pain would be less severe than described in this patient. The diagnosis that fits the clinical description and the laboratory findings is acute pancreatitis. This disorder may be more common during pregnancy, with an incidence of 1 in 100 to 1 in 10,000 pregnancies. Cholelithiasis, chronic alcoholism, infection, abdominal trauma, some medications, and pregnancy-induced hypertension are known predisposing factors. Patients with pancreatitis are usually in acute distress—the classic finding is a person who is rocking with knees drawn up and trunk flexed in agony. Fever, tachypnea, hypotension, ascites, and pleural effusion may be observed. Hypotonic bowel sounds, epigastric tenderness, and signs of peritonitis may be demonstrated on examination.

Leukocytosis, hemoconcentration, and abnormal liver function tests are common laboratory findings in acute pancreatitis. However, the most important laboratory finding is an elevation of serum amylase levels, which appears 12 to 24 h after onset of clinical disease. Values may exceed 200 U/dL (normal values are 50 to 160 U/dL). A useful diagnostic tool in the pregnant patient with only modest elevation of amylase values is the amylase-creatinine ratio. In patients with acute pancreatitis, the ratio of amylase clearance to creatinine clearance is always greater than 5 to 6%.

Treatment considerations for the pregnant patient with acute pancreatitis are similar to those in nonpregnant patients. Intravenous hydration, nasogastric suction, enteric rest, and correction of electrolyte imbalance and of hyperglycemia are the mainstays of therapy. Careful attention to tissue perfusion, volume expansion, and transfusions to maintain a stable cardiovascular performance are critical. Gradual recovery occurs over 5 to 6 days.

7-7. The answer is e. (*Tierney, 42/e, pp 840–844.*) The patient presents with euvolemic hyponatremia secondary to **primary polydipsia** (compulsive water consumption). Since the hyponatremia developed gradually in the absence of neurologic symptoms (i.e., seizures), it should not be corrected rapidly. The appropriate rate of correction should be 12 meq/24 h to prevent central pontine myelinolysis (CPM), which is an osmotically induced demyelination due to overly rapid correction of serum sodium. Patients develop paraplegia, quadriplegia, and coma.

7-8. The answer is d. (*Kaplan, 8/e, pp 520–523.*) Brief psychotic disorder is characterized by the sudden appearance of delusions, hallucinations, and disorganized speech or behavior, usually following a severe stressor. The episode lasts at least 1 day and less than 1 month and is followed by full spontaneous remission. For the woman in the question, the psychotic episode was clearly precipitated by the death of her children. Schizophreniform disorder is differentiated from brief psychotic disorder by temporal factors (in schizophreniform disorder, symptoms are required to last more than 1 month) and lack of association with a stressor. Posttraumatic stress disorder has a more chronic course and is characterized by affective, dissociative, and behavioral symptoms.

7-9. The answer is d. *(Behrman, 16/e, pp 1424–1428. McMillan, 3/e, pp 1405–1417. Rudolph, 21/e, pp 909–913.)* The presentation of infective endocarditis can be quite variable, ranging from prolonged fever with few other symptoms to an acute and severe course with early toxicity. A high index of suspicion is necessary to make the diagnosis quickly. Identification of the causative organism (frequently *Streptococcus* sp. or *Staphylococcus* sp.) through multiple blood cultures is imperative for appropriate treatment. Echocardiography may identify valvular vegetations and can be predictive of impending embolic events. Treatment usually consists of 4 to 6 weeks of appropriate antimicrobial therapy. Bed rest should be instituted only for heart failure. Antimicrobial prophylaxis prior to and after dental cleaning is indicated.

7-10. The answer is d. *(Ebert, pp 334–337.)* Specific phobias are characterized by an unreasonable or excessive fear of an object, an animal, or a situation (flying, being trapped in close spaces, heights, blood, spiders, etc.). Since the exposure to the feared situation, animal, or object causes an immediate surge of anxiety, patients carefully avoid the phobic stimuli. The diagnosis of specific phobia requires the presence of reduced functioning and interference with social activities and relationships due to the avoidant behavior, anticipatory anxiety, and distress caused by the exposure to the feared stimulus. In social phobias and performance anxiety, patients fear social interactions (in general or limited to specific situations) and public performance (public speaking, acting, playing an instrument), respectively. In generalized anxiety disorder, the anxiety is more chronic and less intense than in a phobic disorder and is not limited to a specific situation or item. Agoraphobic patients fear places where escape may be difficult or help may not be available in case the patient has a panic attack. Agoraphobic patients are often prisoners in their own homes and depend on a companion when they need to go out.

7-11. The answer is a. *(Bradley, p 1712.)* Several modest advances in the treatment of Alzheimer's disease have occurred in the past decade. Recognition of the fact that there is a cholinergic deficit in the brains of patients with Alzheimer's disease has led to the development of acetylcholinesterase inhibitors designed to augment the cholinergic neurotransmitter system. Two different agents that have been used in the United States are tacrine, which can cause hepatic dysfunction, and donepezil, which is better tolerated. The effects are modest and act to slow cognitive decline as assessed by scales of cognitive function. There is still no cure for Alzheimer's disease.

7-12. The answer is d. *(Schwartz, 7/e, pp 59–61.)* The patient presented in the question is suffering from acute, life-threatening respiratory acidosis that has been compounded, if not produced, by the injudicious adminis-tration of a central nervous system depressant. While hypoxemia must also be corrected, the immediate task is to correct the acidosis caused by carbon dioxide accumulation. Both disturbances can be resolved by skillful endo-tracheal intubation and ventilatory support. Sodium bicarbonate and high-flow nasal oxygen would both be inappropriate. Bicarbonate should not be administered because buffer reserves are already adequate (serum bicar-bonate is still 34 meq/L based on the Henderson-Hasselbalch equation). Nasal oxygen administration is not warranted because both acidemia and hypoxemia are themselves potent stimulants to spontaneous ventilation. Headache, confusion, and papilledema are all signs of acute carbon dioxide retention and do not imply the presence of a structural intracranial lesion.

7-13. The answer is d. *(Behrman, 16/e, pp 512–513. McMillan, 3/e, pp 325–332. Rudolph, 21/e, pp 140–143.)* The infant presented in the question has necrotizing enterocolitis (NEC), a potentially life-threatening disease of the neonate. It is more common in premature infants, but has been described in term infants as well. Although several organisms have been isolated from NEC patients, no clear cause for this condition has been iden-tified. Patients present with feeding intolerance and a distended abdomen. About a quarter have grossly bloody stool. Pneumatosis intestinalis is found on plain radiograph of the abdomen and is diagnostic for NEC in this age group. Management depends initially on perforation; if there is no evidence of free peritoneal air, the infant should be put on bowel rest with nasogastric decompression, and systemic antibiotics are initiated. Elec-trolytes and vital signs should be monitored closely, and serial abdominal films should be performed to evaluate for perforation. If free air is identi-fied on plain radiographs or if the infant clinically worsens with medical management, surgical consultation is required. An exploratory laparotomy is usually performed, and any necrotic gut is removed. Occasionally, removal of necrotic gut will result in an infant without adequate intestinal surface area to absorb nutrition, a condition known as *short bowel syndrome.*

7-14. The answer is c. (*Droegemueller, 3/e, pp 578–580. Beckmann, 4/e, pp 393–394.*) Approximately 15 to 20% of women develop urinary tract infections (cystitis) at some point during their lives. Cystitis is diagnosed when a clean-catch urine sample has a concentration of at least 100,000 bacteria per milliliter of urine and when the patient suffers the symptoms of dysuria, frequency, urgency, and pain. The most common etiology of urinary tract infections is *E. coli.* Treatment of a urinary tract infection involves obtaining a culture and starting a patient on an antibiotic regimen of sulfa or nitrofurantoin, which has good coverage against *E. coli* and is relatively inexpensive. Patients treated for a urinary tract infection should have a follow-up culture done 10 to 14 days after the initial diagnosis to document a cure. Women who experience recurrent urinary tract infections with intercourse benefit from voiding immediately after intercourse and/or prophylactic treatment with an antibiotic effective against *E. coli.*

7-15. The answer is b. (*Tierney, 42/e, pp 1311–1313.*) The patient's symptomatology is most consistent with **mononucleosis.** A monospot test (IgM or **heterophile test**) must be ordered to confirm the diagnosis of EBV mononucleosis syndrome. If the heterophile test is negative, the most likely etiology of the mononucleosis is CMV. **Atypical lymphocytes** may be seen transiently in EBV, CMV, toxoplasmosis, drug reactions, viral hepatitis, rubella, mumps, and rubeola. Mononucleosis is transmitted through saliva.

7-16. The answer is b. (*Tierney, 42/e, p 1357.*) Fever, regional adenopathy, and a painless ulcer covered by a black eschar and surrounded by extensive nonpitting edema is a presentation most consistent with **cutaneous anthrax.** Patients with **leprosy** present with pale, anesthetic, and erythematous macular or nodular skin lesions. **Cat-scratch disease** is an acute infection of children and young adults transmitted by cats through a scratch or bite. Patients develop a papule or ulcer at the site of the inoculation and weeks later develop fever, malaise, headache, and regional lymphadenopathy. Patients with **smallpox** present with generalized macular or papular-vesicular-pustular eruptions, with the greatest concentration of the rash being on the face and the distal extremities, especially the palms. Although spider bites are rare, the bite of the **brown recluse spider** may cause a severe necrotic reaction and death due to intravascular hemolysis.

7-17. The answer is e. *(Goldman, 21/e, pp 405–406.)* **Bronchiectasis** is an acquired disease that causes abnormal dilatation of the bronchi leading to pooling of secretions in the airways and recurrent infections. Patients typically present with cough and production of purulent sputum. Lung auscultation may be normal or remarkable for wheezes, rhonchi, or crackles. Chest radiograph may be normal, but occasionally the damaged, dilated airways will appear as **tram tracks** or **ring shadows.** Bronchiectasis may be a sequela of foreign body aspiration, cystic fibrosis, rheumatic diseases (rheumatoid arthritis, Sjögren's disease), pulmonary infections (tuberculosis, pertussis, *Mycoplasma*), AIDS, or allergic bronchopulmonary aspergillosis (ABPA).

7-18. The answer is a. *(Schwartz, 7/e, pp 1678–1689.)* This patient's thyroid scan shows a discrete area of decreased radioactive iodine uptake with the remainder of the gland accepting iodine normally. This means the tissue that composes the nodule is not endocrinologically active for thyroid hormone. The two major mass lesions of the thyroid that can produce this pattern are a nonfunctioning follicular adenoma and a carcinoma. Carcinomas seldom produce thyroid hormone. Adenomas may be very active (toxic) and suppress the remaining gland. Most thyroid adenomas, however, are not hormone-producing and appear as cold nodules on thyroid scan. Graves' disease produces a diffusely hyperactive gland without nodularity. de Quervain's thyroiditis presents as a painful, swollen thyroid gland rather than as a discrete nodule. A large parathyroid adenoma could conceivably displace the thyroid gland and produce a pattern similar to the one shown, but it would be unusual. A localized infectious process also could produce such a pattern. The essential point is that a cold thyroid nodule may represent a carcinoma, and needle biopsy or surgical excision is indicated to rule out this possibility.

7-19. The answer is b. *(Behrman, 16/e, pp 32, 458, 516, 1499. McMillan, 3/e, pp 186–187, 192–193, 197, 2224. Rudolph, 21/e, p 207.)* There is loss of body weight of 1.5 to 2% per day for the first 5 days of life for a normal newborn infant as excessive fluid is excreted. This would tend to produce an increase in hematocrit, but, to the contrary, the hematocrit falls as an adaptation to an environment of higher oxygen. Infants usually have several meconium stools during the first day or two of life, changing to soft yellow stools at 1 to 2 days of life. As the hematocrit falls, there is a corresponding increase in serum bilirubin that peaks around 3 to 5 days of life. Temperature should not change; temperature instability in a term infant is frequently a sign of serious infection.

7-20. The answer is a. (*Braunwald, 15/e, pp 1506–1508.*) Although a difficult diagnosis to make, primary pulmonary hypertension is the most likely diagnosis in this young woman who has used appetite suppressants. There has been a recent increase in primary pulmonary hypertension in the United States associated with fenfluramines. The predominant symptom is dyspnea, which is usually not apparent in the previously healthy young woman until the disease has advanced. When signs of pulmonary hypertension are apparent from physical findings, chest x-ray, or echocardiography, the diagnosis of recurrent pulmonary embolus must be ruled out. In this case, a normal perfusion lung scan makes pulmonary angiography unnecessary. Restrictive lung disease should be ruled out with pulmonary function testing. An echocardiogram will show right ventricular enlargement and a reduction in the left ventricle size consistent with right ventricular pressure overload.

7-21. The answer is c. (*Victor, p 1572.*) The markedly elevated sedimentation rate, anemia, weight loss, and malaise in a person of this age suggest polymyalgia rheumatica, although the same complaints in someone 20 years younger could not be explained on the basis of this disorder. Fever may also be evident in the affected person. This constellation of symptoms also suggests an occult neoplasm or infection, and investigations should be conducted to reduce the likelihood of overlooking one of these diseases. Polymyalgia rheumatica is an arteritis of the elderly and is improbable in someone less than 60 years of age. The normal CPK activity markedly reduces the likelihood that this myalgia is the result of polymyositis or dermatomyositis. The new onset of rheumatoid arthritis at this age is also improbable. A hyperthyroid myopathy in the face of a normal T_4 level is possible on the basis of an elevated T_3 level, but it is also much less likely than polymyalgia rheumatica in this age group.

7-22. The answer is c. (*Kaplan, 8/e, p 1237.*) Reactive attachment disorder is the product of a severely dysfunctional early relationship between the principal caregiver and the child. When caregivers consistently disregard the child's physical or emotional needs, the child fails to develop a secure and stable attachment with them. This failure causes a severe disturbance of the child's ability to relate to others, manifested in a variety of behavioral and interpersonal problems. Some children are fearful, inhibited, withdrawn, and apathetic; others are aggressive, disruptive, and disorganized with low frustration tolerance and poor affect modulation. This condition is often confused with ODD or ADHD.

7-23. The answer is b. *(Behrman, 16/e, pp 513–517. McMillan, 3/e, pp 197–206. Rudolph, 21/e, pp 164–169.)* The development of jaundice in a healthy full-term baby may be considered the result of a normal physiologic process if the time of onset and duration of the jaundice and the pattern of serially determined serum concentrations of bilirubin are in conformity with currently accepted safe criteria. Physiologic jaundice becomes apparent on the second or third day of life, peaks to levels no higher than about 12 mg/dL on the fourth or fifth day, and disappears by the end of the week. The rate of rise is less than 5 mg/dL per 24 h and levels of conjugated bilirubin do not exceed about 1 mg/dL. Concern about neonatal jaundice relates to the risk of the neurotoxic effects of unconjugated bilirubin. The precise level and duration of exposure necessary to produce toxic effects are not known, but bilirubin encephalopathy, or kernicterus, is rare in term infants whose bilirubin level is kept below 18 to 20 mg/dL. Certain risk factors affecting premature or sick newborns increase their susceptibility to kernicterus at much lower levels of bilirubin. The diagnosis of physiologic jaundice is made by excluding other causes of hyperbilirubinemia by means of history, physical examination, and laboratory determinations. Jaundice appearing in the first 24 h is usually a feature of hemolytic states and is accompanied by an indirect hyperbilirubinemia, reticulocytosis, and evidence of red-cell destruction on smear. In the absence of blood group or Rh incompatibility, congenital hemolytic states (e.g., spherocytic anemia) or G6PD deficiency should be considered. With infection, hemolytic and hepatotoxic factors are reflected in the increased levels of both direct and indirect bilirubin.

Studies should include maternal and infant Rh types and blood groups and Coombs tests to detect blood group or Rh incompatibility and sensitization. Measurements of total and direct bilirubin concentrations help to determine the level of production of bilirubin and the presence of conjugated hyperbilirubinemia. Hematocrit and reticulocyte count provide information as to the degree of hemolysis and anemia, and a complete blood count screens for the possibility of sepsis and the need for cultures. Examination of the blood smear is useful in differentiating common hemolytic disorders. Except for determinations of total and direct bilirubin, tests of liver function are not particularly helpful in establishing the cause of early-onset jaundice. Transient elevations of transaminases (AST and ALT) related to the trauma of delivery and to hypoxia have been noted. Biliary atresia and neonatal hepatitis can be accompanied by elevated levels of transaminase but characteristically present as chronic cholestatic jaundice with mixed hyperbilirubinemia after the first week of life.

7-24. The answer is e. (*ACOG, Committee Opinion 246.*) The leading causes of death in women ages 40 to 64 are the following in order of decreasing incidence: cancer, diseases of the heart, cerebrovascular diseases, accidents, chronic obstructive pulmonary disease, diabetes mellitus, chronic liver disease and cirrhosis, and pneumonia and influenza.

7-25. The answer is e. (*Greenfield, 2/e, pp 1148–1150.*) Epidermoid cancers of the anal canal metastasize to inguinal nodes as well as to the perirectal and mesenteric nodes. The results of local radical surgery have been disappointing. Combined external radiation (dose range 3500 to 5000 cG) with synchronous chemotherapy (fluorouracil and mitomycin) is now recommended as the means for controlling the disease. Radical surgical approaches are now generally reserved for treatment failures and recurrences.

7-26. The answer is c. (*Seidel 5/e, p 198.*) The best treatment for pressure ulcers is prevention by frequent turning. The grading for pressure ulcers is as follows:

Stage 1 = Skin is red but not broken
Stage 2 = Damage through the epidermis and dermis
Stage 3 = Damage through to the subcutaneous tissue
Stage 4 = Muscle and possible bone involvement

7-27. The answer is c. (*Victor, pp 844–846.*) Wallenberg, or lateral medullary, syndrome is due to infarction involving some or all of the structures located in the lateral medulla, including the nucleus and descending tract of the fifth nerve, the nucleus ambiguus, lateral spinothalamic tracts, inferior cerebellar peduncle, descending sympathetic fibers, vagus, and glossopharyngeal nerves. The patient with Wallenberg syndrome has ipsilateral ataxia and ipsilateral Horner syndrome. The trigeminal tract damage may produce ipsilateral loss of facial pain and temperature perception and ipsilateral impairment of the corneal reflex. The lateral spinothalamic damage produces pain and temperature disturbances contralateral to the injury in the limbs and trunk. Dysphagia and dysphonia often develop with damage to the ninth and tenth nerves.

7-28. The answer is a. (*Behrman, 16/e, pp 1434–1435. McMillan, 3/e, pp 1389–1397. Rudolph, 21/e, pp 1860–1861.*) The findings of pallor, dyspnea, tachypnea, tachycardia, and cardiomegaly are common in congestive heart failure regardless of the cause. The most common causes of myocarditis include adenovirus and coxsackievirus B, although many other viruses can cause this condition. The constellation of findings in the question point to myocarditis as the etiology of this patient's condition. The lack of echocardiographic findings other than ventricular and left atrial dilatation and poor ventricular function is inconsistent with both glycogen storage disease of the heart, in which there is muscle thickening, and pericarditis, since there is no pericardial effusion. It is also not consistent with an aberrant origin of the left coronary artery, although the origin of the coronary arteries can be more easily missed. On electrocardiogram, the voltages of the ventricular complexes seen with aberrant origin of the left coronary artery are not diminished, and a pattern of myocardial infarction can be seen. Voltages from the left ventricle are usually high in endocardial fibroelastosis, and both right and left ventricular forces are high in glycogen storage disease of the heart.

7-29. The answer is c. (*Cunningham, 21/e, pp 26–29, 891–892, 1114*). Measurement of the fetal crown-rump length is the most accurate means of estimating gestational age. In the first trimester, this ultrasound measurement is accurate to within 3 to 5 days. Estimating the uterine size on physical exam can result in an error of 1 to 2 weeks in the first trimester. Quantification of serum HCG cannot be used to determine gestational age because at any gestational age the HCG number can vary widely in normal pregnancies. A single serum progesterone level cannot be used to date a pregnancy; however, it can be used to establish that an early pregnancy is developing normally. Serum progesterone levels less than 5 ng/mL usually indicate a nonviable pregnancy, while levels greater than 25 ng/mL indicate a normal intrauterine pregnancy. Progesterone levels in conjunction with quantitative HCG levels are often used to determine the presence of an ectopic pregnancy.

7-30. The answer is d. *(Kaplan, 8/e, pp 397–399.)* A diagnosis of alcohol dependence requires the presence of compulsive drinking with ineffective attempts to stop or cut down; evidence of a severe impairment of occupational, social, and family life due to the great deal of time the patient spends procuring and consuming alcohol or recovering from its effects; persistent excessive drinking despite the problems alcohol causes; and physical symptoms and signs of withdrawal and tolerance.

7-31. The answer is e. *(Behrman, 16/e, pp 1586–1587. McMillan, 3/e, pp 2201–2206. Rudolph, 21/c, pp 1696–1698.)* Hemolytic uremic syndrome is characterized by an acute microangiopathic hemolytic anemia, thrombocytopenia from increased platelet utilization, and renal insufficiency from vascular endothelial injury and local fibrin deposition. Ischemic changes result in renal cortical necrosis and damage to other organs such as colon, liver, heart, brain, and adrenal. Laboratory findings associated with hemolytic-uremic syndrome include low hemoglobin level, decreased platelet count, hypoalbuminemia, and evidence of hemolysis on peripheral smear (burr cells, helmet cells, schistocytes). Urinalysis reveals hematuria and proteinuria. A marked reduction of renal function leads to oliguria and rising levels of blood urea nitrogen (BUN) and creatinine. Gastrointestinal bleeding and obstruction, ascites, and central nervous system findings such as somnolence, convulsions, and coma can occur. In the past decade, infection by the verotoxin-producing *Escherichia coli* 0157:H7 has been implicated as a cause of hemolytic-uremic syndrome. This organism is epizootic in cattle. Outbreaks associated with undercooked contaminated hamburgers have been reported in several states. Roast beef, cow's milk, and fresh apple cider have been implicated as well. The Coombs test is not positive in this type of hemolytic anemia.

7-32. The answer is c. *(Braunwald, 15/e, p 329.)* Because the clinical signs of neurologic deterioration and a petechial rash have occurred in the setting of fracture and hypoxia, fat embolism is the most likely diagnosis. This process occurs when neutral fat is introduced into the venous circulation after bone trauma or fracture. The latent period is 12 to 36 hours, usually earlier than a pulmonary embolus would occur after trauma.

7-33. The answer is b. *(Seidel, 5/e, pp 551–552.)* The kidneys normally extend from T12 to L3 (11 cm long). The right kidney is lower than the left kidney due to the liver above it. The left kidney is usually not palpable. Bilateral large kidneys suggest polycystic kidney disease or bilateral hydronephrosis. **Polycystic kidney disease (PKD)** is the most common inherited disorder in the United States and may be autosomal dominant (ADPKD) due to a defect on the short arm of chromosome 16. Patients develop hypertension and renal cysts and often require dialysis or transplantation by the age of 40. Extrarenal manifestations of ADPKD include mitral valve prolapse, berry aneurysms of the circle of Willis, diverticulosis, diverticulitis, and liver cysts. **Medullary sponge kidney** is a benign condition seen in older patients (40 to 50) that almost never leads to renal failure. **Horseshoe kidney** is a kidney that can be palpated crossing the midline. **Renal carcinoma** often presents as a hard mass. Patients with **bilateral hydronephrosis** typically have signs of infection, such as fever, hematuria, and dysuria.

7-34. The answer is e. *(Cunningham, 21/e, pp 184–185. Beckmann, 4/e, pp 57–58.)* Late in pregnancy, when the mother assumes the supine position, the gravid uterus compresses the inferior vena cava and decreases venous return to the heart. This results in decreased cardiac output and symptoms of dizziness, light-headedness, and syncope. This significant arterial hypotension resulting from inferior vena cava compression is known as supine hypotensive syndrome or inferior vena cava syndrome. Therefore, it is not recommended that women remain in the supine position for any prolonged period of time in the latter part of pregnancy. When patients describe symptoms of the supine hypotensive syndrome, there is no need to proceed with additional cardiac or pulmonary workup.

7-35. The answer is c. *(Victor, p 335.)* This is a common presentation for primary generalized epilepsy of childhood. An electroencephalogram showing the classic 3-Hz spike-and-wave pattern would confirm this diagnosis. Brain MRI and CT are useful for evaluating brain anatomy. Anatomic problems can cause seizures, but these tests will not tell anything about brain electrical activity. Lumbar puncture is useful for measuring cere-brospinal fluid pressure and looking for central nervous system inflammation or infection. Central nervous system inflammation or infection may cause seizures. Nerve conduction study is useful to evaluate peripheral nerve injuries such as nerve entrapment.

7-36. The answer is d. *(Braunwald, 15/e, p 2054–2056.)* Metastatic tumors rarely cause diabetes insipidus, but of the tumors that may cause it, carcinoma of the breast is by far the most common. In this patient, the diagnosis of diabetes insipidus is suggested by hypernatremia and low urine osmolality. Psychogenic polydipsia is an unlikely diagnosis since serum sodium is usually mildly reduced in this condition. Renal glycosuria would be expected to induce a higher urine osmolality than this patient has because of the osmotic effect of glucose. While nephrocalcinosis secondary to hypercalcemia may produce polyuria, hypercalciuria does not. Finally, the findings of inappropriate antidiuretic hormone syndrome are the opposite of those observed in diabetes insipidus and thus are incompatible with the clinical picture in this patient.

7-37. The answer is c. *(Behrman, 16/e, pp 1142–1143. McMillan, 3/e, pp 1652–1655. Rudolph, 21/e, pp 1407–1408.)* The usual presentation of intussusception is that of an infant between 4 and 10 months of age who has a sudden onset of intermittent colicky abdominal pain. The child can appear normal when the pain abates, but as it recurs with increasing frequency, the child can begin to vomit and become progressively more obtunded. The passage of stool containing blood and mucus, and resembling currant jelly, is often observed. Early examination of the abdomen can be unremarkable, but as the problem persists, a sausage-shaped mass in the right upper quadrant is frequently palpated. A contrast enema examination under fluoroscopic control can be therapeutic as well as diagnostic when the hydrostatic effects of the column of air serve to reduce the intussusception. Early diagnosis prevents bowel ischemia. The cause of most intussusceptions is unknown, but a Meckel's diverticulum or polyp can serve as a lead point.

7-38. The answer is c. *(Rowland, pp 552–553.)* Abetalipoproteinemia (Bassen-Kornzweig syndrome) usually becomes symptomatic during early childhood. The peripheral blood smear will exhibit abnormally shaped erythrocytes (acanthocytes), and the plasma lipid profile will reveal a very low cholesterol and triglyceride content. Acanthocytes are spiked or crenated RBCs. These are an unusual hematologic finding in patients with ataxia and are often diagnostic of abetalipoproteinemia. Autopsy examination of the CNS in patients with abetalipoproteinemia reveals posterior column and spinocerebellar tract degeneration. The initial complaints are similar to the spinocerebellar signs of Friedreich's disease. Position sense is lost and extensor plantar responses develop as the disease progresses. As is true for Friedreich's disease, dementia is not an obvious part of the syndrome. Deficits accumulate over the course of years. Vitamin E supplementation may retard the disease's progression. The differential diagnosis of retinitis pigmentosa is broad, and includes many other conditions besides abetalipoproteinemia: mitochondrial diseases, Bardet-Biedl syndrome, Laurence-Moon syndrome, Friedreich's ataxia, and Refsum's disease. It may also occur alone as a hereditary disorder linked to chromosome 3. It is characterized by a degeneration of all layers of the retina. Because it is a noninflammatory condition, retinitis is actually something of a misnomer.

7-39. The answer is a. *(Tierney, 42/e, p 314.)* The patient has a **functional** or **innocent** heart murmur. These are nonpathologic murmurs generated by flow abnormalities (systolic ejection), not structural heart abnormalities. Functional murmurs are extremely common in children (>50% of children) and may be found in 50% of patients >50 years old (aortic sclerosis). Functional murmurs are the most common kinds of murmurs encountered by physicians.

7-40. The answer is b. *(Braunwald, 15/e, pp 754–755.)* This patient with gram-negative bacteremia has developed disseminated intravascular coagulation, as evidenced by multiple-site bleeding, thrombocytopenia, fragmented red blood cells on peripheral smear, prolonged PT and PTT, and reduced fibrinogen levels from depletion of coagulation proteins. Initial treatment is directed at correcting the underlying disorder—in this case infection. Although heparin was formerly recommended for the treatment of DIC, it is now used rarely and only in unusual circumstances (such as acute promyelocytic leukemia). For the patient who continues to bleed, supplementation of platelets and clotting factors (with fresh frozen plasma or cryoprecipitate) may help control life-threatening bleeding. Red cell fragmentation and low platelet count can be seen in microangiopathic disorders such as TTP, but in these disorders the coagulation pathway is not activated. Therefore in TTP the prothrombin time and partial thromboplastin time as well as the plasma fibrinogen levels will be normal.

7-41. The answer is a. *(Ebert, p 441.)* Sleep apnea is the cessation of breathing during sleep for 10 s or more. In obstructive sleep apnea, breathing stops due to airway blockage, while in central sleep apnea the breathing stops due to an absence of respiratory efforts secondary to a neurological dysfunction. Features associated with obstructive sleep apnea are excessive daytime somnolence, snoring, restless sleep, and nocturnal awakening with gasping for air. Patients often wake up in the morning with dry mouth and headache. Predisposing factors are maleness, middle age, obesity, hypothyroidism, and various malformations of the upper airways. Narcolepsy is characterized by irresistible urges to fall asleep for brief periods during the day, regardless of the situation. Nocturnal myoclonus refers to stereotyped, repetitive movements of the legs during sleep, accompanied by brief arousal and sleep disruption.

7-42. The answer is b. *(Braunwald, 15/e, p 464.)* The signs and symptoms described are most consistent with scurvy (vitamin C deficiency). This syndrome can occur in older patients who are poorly nourished. Perifollicular papules develop when hairs become fragmented and buried in the follicle. Capillary fragility occurs, and bleeding into soft tissue is common. Pellagra (vitamin B_3 deficiency) causes a dermatitis that is symmetrical and related to photosensitivity. Beriberi (vitamin B_1 deficiency) does not typically cause a rash, but presents with high-output cardiac failure, peripheral neuropathy, and Wernicke's encephalopathy. The perifollicular nature of the bleeding described in this patient does not suggest a traumatic etiology.

7-43. The answers are 138-c, 139-a. *(Sabiston, 15/e, p 308.)* Tension pneumothorax is a life-threatening problem requiring immediate treatment. A lung wound that behaves as a ball or flap valve allows escaped air to build up pressure in the intrapleural space. This causes collapse of the ipsilateral lung and shifting of the mediastinum and trachea to the contralateral side, in addition to compression of the vena cava and contralateral lung. Sudden death may ensue because of a decrease in cardiac output; hypoxemia; and ventricular arrhythmias. To accomplish rapid decompression of the pleural space, a large-gauge needle should be passed into the intrapleural cavity through the second intercostal space at the midclavicular line. This may be attached temporarily to an underwater seal with subsequent insertion of a chest tube after the life-threatening urgency has been relieved. Tension pneumothorax produces characteristic x-ray findings of ipsilateral lung collapse, mediastinal and tracheal shift, and compression of the contralateral lung. Occasionally, adhesions prevent complete lung collapse, but the tension pneumothorax is evident because of the mediastinal displacement. A pleural effusion would not be expected acutely in the absence of associated intrapleural blood.

7-44. The answer is c. (*Fitzpatrick, 4/e, pp 528–538.*) **Mycosis fungoides,** also called cutaneous T cell lymphoma (CTCL), is a neoplastic disease of the helper T cells that first manifests in the skin but eventually spreads to the lymph nodes and internal organs. The scaly plaques of this disease disappear with sun exposure, mimicking psoriasis. Multiple biopsies and a careful examination for adenopathy are required to make the diagnosis. **Lichen planus** is an inflammatory dermatosis with unknown etiology that involves the skin and mucous membranes. **Pityriasis rosea** is seen in patients under the age of 40 and is more common in the spring and fall months. Its characteristic course begins with a single bright red **herald** or primary patch, usually on the trunk, followed 1 to 2 weeks later by similar nonpruritic (may be mildly itchy) plaques distributed in a **Christmas tree** pattern. The disorder is self-limited and remits within 6 weeks. **Seborrheic keratosis** is a benign epithelial tumor seen in individuals over the age of 30. It typically appears as brown plaques, papules, or nodules with a stuck-on appearance and has a predilection for the face, trunk, and upper extremities. **Kaposi's sarcoma (KS)** is a multisystem vascular neoplasm that may be seen in elderly males of eastern European heritage (Mediterranean and Ashkenazi Jewish) and predominantly arises in the legs. The papules and nodules of KS are usually violaceous. The disease is also seen in patients who are immunocompromised due to transplant, chemotherapy, or HIV and is thought to be due to herpesvirus type 8 (HHV-8).

7-45. The answer is e. (*Behrman, 16/e, pp 1268–1271. McMillan, 3/e, pp 1256–1258. Rudolph, 21/e, pp 1937–1941.*) A nasopharyngeal airway, the use of nasal CPAP, and tonsillectomy and adenoidectomy can be effective treatments for obstructive sleep apnea (OSA). However, the diagnosis of OSA should first be made by polysomnography (sleep study) to exclude other causes of snoring. Administering oxygen may decrease the respiratory drive in severe OSA, and thus should be used only with caution. Irradiation should not be used for fear of development of malignancy, particularly of the thyroid.

7-46. The answer is e. *(Cunningham, 21/e, pp 630–634.)* Any patient who gives a history of vaginal bleeding in the third trimester should undergo an ultrasound exam as the first step in evaluation to rule out the presence of a placenta previa. A digital or speculum exam performed in the presence of a placenta previa can precipitate a hemorrhage. There is no indication to work the patient up for infection in the case described here; therefore, an amniocentesis is not indicated. She should not be sent home even though the bleeding has resolved. She first needs to undergo an ultrasound and should be monitored for uterine contractions and further bleeding prior to being discharged.

7-47. The answer is a. *(Kaplan, 8/e, p 422.)* Cocaine inhibits the normal reuptake of norepinephrine and dopamine, causing an increase of the concentration of these neurotransmitters in the synaptic cleft. This mechanism is responsible for the euphoria and sense of well-being that follow cocaine use, but it also causes excessive sympathetic activation and diffuse vasoconstriction. High blood pressure, mydriasis, cardiac arrhythmias, coronary artery spasms, and myocardial infarcts are all seen with cocaine intoxication. Other toxic effects of cocaine include headaches, ischemic cerebral and spinal infarcts, subarachnoid hemorrhages, and seizures. Ritalin, heroin, PCP, and LSD intoxications present with different symptoms and signs.

7-48. The answer is d. *(Braunwald, 15/e, p 1887.)* Although many glomerular lesions occur in association with HIV, focal sclerosis is by far the commonest etiology of this patient's syndrome. While focal sclerosis is more common in intravenous drug users than homosexuals, the lesion is different than so-called heroin nephropathy. Indinavir toxicity may cause tubular obstruction by crystals and is a cause of renal stones, but does not cause nephrotic syndrome. Analgesic nephropathy is a frequently unrecognized cause of occult renal failure; this entity requires at least 10 years of analgesic use and rarely causes significant proteinuria. Trimethoprim-sulfamethoxazole may cause acute interstitial nephritis, but there is no fever, rash, WBC casts, or eosinophils in the urinalysis.

7-49. The answer is e. (*Victor, p 287.*) Oculomotor fibers that have been damaged reversibly may regenerate and connect to the wrong target. This aberrant regeneration is seen most often with lesions that chronically compress the third nerve. Aneurysms, cholesteatomas, and neoplasms should be suspected in the person exhibiting this type of disturbance.

7-50. The answer is b. (*Schwartz, 7/e, pp 966–968.*) Abdominal pain out of proportion to findings on physical examination is characteristic of intestinal ischemia. The etiology of ischemia may be embolic or thrombotic occlusion of the mesenteric vessels or nonocclusive ischemia due to a low cardiac index or mesenteric vasospasm. Differentiation among these etiologies is best made by mesenteric angiography. While not without serious risks, angiography also offers the possibility of direct infusion of vasodilators into the mesenteric vasculature in the setting of nonocclusive ischemia. This patient, with a recent myocardial infarction and a low cardiac index, is at risk for embolism of clot from a left ventricle mural thrombus as well as low-flow mesenteric ischemia. If embolism or thrombosis is found angiographically (usually involving the superior mesenteric artery), operative embolectomy or vascular bypass is indicated to restore flow. If occlusive disease cannot be demonstrated, efforts should be made to simultaneously increase cardiac output with inotropic agents and dilate the mesenteric vascular bed by angiographic instillation of papaverine, nitrates, or calcium channel blockers. Computed tomography is not helpful in delineating the cause of intestinal ischemia because it does not provide a sufficiently detailed image of the mesenteric vessels. Laparoscopy might secure the diagnosis of intestinal ischemia, but requires administering general anesthesia and would shed no light on the etiology of this patient's problem. Flexible sigmoidoscopy, while useful in patients with ischemic colitis, has no role in the workup of mesenteric ischemia, which primarily involves the small intestine and right colon. Serum lactate is helpful in raising the suspicion of intestinal ischemia, but no absolute level should be used to decide whether or not to explore a patient.

BLOCK 8

Answers

8-1. The answer is c. *(Cunningham, 20/e, pp 4, 538, 763, 1235.)* A disadvantage of home delivery is the lack of facilities to control postpartum hemorrhage. The woman described in the question delivered a large baby, suffered multiple soft tissue injuries, and went into shock, needing 9 units of blood by the time she reached the hospital. Sheehan syndrome seems a likely possibility in this woman. This syndrome of anterior pituitary necrosis related to obstetric hemorrhage can be diagnosed by 1 week postpartum, as lactation fails to commence normally. Although many modern women choose hormonal therapy to prevent lactation, the woman described in the question was intent on breast-feeding and so would not have received suppressant. She therefore could have been expected to begin lactation at the usual time. Other symptoms of Sheehan syndrome include amenorrhea, atrophy of the breasts, and loss of thyroid and adrenal function. The other presented choices for late sequelae are rather far-fetched. Hemochromatosis would not be expected to occur in this healthy young woman, especially since she did not receive prolonged transfusions. Cushing, Simmonds, and Stein-Leventhal syndromes are not known to be related to postpartum hemorrhage. It is important to note that home delivery is not a predisposing factor to postpartum hemorrhage.

8-2. The answer is c. *(Braunwald, 15/e, pp 1969–1974.)* Sarcoidosis is a systemic illness of unknown etiology. Many patients have respiratory symptoms, including cough and dyspnea. Hilar and peripheral lymphadenopathy is common, and 20 to 30% of patients have hepatomegaly. The chest x-ray shows symmetrical hilar lymphadenopathy. The diagnostic method of choice is transbronchial biopsy, which will show a mononuclear cell granulomatous inflammatory process. While liver and scalene node biopsies are often positive, noncaseating granulomas are so frequent in these sites that they are not considered acceptable for primary diagnosis. ACE levels are elevated in two-thirds of patients, but false-positive values are common in other granulomatous disease processes.

8-3. The answer is c. (*Braunwald, 15/e, pp 1523–1526.*) Sepsis is the most important single cause of adult respiratory distress syndrome. Early in the course of ARDS, patients may appear stable without respiratory symptoms. Tachypnea, hypoxemia, and diffuse infiltrates gradually develop. It may be difficult to distinguish the process from cardiogenic pulmonary edema, especially in patients who have been given large quantities of fluid. This young patient with no evidence of volume overload would be strongly suspected of having ARDS. The pulmonary capillary wedge pressure would be normal or low in ARDS, but elevated in left ventricular failure. ARDS is a complication of sepsis, but blood cultures may or may not be positive. Neither CT of the chest nor ventilation-perfusion scan would be specific enough to help in diagnosis of ARDS.

8-4. The answer is d. (*Thoren, Anesth Analg 67:687–694, 1988.*) Thoracic epidural narcotics have become an increasingly popular means of postoperative pain relief in thoracic and upper abdominal surgery. Local action on γ opiate receptors ensures pain relief and consequent improvement in respiration without vasodilation or paralysis. The less lipid-soluble opiates are effective for long periods. Their slow absorption into the circulation also ensures a low incidence of centrally mediated side effects, such as respiratory depression or generalized itching. When these do occur, the intravenous injection of an opiate antagonist is an effective antidote. The locally mediated analgesia is not affected. One poorly understood side effect, which is apparently unrelated to systemic levels, is a profound reduction in gastric activity. This may be an important consideration after thoracic surgery when an early resumption of oral intake is anticipated.

8-5. The answer is d. (*Ebert, pp 475–477.*) The patient's history and presenting symptoms are classic for the diagnosis of borderline personality disorder. Patients with borderline personalities present with a history of a pervasive instability of mood, relationships, and self-image beginning by early adulthood. Their behavior is often impulsive and self-damaging; their sexuality is chaotic; sexual orientation may be uncertain; and anger is intense and often acted out. Recurrent suicidal gestures are common. The shifts of mood usually last from a few hours to a few days. Patients often describe chronic feelings of boredom and emptiness.

8-6. The answer is b. (*Ebert, pp 401–405.*) During periods of REM sleep, men experience penile erections defined as nocturnal penile tumescence (NPT). NPT studies can be helpful in differentiating patients with organic erectile problems from patients with psychogenic impotence. However, these findings are not absolute since many men have both organic and psychological causes for their impotence and nocturnal erections may be decreased or absent in depression. Since this patient has NPT, it is likely that his impotence stems from a psychogenic determinant, which may be reversible with treatment.

8-7. The answer is a. (*Victor, pp 1285–1286.*) Cyclosporine and tacrolimus (FK 506) may both induce a syndrome resembling hypertensive encephalopathy, which has been called by some reversible posterior leukoencephalopathy, although it involves more than white matter and may also occur in the anterior frontal regions. In the setting of cyclosporine use, patients may develop headache, visual dysfunction related to occipital lobe dysfunction, confusion, and seizures. Usually there is associated hypertension. The visual loss may include cortical blindness or scotomas. Imaging may show bilateral, more or less symmetrical signal changes in the white matter and occasionally the cortex of the occipital and parietal lobes.

8-8. The answer is c. (*Behrman, 16/e, p 1266. McMillan, 3/e, pp 572–573, 1299–1301. Rudolph, 21/e, p 1944.*) Suppurative infection of the chain of lymph nodes between the posterior pharyngeal wall and the prevertebral fascia leads to retropharyngeal abscesses. The most common causative organisms are *Staphylococcus aureus*, group A β-hemolytic streptococci, and oral anaerobes. Presenting signs and symptoms include a history of pharyngitis, abrupt onset of fever with severe sore throat, refusal of food, drooling, and muffled or noisy breathing. A bulge in the posterior pharyngeal wall is diagnostic, as are radiographs of the lateral neck that reveal the retropharyngeal mass. Palpation (with adequate provision for emergency control of the airway in case of rupture) reveals a fluctuant mass. Treatment should include incision and drainage if fluctuance is present.

8-9. The answer is d. (*Schwartz, 7/e, pp 448, 499.*) The cause of malignant hyperthermia is unknown, but it is associated with inhalational anesthetic agents and succinylcholine. It may develop in an otherwise healthy person who has tolerated previous surgery without incident. It should be suspected in the presence of a history of unexplained fever, muscle or connective tissue disorder, or a positive family history (evidence suggests an autosomal dominant inheritance pattern). In addition to fever during anesthesia, the syndrome includes tachycardia, increased O_2 consumption, increased CO_2 production, increased serum K^+, myoglobinuria, and acidosis. Rigidity rather than relaxation following succinylcholine injection may be the first clue to its presence. Treatment of malignant hyperthermia should include prompt conclusion of the operative procedure and cessation of anesthesia, hyperventilation with 100% oxygen, and administration of intravenous dantrolene. The urine should be alkalinized to protect the kidneys from myoglobin precipitation. If reoperation is necessary, the physician should premedicate heavily, alkalinize the urine, and avoid depolarizing agents such as succinylcholine. Pretreatment for 24 h with dantrolene is helpful; it is thought to act directly on muscle fiber to attenuate calcium release.

8-10. The answer is a. (*Victor, pp 286–287.*) An abducens dysfunction with lateral rectus palsy may develop in children with increased intracranial pressure or with direct damage to the brainstem. With a brainstem glioma, both brainstem damage and increased intracranial pressure may develop secondary to the tumor. The adult who develops an acute abducens palsy is also at high risk for tumor. Metastatic lesions from the nasopharynx are especially likely in the adult, but vascular disease is also a significant cause of ocular motor dysfunction in adults, especially in the elderly.

8-11. The answer is e. (*Schwartz, 7/e, pp 1275–1277.*) The history, x-ray, and clinical findings are typical of a postoperative cecal volvulus, a condition in which the cecum is twisted on its mesentery (often, after aneurysm resection, a neomesentery) and becomes acutely obstructed. At 12 cm, the cecum is in imminent danger of perforation. Particularly in the presence of a prosthetic graft, cecal perforation is a catastrophe. Urgent decompression is needed. To attempt colonoscopic decompression would necessitate insufflation of additional air and increase the stress on the already compromised cecal wall. A transverse colostomy "decompression" would not decompress the cecum, nor would it provide detorsion of the cecal mesentery to allow restoration of adequate blood supply to the right colon. While untwisting the cecum and fixing it to the lateral abdominal wall (to inhibit recurrence) by a decompressing cecostomy might be advocated in some settings, the risk of contaminating the aortic graft would be excessive. Resection of the offending organ with ileotransverse colostomy would be the procedure of choice.

8-12. The answer is a. (*Postgraduate Obstetrics and Gynecology. Droege-mueller, 3/e, pp 474–475, 947–948, 1163–1164. Beckmann, 4/e, p 538–539.*) Vulvar vestibulitis is syndrome of unknown etiology. To make the diagnosis of this disorder, the following three findings must be present: (1) severe pain on vestibular touch or attempted vaginal entry, (2) tenderness to pressure localized within the vulvar vestibule, and (3) visible findings confined to vulvar erythema of various degrees. To treat vulvar vestibulitis, the first step is to avoid tight clothing, tampons, hot tubs, and soaps, which can all act as vulvar irritants. Topical treatments include lidocaine, estrogen, and steroids. Tricyclic antidepressants and intralesional interferon injections have also been used. For women refractory to medical therapy, surgical excision of the vestibular mucosa may be helpful. Valtrex (valacyclovir) is an antiviral medication used in the treatment of genital herpes and is not indicated for vulvar vestibulitis. Contact dermatitis is an inflammation and irritation of the vulvar skin due to a chemical irritant. The vulvar skin is usually red, swollen, and inflamed and may become weeping and eczemoid. Women with a contact dermatitis usually experience chronic vulvar tenderness, burning, and itching that can occur even when they are not engaging in intercourse. Atrophic vaginitis is a thinning and ulceration of the vaginal mucosa that occurs as a result of hypoestrogenism; thus this condition is usually seen in postmenopausal women not on any hormone replacement therapy. Lichen sclerosus is another atrophic condition of the vulva. It is characterized by diffuse, thin whitish epithelial areas on the labia majora, minora, clitoris, and perineum. In severe cases, it may be difficult to identify normal anatomic landmarks. The most common symptom of lichen sclerosus is chronic vulvar pruritus. Vulvar intraepithelial neoplasia (VIN) are precancerous lesions of the vulva that have a tendency to progress to frank cancer. Women with VIN complain of vulvar pruritus, chronic irritation, and raised lesions. These lesions are most commonly located along the posterior vulva and in the perineal body and have a whitish cast and rough texture.

8-13. The answer is c. *(Schwartz, 7/e, pp 1181–1182.)* Most enterocutaneous fistulas result from trauma sustained during surgical procedures. Irradiated, obstructed, and inflamed intestine is prone to fistulization. Complications of fistulas include fluid and electrolyte depletion, skin necrosis, and malnutrition. Fistulas are classified according to their location and the volume of output, because these factors influence prognosis and treatment. When the patient is stable, a barium swallow is obtained to determine (1) the location of the fistula, (2) the relation of the fistula to other hollow intraabdominal organs, and (3) whether there is distal obstruction. Proximal small-bowel fistulas tend to produce a high output of intestinal fluid and are less likely to close with conservative management than are distal, low-output fistulas. Small-bowel fistulas that communicate with other organs, particularly the ureter and bladder, may need aggressive surgical repair because of the risk of associated infections. The presence of obstruction distal to the fistula (e.g., an anastomotic stricture) can be diagnosed by barium contrast study and mandates correction of the obstruction. When these poor prognostic factors for stabilization and spontaneous closure are observed, early surgical intervention must be undertaken. The patient in the question, however, appears to have a low-output, distal enterocutaneous fistula. Control of the fistulous drainage should be provided by percutaneous intubation of the tract with a soft catheter. This is usually accomplished under fluoroscopic guidance. Antispasmodic drugs have not been proved effective; somatostatin has been used with mixed success in the setting of high-output (greater than 500 mL/day) fistulas. There is no indication for antibiotics in the absence of sepsis. Total parenteral nutrition (TPN) is given to maintain or restore the patient's nutritional balance while minimizing the quantity of dietary fluids and endogenous secretions in the gastrointestinal tract. A period of 4 to 6 weeks of TPN therapy is warranted to allow for spontaneous closure of a low-output distal fistula. Should conservative management fail, surgical closure of the fistula is performed.

8-14. The answer is a. *(Kaplan, 8/e, p 630.)* A conversion disorder usually presents in a monosymptomatic manner, acutely, and simulating a physical disease. The sensory or motor symptoms present are not fully explained by any known pathophysiology. The diagnostic features are such that the physical symptom is incompatible with known physiological mechanisms or anatomy. Usually an unconscious psychological stress or conflict is present. In hypochondriasis, a patient is overly concerned that he or she has an illness or illnesses; this conviction can temporarily be appeased by physician reassurance, but the reassurance generally does not last long. Factitious disorder usually presents with physical or mental symptoms that are induced by the patient to meet the psychological need to be taken care of (primary gain). Malingering is similar to factitious disorder in that symptoms are faked, but the reason in malingering is for some secondary gain, such as getting out of jail. In delusional disorder with somatic delusions, the patient has an unshakable belief that he or she has some physical defect or a medical condition.

8-15. The answer is e. *(Kaplan, 8/e, p 1070.)* Discontinuation of the antipsychotic medication or a dosage decrease are the initial interventions recommended when tardive dyskinesia is first diagnosed. If discontinuation is not possible and dosage decrease is not effective, clozapine has been proved effective in ameliorating and suppressing the symptoms of tardive dyskinesia.

8-16. The answer is b. *(Behrman, 16/e, pp 1105, 1138–1141. McMillan, 3/e, pp 313–315, 1637–1639, 2281–2282. Rudolph, 21/e, pp 1368–1370.)* The radiograph demonstrates a stool-filled megacolon. Hirschsprung disease is usually suspected in the chronically constipated child despite the fact that 98% of such children have functional constipation. Finding a dilated, stool-filled anal canal with poor tone on the physical examination of a well-grown child supports the diagnosis of functional constipation. The difficulty in treating functional constipation once it has been established emphasizes the need for prompt identification and treatment of problems with defecation and for counseling of parents regarding proper toileting behavior. The extensive workup of this patient would likely be negative and expensive, and is not indicated.

8-17. The answer is b. *(Tierney, 42/e, pp 674–677.)* **Fibroadenomas** are the most common benign neoplasms of the breast. They are well demarcated, rubbery, mobile, and nontender. **Benign cysts** are the most common cause of breast lumps and tend to occur in association with other cysts. They are round, mobile, and soft with a cystic consistency. They are tender premenstrually, become smaller immediately after menses, and regress after menopause. **Breast abscesses** are localized and are tender, swollen, erythematous, and fluctuant. **Malignant lesions** are painless, irregular in contour and shape, hard, nonmobile, and not well demarcated.

8-18. The answer is c. (*Tierney, 42/e, p 581.*) The finding of a palpable supraclavicular node, whether right or left, may indicate metastatic involvement due to ipsilateral breast or lung cancers. Additionally, if located on the left side, a palpable supraclavicular node may also represent intraabdominal or intrapelvic malignancies (**Trosier's node**). A large left supraclavicular node representing metastasis from a gastric carcinoma is specifically referred to as **Virchow's node.** In this patient, the best next step would be to order a mammogram, since her last study was 3 years ago.

8-19. The answer is a. (*Braunwald, 15/e, pp 2454–2457.*) This patient's episode of transient blindness was likely due to optic neuritis. This transient loss of vision in one eye occurs in about 25 to 40% of multiple sclerosis patients. (A similar presentation can occur in SLE, sarcoidosis, or syphilis.) In addition, the patient gives a history of a relapsing-remitting process. There are abnormal signs of cerebellar and upper motor neuron disease. Signs and symptoms therefore suggest multiple lesions, making multiple sclerosis the most likely diagnosis. There are no systemic symptoms to suggest SLE. B_{12} deficiency could not explain all of the neurologic findings, i.e., visual loss and cerebellar dysmetria. Objective physical exam data rules out hypochondriasis—a diagnosis sometimes inappropriately given to the MS patient.

8-20. The answer is c. (*Victor, p 1135.*) The on-off effect is commonly seen in persons who have had Parkinson's disease for several years. Maintaining more stable levels of anti-Parkinsonian medication in the blood does not eliminate this phenomenon of abruptly worsening and remitting symptoms. Variability in the responsiveness of the CNS to the medication, rather than in the medication levels, underlies the phenomenon.

8-21. The answer is b. (*Kaplan, 8/e, pp 508–509.*) Schizoaffective disorder is diagnosed when the required criteria for schizophrenia are met (delusions, hallucination, disorganized speech or behavior, and/or negative symptoms; duration of the disturbance, including prodromal and residual period, of at least 6 months with at least 1 month of active symptoms) and the patient experiences at some point in the course of the illness a major depressive episode or a manic episode. The woman in the question meets all these criteria. She has continuing psychotic symptomatology, interspersed with episodes of a major mood disorder. Notably, she has never had the mood symptoms without the psychotic symptoms, ruling out major depression with psychosis as the diagnosis. Delusional disorder is not accompanied by decline in functions or significant affective symptoms. Individuals with schizoid personality disorder do not experience psychotic symptoms. Bipolar disorder is differentiated from schizoaffective disorder by the absence of periods of psychosis accompanied by prominent affective symptoms.

8-22. The answer is c. *(Beckmann, 4/e, pp 387–388.)* The degree or severity of pelvic relaxation is rated on a scale of 1 to 3, based on the descent of the organ or structure involved. First-degree prolapse involves descent limited to the upper two-thirds of the vagina. Second-degree prolapse is present when the structure is at the vaginal introitus. In cases of third-degree prolapse, the structure is outside the vagina. Total procidentia of the uterus is the same as a third-degree prolapse, which means that the uterus would be located outside the body.

8-23. The answer is d. *(Greenfield, 2/e, pp 1640–1642.)* This case illustrates two (among many) conditions that lead to the anterior compartment syndrome, namely, acute arterial occlusion without collateral inflow and rapid reperfusion of ischemic muscle. Treatment for a compartment syndrome is prompt fasciotomy. Assessing a compartment syndrome and proceeding with fasciotomy are generally based on clinical judgment. Inability to dorsiflex the toes is a grave sign of anterior compartment ischemia. EMG studies and compartment pressure measurements would probably be abnormal, but are unnecessary in view of the known findings and would delay treatment. Mere elevation of the leg would be an ineffective means of relieving compartment pressure, although elevation should accompany fasciotomy. Application of a splint has no role in the acute management of this problem.

8-24. The answer is b. *(Bradley, p 1455.)* Clinical trials have shown that intravenous methylprednisolone for an attack of optic neuritis reduces the likelihood of developing MS over 2 years from 16.7% to 7.5%. It also is associated with a better outcome than oral prednisone. Intravenous methylprednisolone is thus recommended by most experts as appropriate therapy for acute exacerbations of MS involving more than sensory manifestations alone.

8-25. The answer is b. *(Behrman, 16/e, p 1928. McMillan, 3/e, pp 1875–1878, 1993–1995, 2004–2005. Rudolph, 21/e, pp 668, 2323–2324.)* The cherry-red spot represents the center of a normal retinal macula that is surrounded by ganglion cells in which there is an abnormal accumulation of lipid. This alters the surrounding retinal color so that it is yellowish or grayish white and is seen more often in such disorders as GM_1 generalized gangliosidosis type 1, Sandhoff disease, and Niemann-Pick disease type A, in which there is lipid material deposited in the ganglion cells. Generalized gangliosidosis type 1 (Type 1 GM_1 gangliosidosis) presents as noted in the question, with symptoms often present at birth; these infants have a complete lack of acid beta-galactosidase activity. Other findings with generalized gangliosidosis type 1 (and not listed in the question) include gingival hyperplasia, hernias, joint stiffness, dorsal kyphosis, and edema of the extremities. Hexosaminidase A deficiency (GM_2 gangliosidosis, type 1 or Tay-Sachs disease) presents as psychomotor retardation and hypotonia beginning at about 6 to 12 months of age; the children are usually normal at birth. A pronounced startle reflex and severe hyperacusis, seizures, loss of vision (with cherry-red macular spots), and macrocephaly are seen. Reduced activity of alpha-galactosidase (Fabry's disease) presents in older children as acroparesthesia (numbness or tingling in one or more extremities), intermittent painful crisis of the extremities or the abdomen, frequently low-grade fevers, and sometimes cataracts. Patients with Rett syndrome (the etiology of which has been traced to a defective gene called MeCP2 on the X chromosome) present as normal children at birth, but then have a rapid decline in motor and cognitive functions beginning between 6 and 18 months of age. Affected girls demonstrate loss in the use of their hands and loss in their ability to communicate and socialize. Metachromatic leukodystrophy (deficient activity of galactosyl-3-sulfate-ceramide sulfatase) has its onset between 1 and 2 years of age, notable for progressive ataxia, weakness, and peripheral neuropathy. In this disorder, gray macular lesions can be seen that look somewhat similar to cherry-red spots.

8-26. The answer is c. *(Mishell, 3/e, pp 330–339.)* Although there is an increased risk of spontaneous abortion, and a small risk of infection, an intrauterine pregnancy can occur and continue successfully to term with an IUD in place. However, if the patient wishes to keep the pregnancy and if the string is visible, the IUD should be removed in an attempt to reduce the risk of infection, abortion, or both. Although the incidence of ectopic pregnancies with an IUD was at one time thought to be increased, it is now recognized that in fact the overall incidence is unchanged. The apparent increase is the result of the dramatic decrease in intrauterine implantation without affecting ectopic implantation. Thus, while the overall probability of pregnancy is dramatically decreased, when a pregnancy does occur with an IUD in place, there is a higher probability that it will be an ectopic one. With this in mind, in the absence of signs and symptoms suggestive of an ectopic pregnancy, especially after ultrasound documentation of an intrauterine pregnancy, laparoscopy is not indicated. The incidence of heterotopic pregnancy, in which intrauterine and extrauterine implantation occur, is no higher than approximately 1 in 2500 pregnancies.

8-27. The answer is d. (*Osborn, pp 192–194.*) Cerebral amyloid angiopathy (CAA), or congophilic angiopathy, is the most common cause of lobar hemorrhage in elderly patients without hypertension. The deposition of β-amyloid protein (the same as that found in Alzheimer's disease) in brain blood vessels leads to disruption of the vessel walls, which predisposes them to hemorrhage. Patients are usually over age 70 and may present with multiple cortical hemorrhages with or without a history of dementia. At times, additional hemorrhages may be seen only on special imaging techniques, such as gradient echo MRI, which magnifies the effects of hemosiderin in regions of prior hemorrhage.

8-28. The answer is c. (*Greenfield, 2/e, p 1236.*) Hematomas of the rectus sheath are more common in women and present most often in the fifth decade. A history of trauma, sudden muscular exertion, or anticoagulation can usually be elicited. The pain is of sudden onset and is sharp in nature. The hematoma is most common in the right lower quadrant, and irritation of the peritoneum leads to fever, leukocytosis, anorexia, and nausea. The diagnosis can be established preoperatively with an ultrasound or CT scan showing a mass within the rectus sheath. Management is conservative unless symptoms are severe and bleeding persists, in which case surgical evacuation of the hematoma and ligation of bleeding vessels is required.

8-29. The answer is c. (*Moosa, Arch Surg 125:1028–1031, 1990. Schwartz, 7/e, p 1446.*) This scenario is typical for a patient with iatrogenic injury of the common bile duct. These injuries commonly occur in the proximal portion of the extrahepatic biliary system. The transhepatic cholangiogram documents a biliary stricture, which in this clinical setting is best dealt with surgically. Choledochoduodenostomy generally cannot be performed because of the proximal location of the stricture. The best results are achieved with end-to-side choledochojejunostomy (Roux-en-Y) performed over a stent. Percutaneous transhepatic dilatation has been attempted in select cases, but follow-up is too short to make an adequate assessment of this technique. Primary repair of the common bile duct may result in recurrent stricture.

8-30. The answer is a. (*Braunwald, 15/e, pp 1349–1350.*) The classic symptoms of aortic stenosis are exertional dyspnea, angina pectoris, and syncope. Physical findings include a narrow pulse pressure and systolic murmur as described in option a (rather than the aortic insufficiency murmur of option b, the mitral regurgitation murmur of option c, or the mitral valve prolapse click of option d).

8-31. The answer is a. (*Victor, pp 187–189.*) This patient has common migraine. Of the agents listed, only ergotamine tartrate is generally considered of use to abort a headache. Verapamil and amitriptyline hydrochloride may be used as prophylactic (preventative) therapy. Phenobarbital is an anticonvulsant and is not typically used to treat migraine. Nitroglycerine can actually precipitate headaches in susceptible individuals. Nausea is a frequent accompaniment of migraine. Metoclopramide hydrochloride (Reglan) may be effective in relieving the nausea, but it also reduces gastric stasis, which can retard absorption of oral medications. Certain antiemetics, such as prochlorperazine, may relieve nausea and also provide relief from the headache itself. Additional agents that might be of benefit in abortive therapy include ibuprofen, aspirin, acetaminophen, isomeheptene (Midrin), ergotamine, or a triptan. The triptans are a group of medications that act as agonists at serotonergic receptors (specifically, the 5HT-1 receptors), and they have been found to be very effective at stopping migraine headaches.

8-32. The answer is d. (*Ebert, p 205.*) Alzheimer's disease is the most common dementing disorder in North America, Europe, and Scandinavia. Typical symptoms are progressive memory loss, aphasia, anomia (inability to recall the name of objects), apraxia (inability to perform voluntary motor activity in the absence of motor and sensory deficits), and agnosia (inability to process and understand sensory stimuli in the absence of sensory deficits). Motor functions are spared until the very end. Personality is preserved in the early stages of the disorder, but considerable deterioration follows in later stages.

8-33. The answer is e. *(Victor, pp 927–928.)* Anosmia is one of the more common long-term cranial nerve deficits after head injury, though it is present in only 6% in one series. It is often associated with ageusia (loss of taste). It can be very disabling and discouraging to patients. Approximately one-third of patients recover. It is caused by avulsion of olfactory nerve rootlets due to acceleration-deceleration injury at the cribriform plate. Damage may be unilateral or bilateral.

8-34. The answer is d. *(Tierney, 42/e, pp 487–489.)* The patient most likely has **polycythemia vera.** This is an acquired myeloproliferative disorder characterized by a primary erythrocytosis, but there is overproduction of all three cell lines. Hematocrits are >54% in males and >51% in females. Patients present with symptoms related to an increase in blood volume and viscosity. Pruritus after a warm bath or shower is due to histamine release by basophils. Splenomegaly exists in virtually every patient with polycythemia vera. The treatment of choice for polycythemia vera is phlebotomy. Spurious polycythemia or **Gaisbock syndrome** is due to a contracted plasma volume (diuretic use); secondary polycythemia may be due to smoking, high altitudes, cardiac or pulmonary disease, or erythropoietin-secreting cysts or tumors. Patients with **chronic myelogenous leukemia (CML)** typically have a leukocytosis and the Philadelphia chromosome. Patients with **essential thrombocythemia** have platelet counts >2 million/μL. Patients with **myelofibrosis** have splenomegaly, dry bone marrow taps, and peripheral blood smears showing abnormal and bizarre morphologies and immature forms.

8-35. The answer is a. *(Ebert, p 579.)* Separation anxiety disorder is characterized by manifestations of distress when the child has to be separated from loved ones. The distress often leads to school refusal, refusal to sleep alone, multiple somatic symptoms, and complaints when the child is separated from loved ones, and at times may be associated with full-blown panic attacks. The child is typically afraid that harm will come either to loved ones or to him- or herself during the time of separation. This is normal behavior in children 1 to 3 years old, after which it is thought to be pathological.

8-36. The answer is d. *(Behrman, 16/e, pp 1275–1278. McMillan, 3/e, pp 1307–1311. Rudolph, 21/e, pp 1275–1276.)* The signs of illness described are those involving the airway above the point at which the trachea enters the neck and leaves the thorax, as in croup syndrome. Intrathoracic airway diseases, such as asthma or bronchiolitis, produce breathing difficulty on expiration, with expiratory wheezing, prolonged expiration, and signs of air trapping due to the increased narrowing during expiration as the airways are exposed to the same intrathoracic pressure changes as the alveoli. The extrathoracic airway, to the contrary, tends to collapse on inspiration, producing the characteristic findings this patient demonstrates.

Agents causing croup include parainfluenza types I and III, influenza A and B, RSV, and occasionally, other viruses. Treatment is usually supportive, but racemic epinephrine and corticosteroids reduce the length of time in the emergency room and hospitalizations.

8-37. The answer is d. *(Behrman, 16/e, pp 1289–1290, McMillan, 3/e, pp 621–622. Rudolph, 21/e, pp 366–367.)* Hydrocarbons with low viscosity and high volatility are the most likely agents to cause respiratory symptoms. Gasoline, kerosene, and furniture polish (which contain hydrocarbons) are common agents responsible for hydrocarbon aspiration. Hydrocarbon aspiration can produce dyspnea, cyanosis, and respiratory failure. Treatment is symptomatic, sometimes requiring intubation and mechanical ventilation. Induction of emesis is contraindicated, as this may cause further aspiration. Placement of a nasogastric tube is used only in high-volume ingestions or when the hydrocarbon is mixed with another toxin. Charcoal is not useful, and no intravenous binding agent is available.

8-38. The answer is c. *(Braunwald, 15/e, pp 2098–2099.)* This patient's symptoms of weakness, fatigue, and weight loss in combination with signs of hypotension and extensor hyperpigmentation are all consistent with Addison's disease (adrenal insufficiency). Tuberculosis can involve the adrenal glands and result in adrenal insufficiency. Measurement of serum cortisol baseline and then stimulation with ACTH will confirm the clinical suspicion. The ACTH stimulation test is used to determine the adrenal reserve capacity for steroid production. Cortisol response is measured 60 min after cosyntropin is given intramuscularly or intravenously.

8-39. The answer is d. *(Schwartz, 7/e, pp 771–780.)* The boundaries of the mediastinum are the thoracic inlet, the diaphragm, the sternum, the vertebral column, and the pleura bilaterally. The mediastinum itself is divided into three portions delineated by the pericardial sac: the anterosuperior and posterosuperior regions are in front of and behind the sac, respectively, while the middle region designates the contents of the pericardium. Mediastinal masses occur most frequently in the anterosuperior region (54%) and less often in the posterosuperior (26%) and middle (20%) regions. Cysts (pericardial, bronchogenic, or enteric) are the most common tumors of the middle region; neurogenic tumors are the most common (40%) of the primary tumors of the posterior mediastinum. The primary neoplasms of the mediastinum in the anteroposterior region are thymomas (31%), lymphomas (23%), and germ cell tumors (17%). More commonly, though, a mass in this area represents the substernal extension of a benign substernal goiter. Diagnosis may be made by visualization of an enhancing structure on CT; radioactive iodine scanning is useful in management because it may make the diagnosis if the mediastinal tissue is functional and will also document the presence of functioning cervical thyroid tissue to prevent removal of all functional thyroid tissue during mediastinal excision.

8-40. The answer is b. *(Tierney, 42/e, pp 1369–1370.)* The clinical presentation is most consistent with **Legionnaires' disease.** Patients are usually elderly or immunocompromised or have chronic lung disease. Air conditioners, whirlpools, water-using machinery, and cooling towers have been linked to outbreaks of the disease. Clinical signs of the disease include fever, relative bradycardia, abdominal complaints, scanty cough, and laboratory abnormalities. Pontiac fever is an acute, self-limited, flulike illness due to *Legionella,* but it does not cause pneumonia. Psittacosis (*Chlamydia*) is pneumonia associated with the handling of birds.

8-41. The answer is b. *(Tintinalli, 5/e, pp 554–555.)* Complications of **diverticular disease** include diverticulitis and gastrointestinal bleeding. **Diverticulitis** is an acute inflammatory process caused by bacteria in a diverticulum (outpouching of the mucosa or submucosa). It may occur in up to 50% of patients with diverticulosis. The patient most likely has diverticulitis, which is usually left-sided since the diameter of the sigmoid colon is the smallest of the colon (higher wall tension and intraluminal pressure in this area are probably responsible for the diverticular formation). The palpable mass reflects adherent loops of bowel. Peritonitis often results in involuntary guarding (abdominal rigidity due to reflex muscle spasm from the peritoneal irritation). Decreased bowel sounds may be heard in peritonitis or in any condition that causes an ileus (absence of peristalsis). Tenderness upon abrupt withdrawal of the hand (rebound tenderness or **Blumberg sign**) occurs because when the abdominal wall passively springs back into place, it carries with it the inflamed peritoneum. The **referred rebound test** is conducted in the same way but in a location away from the area of tenderness. The patient will experience pain in the area of stated tenderness rather than the site where the test is performed.

8-42. The answer is b. (*Scott, 8/e, p 613.*) Dysmenorrhea is considered secondary if associated with pelvic disease such as endometriosis, uterine myomas, or pelvic inflammatory disease. Primary dysmenorrhea is associated with a normal pelvic examination and with ovulatory cycles. The pain of dysmenorrhea is usually accompanied by other symptoms (nausea, fatigue, diarrhea, and headache) which may be related to excess of prostaglandin $F_{2\alpha}$. The two major drug therapies effective in dysmenorrhea are oral contraceptives and antiprostaglandins. GnRH analogues are used in several gynecologic conditions, but would not be first-line therapy for primary dysmenorrhea. Danazol is used for the treatment of endometriosis and ergot derivatives for hyperprolactinemia. Analgesics such as codeine or narcotics would generally be employed only in very severe cases when no other treatment provides adequate relief. Treatment will reduce the number of women incapacitated by menstrual symptoms to about 10% of those treated. Contrary to past beliefs, psychological factors play only a minor role in dysmenorrhea.

8-43. The answer is d. (*Stoudemire, 3/e, p 556.*) Behavioral therapy techniques such as exposure and response prevention and desensitization are very effective in adults and adolescents with a diagnosis of OCD. OCD has a lifetime prevalence of between 0.2 and 1.2% in children. Children as young as 2 have been diagnosed with the disorder. Contrary to the case in adult-onset OCD, obsessions and compulsion are often ego-syntonic in childhood OCD.

8-44. The answer is a. (*Victor, pp 12–19.*) The differential diagnosis is rather broad at this point. You should look for an infectious or malignant mass with a contrast-enhanced CT or MRI. A noncontrast head CT is less sensitive for abscess or tumor. A lumbar puncture should only be done after you are sure that there is not significant mass effect. This patient has an acute problem, which should be addressed now. Antiretroviral therapy will help him in the long term, but does not need to be initiated in the emergency room. Intravenous heparin is a treatment for embolic stroke. Embolic stroke is unlikely in this case, and further evaluation is needed before treatment with intravenous heparin is considered.

8-45. The answer is a. (*Ebert, p 216.*) Multiple cerebral infarcts cause a progressive dementia (usually described as stepwise), focal neurological signs, and often neuropsychiatric symptoms such as depression, mood lability (but usually not elated mood), and delusions. Loose associations, catatonic posturing, and bizarre proverb interpretations occurring with affective symptoms are typical of schizoaffective disorder. In delirium, one would expect to see the waxing and waning of consciousness over time, including problems with orientation to person, place, and time.

8-46. The answer is c. (*Greenfield, 2/e, pp 779–787.*) Benign gastric ulcers have a peak incidence in the fifth decade, with male predominance. About 95% of gastric ulcers are located near the lesser curvature. It should be recognized that up to 16% of patients with gastric carcinoma pass a 12-week healing trial and that benign ulcers may enlarge during medical therapy. Therefore, the possibility of malignancy must be assessed by biopsy despite a 5 to 10% false-negative rate. Six weeks of medical therapy will heal many gastric ulcers, but a recurrence rate as high as 63% and the serious consequence of complications in this older group of patients warrant surgery for recurrent or nonhealing ulcers. A distal gastrectomy with gastroduodenostomy is usually feasible in the absence of duodenal disease. Vagotomy, while advocated by some, is generally not included. Local excision with definitive distal resection or vagotomy and pyloroplasty is appropriate for a proximal ulcer that would otherwise require a subtotal gastrectomy.

8-47. The answer is a. (*Speroff, 6/e, p 544.*) This patient has polycystic ovarian syndrome (PCOS), diagnosed by the clinical picture, abnormally high LH-to-FSH ratio (which should normally be approximately 1:1), and elevated androgens but normal DHAS. DHAS is a marker of adrenal androgen production; when normal, it essentially excludes adrenal sources of hyperandrogenism. Several medications have been used to treat hirsutism associated with PCOS. For many years contraceptives were the most frequently used agents; they can suppress hair growth in up to two-thirds of treated patients. They act by directly suppressing ovarian steroid production and increasing hepatic binding globulin production, which binds circulating hormone and lowers the concentration of metabolically active (free unbound) androgen. However, clinical improvement can take as long as 6 months to manifest. Other medications that have shown promise include medroxyprogesterone acetate, spironolactone, cimetidine, and GnRH agonists, which suppress ovarian steroid production. However, GnRH analogues are expensive and have been associated with significant bone demineralization after only 6 months of therapy in some patients. Surgical wedge resection is no longer considered an appropriate therapy for PCOS given the success of pharmacologic agents and the ovarian adhesions that were frequently associated with this surgery.

8-48. The answer is e. (*Victor, pp 171, 1317–1318.*) This patient probably has a spinal cord infarction from an anterior spinal artery occlusion. The posterior cord may be spared, preserving joint proprioception. Bilateral lower extremity deficits without cranial nerve or mental status findings would be an exceedingly unusual cerebral stroke presentation. There is no information, such as psychological stressors or a non-physiologic exam, to suggest a conversion disorder in this case. Multiple sclerosis causes neurological deficits over space and time. In this case we have a single deficit at a single point in time. History of metastatic cancer or trauma might make the physician suspect spinal cord compression.

8-49. The answer is e. (*Behrman, 16/e, p 505. McMillan, 3/e, p 259. Rudolph, 21/e, pp 179–181.*) Transient tachypnea of the newborn is usually seen after a normal vaginal or, especially, after a cesarean delivery. These patients have tachypnea, retractions, grunting, and sometimes, cyanosis. The chest examination is usually normal; the chest radiograph demonstrates prominent pulmonary vascular markings with fluid in the fissures and hyperexpansion (flat diaphragms). Therapy is supportive, with maintenance of normal oxygen saturation. Resolution usually occurs in the first 3 days of life.

8-50. The answer is c. *(Kane, 4/e, p 169.)* This patient presents with typical characteristics of a bereavement reaction. Symptoms of guilt, insomnia, and loss are occurring within 1 year of the spouse's death. There are no symptoms of a major depression. It is not uncommon to have transient hallucinations of hearing the spouse's voice; this does not represent psychosis and does not require medication. Antidepressants can usually be avoided, and indeed may interfere with the process of adjustment. Counseling and supportive services such as widows' groups facilitate the transition period. The physician should be aware of any clues to decline in health, common during this period. The patient should be followed for suicidal ideation.

Bibliography

American College of Obstetricians and Gynecologists: *Primary and Preventive Care: Periodic Assessments.* Committee Opinion 246, December 2000.

American College of Obstetricians and Gynecologists: *Circumcision.* Committee Opinion 260, October 2001.

American College of Obstetricians and Gynecologists: *Vaginal Birth After Previous Cesarean Delivery.* Practice Bulletin 5, July 1999.

American College of Obstetricians and Gynecologists: *Thrombocytopenia in Pregnancy.* Practice Bulletin 6, September 1999.

American College of Obstetricians and Gynecologists: *Operative Vaginal Delivery.* Practice Bulletin 17, June 2000.

American College of Obstetricians and Gynecologists: *Fetal Heart Rate Patterns: Monitoring, Interpretation, and Management.* Technical Bulletin 207, July 1995.

Beckmann CRB, et al (eds): *Obstetrics and Gynecology,* 4/e. Philadelphia, Lippincott, Williams & Wilkins, 2002.

Behrman RE, Kliegman RM, Jenson HB (eds): *Nelson Textbook of Pediatrics,* 16/e. Philadelphia, WB Saunders Co., 2000.

Bradley W, et al (eds): *Neurology in Clinical Practice,* 4/e. Boston, Butterworth-Heinemann, 2000.

Braunwald E, Fauci AS, Kasper DL, Hauser SL, et al (eds): *Harrison's Principles of Internal Medicine,* 15/e. New York, McGraw-Hill, 2001.

Brewster DC, Franklin DP, Cambria RP, et al: Intestinal ischemia complicating abdominal aortic surgery. *Surgery* 109:447–454, 1991.

Cunningham FG, et al (eds): *Williams Obstetrics,* 20/e. Stamford, CT, Appleton & Lange, 1997

Cunningham FG, et al (eds): *Williams Obstetrics,* 21/e. New York, McGraw-Hill, 2001.

Droegemueller, et al (eds): *Comprehensive Gynecology,* 3/e. St. Louis, Mosby, 1997.

Ebert MH, Loosen PT, Nurcombe B (eds): *Current Diagnosis and Treatment in Psychiatry.* New York, Lange/McGraw-Hill, 2000.

Fitzpatrick TB, Johnson RA, Wolff K, Suurmond D: *Color Atlas and Synopsis of Clinical Dermatology,* 4/e. New York, McGraw-Hill, 2001.

Fleisher AC, et al (eds): *Principles and Practice of Ultrasonography in Obstetrics and Gynecology,* 5/e. Stamford, CT, Appleton & Lange, 1996.

Fuster V, Alexander RW, O'Rourke RA, et al (eds): *Hurst's The Heart,* 10/e. New York, McGraw-Hill, 2001.

Gaster B, Holroyd J: St. John's Wort for depression. *Arch Int Med* 160: 152–156, 2000.

Gleicher N, et al (eds): *Principles and Practice of Medical Therapy in Pregnancy,* 3/e. Stamford, CT, Appleton & Lange, 1998.

Goldman L, Bennett JC: *Cecil Textbook of Medicine,* 21/e. Philadelphia, Saunders, 2000.

Gorbach SL, Bartlett JG, Blacklow NR (eds): *Infectious Diseases,* 2/e. Philadelphia, Saunders, 1998.

Greenberg DA, et al: *Clinical Neurology,* 5/e. New York, McGraw-Hill, 2002.

Greenberg JO (ed): *Neuroimaging,* 2/e. New York, McGraw-Hill, 1999.

Greenfield L, et al (eds): *Surgery: Scientific Principles and Practice,* 2/e. Philadelphia, Lippincott-Raven, 1997.

Hankins GDV, et al (eds): *Operative Obstetrics.* Norwalk, CT, Appleton & Lange, 1995.

Harrison's Online: www.harrisonline.com.

Hazzard WR, Blass JP, Ettinger WH et al (eds): *Principles of Geriatric Medicine and Gerontology,* 4/e, New York, McGraw-Hill, 1999.

Hoskins WJ, Perez CA, Young RC (eds): *Principles and Practice of Gynecologic Oncology,* 2/e. Philadelphia, Lippincott, 1997.

Kane RL, Ouslander JG, Abrass IB: Essentials of Clinical Geriatrics, 4/e. New York, McGraw-Hill, 1999.

Kaplan HI, Sadock BJ: *Synopsis of Psychiatry: Behavioral Sciences/Clinical Psychiatry.* 8/e. Philadelphia, Lippincott Williams & Wilkins, 1998.

McMillan JA, DeAngelis CD, Feigin RD, Warshaw JB (eds): *Oski's Pediatrics,* 3/e. Philadelphia, Lippincott Williams & Wilkins, 1999.

Mishell DR, Stenchever MA, Droegemueller W, Herbst AL (eds): *Comprehensive Gynecology,* 3/e. St. Louis, Mosby, 1997.

Moosa AR, Mayer AD, Stabile B: Iatrogenic injury to the bile duct: Who, how, where? *Arch Surg* 125:1028–1031, 1990.

National Cholesterol Education Program, Adult Treatment Panel III.

Osborn AG: *Diagnostic Neuroradiology.* St. Louis, MO, Mosby, 1994.

Patten J: *Neurological Differential Diagnosis,* 2/e. London, Springer-Verlag, 2001.

Postgraduate Obstetrics and Gynecology, 22:25, December 2002.

Ransom SB, Dombrowski MP, McNeeley SG, Moghissi K, Munkarah AR (eds): *Practical Strategies in Obstetrics and Gynecology.* Philadelphia, Saunders, 2000.

Ransom SB, McNeeley SG (eds): *Gynecology for the Primary Care Provider.* Philadelphia, Saunders, 1997.

Reece EA, et al (eds): *Medicine of the Fetus and Mother,* 2/e. Philadelphia, Lippincott, 1999.

Rock JA, Thompson JD (eds): *TeLinde's Operative Gynecology,* 8/e. Philadelphia, Lippincott-Raven, 1997.

Rowland LP (ed): *Merritt's Textbook of Neurology,* 10/e. Baltimore, Williams & Wilkins, 2000.

Rudolph CD, Rudolph AM, Hostetter MK, Lister G, Siegel NJ (eds): *Rudolph's Pediatrics,* 21/e. New York, McGraw-Hill, 2003.

Sabiston DC Jr, et al (eds): *Surgery. The Biological Basis of Modern Surgical Practice,* 15/e. Philadelphia, Saunders, 1997.

Schwartz SI, Shires GT, Spencer FC (eds): *Principles of Surgery,* 7/e. New York, McGraw-Hill, 1999.

Scott JR, et al (eds): *Danforth's Obstetrics and Gynecology,* 8/e. Philadelphia, Lippincott-Raven, 1999.

Seidel HM, Ball JW, Dains JE, Benedict GW: *Mosby's Guide to Physical Examination,* 5/e. St. Louis, MO, Mosby, 2003.

Shuaib A, Goldstein LB (eds): *Management of Acute Stroke.* New York, Marcel Dekker, 1999.

Speroff L, Glass RH, Kase NG (eds): *Clinical Gynecologic Endocrinology and Infertility,* 6/e. Baltimore, Lippincott, Williams & Wilkins, 1999.

Stein JH: *Internal Medicine,* 5/e. Boston, Little, Brown & Company, 1998.

Stobo JD, Hellman DB, Ladenson PW, et al (eds): *The Principles and Practice of Medicine,* 23/e. Stamford, CT, Appleton & Lange, 1996.

Stoudemire A: *Clinical Psychiatry for Medical Students,* 3/e. Philadelphia, Lippincott Williams & Wilkins, 1998.

Thoren T, Wattwil M: Effects on gastric emptying of thoracic epidural analgesia with morphine or bupivacaine. *Anesth Analg* 67:687–694, 1988.

Tierney LM Jr, McPhee SJ, Papadakis MA: *Current Medical Diagnosis and Treatment,* 42/e. New York, McGraw-Hill, 2003.

Tintinalli JE, Kelen GD, Stapczynski JS: *Emergency Medicine: A Comprehensive Study Guide,* 5/e. American College of Emergency Physicians. New York, McGraw-Hill, 2000.

Victor M, et al: *Principles of Neurology,* 7/e. New York, McGraw-Hill, 2001.